Ethics *and* Law

for AUSTRALIAN NURSES

Fifth edition

Every day, registered nurses are required to act and make decisions based on their moral and legal obligations. They must build professional, culturally safe relationships with patients, understand patient rights and the requirements of consent, and prevent and manage clinical mistakes in order to avoid negligence and abuse of power.

Now in its fifth edition, *Ethics and Law for Australian Nurses* guides students through foundational concepts such as personhood, autonomy, trust, consent and vulnerability, and considers a nurse's responsibilities in relation to voluntary assisted dying, abortions and advanced care directives. It explains the Australian legal system and how it relates to nursing practice.

This edition discusses the impact of the COVID-19 pandemic, particularly on elderly Australians, as well as on injury and negligence claims. It includes updated discussions on guardianship, assisted dying, abortion and 'not for resuscitation' orders. This book uses thought-provoking reflective questions to help students broaden their own perspectives and consider various ethical dilemmas, with answers for each question available online. Law and Ethics in Practice case studies show how concepts can be applied in real-world scenarios.

Ethics and Law for Australian Nurses is a comprehensive guide for nurses on providing morally and legally responsible and culturally safe care for patients in Australia.

Kim Atkins is Adjunct Associate Professor of Philosophy at the University of Tasmania, and Education Manager at Laurel House. She was previously a registered nurse and specialised in intensive care nursing for over 20 years.

Bernhard Ripperger is Director, Community Protection in the NSW Department of Communities and Justice. He has worked as a government lawyer for almost 25 years, and has taught philosophy at Macquarie University and the University of Wollongong.

Rebecca Ripperger works in the NSW Department of Communities and Justice. She was previously a registered nurse and worked in the hospital system for over 20 years.

Cambridge University Press acknowledges the Australian Aboriginal and Torres Strait Islander peoples of this nation. We acknowledge the traditional custodians of the lands on which our company is located and where we conduct our business. We pay our respects to ancestors and Elders, past and present. Cambridge University Press is committed to honouring Australian Aboriginal and Torres Strait Islander peoples' unique cultural and spiritual relationships to the land, waters and seas, and their rich contribution to society.

Ethics
and
Law
for
AUSTRALIAN
NURSES
Fifth edition

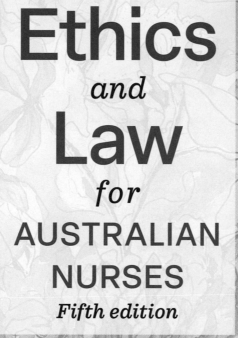

Kim Atkins
Bernhard Ripperger
Rebecca Ripperger

CAMBRIDGE
UNIVERSITY PRESS

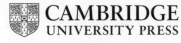

Shaftesbury Road, Cambridge CB2 8EA, United Kingdom

One Liberty Plaza, 20th Floor, New York, NY 10006, USA

477 Williamstown Road, Port Melbourne, VIC 3207, Australia

314–321, 3rd Floor, Plot 3, Splendor Forum, Jasola District Centre, New Delhi – 110025, India

103 Penang Road, #05–06/07, Visioncrest Commercial, Singapore 238467

Cambridge University Press is part of Cambridge University Press & Assessment,
a department of the University of Cambridge.

We share the University's mission to contribute to society through the pursuit of education,
learning and research at the highest international levels of excellence.

www.cambridge.org
Information on this title: www.cambridge.org/highereducation/isbn/9781009236027

First published 2011
Second edition 2014
Third edition 2017
Fourth edition 2020
Fifth edition 2023

Cover designed by Shaun Jury
Typeset by Integra Software Services Pvt. Ltd
Printed in China by C & C Offset Printing Co., Ltd, November 2022

A catalogue record for this publication is available from the British Library

A catalogue record for this book is available from the National Library of Australia

ISBN 978-1-009-23602-7 Paperback

Additional resources for this publication at www.cambridge.org/highereducation/isbn/9781009236027/resources

CONTENTS

4   Consent   93

Kim Atkins

5   Duty of care and professional negligence   121

Bernhard Ripperger

6   Culturally safe nursing practice   150

Kim Atkins

11 Ethics of aged care: Autonomy under threat and the nurse as capacity-builder 264

Rebecca Ripperger

Kim Atkins is Adjunct Associate Professor of Philosophy at the University of Tasmania, and Education Manager at Laurel House (the sexual assault support service for North and North-West Tasmania). She became a registered nurse in 1985 and specialised in intensive care nursing for over 20 years. Kim also has extensive experience in health system management within the Tasmanian Department of Health. Kim completed a PhD in philosophy and taught at Macquarie University. She went on to teach philosophy and ethics in the Bachelor of Arts and Bachelor of Nursing programs at the University of Wollongong and the University of Tasmania. She also runs workshops on values in the workplace, having difficult conversations, and trauma-informed practices. Kim is the author of *Narrative Identity and Moral Identity: A Practical Perspective*, editor of *Self and Subjectivity*, and co-editor of *Practical Identity and Narrative Agency*.

Bernhard Ripperger has worked as a government lawyer in the NSW public sector for almost 25 years. He is currently the Director, Community Protection in the NSW Department of Communities and Justice. In addition to his qualifications in law, he has completed a PhD in philosophy, and has taught philosophy at Macquarie University and the University of Wollongong.

Rebecca Ripperger has a BA (Hons) majoring in philosophy and has worked as a tutor and research assistant in moral and social philosophy at Macquarie University. She became a registered nurse in 1983 and worked in the NSW hospital system for over 20 years. She has worked in the NSW public service, currently in the Department of Communities and Justice, in the area of guardianship for over 15 years. In line with her interest in promoting equity of access to the justice system, Rebecca developed and coordinated the 'Culture of Inclusion' training initiative, which showcases projects that support people with disabilities to engage actively and creatively in the world. She has recently worked for Laurel House Sexual Assault Support Service in Tasmania, developing resources for its disability project, including the development of its Decision-making Guide.

ACKNOWLEDGEMENTS

The authors and Cambridge University Press would like to thank the following for permission to reproduce material in this book.

Figure 1.1: © Getty Images/Phil Boorman; **3.1**: © Getty Images/Westend61; **4.1**: © Getty Images/Marko Geber; **5.1**: © Getty Images/urbancow; **6.1**: © Getty Images/Indeed; **8.1**: © Getty Images/Jonathan Knowles; **9.1**: © Getty Images/Kemal Yildirim; **9.2**, **9.3**: Reproduced with permission from Australian Commission on Safety and Quality in Health Care (2013) Open disclosure principles, elements and process, ACSQHC, Sydney. © Commonwealth of Australia 2013; **10.1**: © Getty Images/IAN HOOTON/SPL; **10.2**: © Getty Images/mikroman6; **11.1**: © Getty Images/fstop123; **11.2**: © Australian Institute of Health and Welfare 2022, reproduced under a CC BY 4.0 licence, https://creativecommons.org/licenses/by/4.0/; **11.3**: © Getty Images/ Larry Williams & Associates; **11.5**: © Australian Institute of Health and Welfare 2021, reproduced under a CC BY 4.0 licence, https://creativecommons.org/licenses/by/4.0/

Table 1.1 and extracts from Code of Conduct for Nurses: Reproduced with permission of the Nursing and Midwifery Board of Australia. ©2018 AHPRA. The Nursing and Midwifery Board of Australia website being the best place to find up to date information, standards and guidelines for nurses and midwives (www.nursingmidwiferyboard.gov.au); **1.2** and extracts from International Council of Nurses Code of Ethics for Nurses: © ICN – International Council of Nurses 2021.

Extract from *Preventing and responding to abuse of older people (Elder Abuse)* (Family and Community Services, NSW Government 2018): © State of New South Wales. For current information go to www.nsw.gov.au. Licensed under Creative Commons 4.0, http://creativecommons.org/licenses/by/4.0.

Extracts from Commonwealth legislation: Sourced from the Federal Register of Legislation and reproduced under Creative Commons Attribution 4.0 International (CC BY 4.0). For the latest information on Australian Government law please go to https://www.legislation.gov.au.

Extracts from New South Wales legislation: Sourced from the New South Wales Legislation website at 21 July 2022. For the latest information on New South Wales Government legislation please go to https://www.legislation.nsw.gov.au. Reproduced under a CC BY 4.0 licence, https://creativecommons.org/licenses/by/4.0/.

Extracts from Queensland legislation: Sourced from the Queensland legislation website at 21 July 2022. For the latest information on Queensland Government legislation please go to https://www.legislation.qld.gov.au. Reproduced under a CC BY 4.0 licence, https://creativecommons.org/licenses/by/4.0/.

Extracts from Victorian legislation: © State of Victoria, Australia. Copyright in all legislation of the Parliament of the State of Victoria, Australia, is owned by the Crown in right of the State of Victoria, Australia. DISCLAIMER: This product or service contains an unofficial version of the legislation of the Parliament of State of Victoria. The State of Victoria accepts no responsibility for the accuracy and completeness of any legislation contained in this product or provided through this service.

Appendix Table Chapter 7: Mandatory Reporting Requirements, Australian Institute of Family Studies (AIFS) on behalf of the Commonwealth of Australia, CC BY 4.0. https://aifs.gov.au/sites/default/files/publication-documents/2006_mandatory_reporting_of_child_abuse_and_neglect_0.pdf; https://aifs.gov.au/copyright; https://creativecommons.org/licenses/by/4.0/.

Every effort has been made to trace and acknowledge copyright. The publisher apologises for any accidental infringement and welcomes information that would redress this situation.

INTRODUCTION

KIM ATKINS

This book has been written specifically for nurses training and practising within Australia, to assist and encourage them to develop a strong and well-defined sense of professional and moral identity. It endeavours to provide an integrated, practical framework for understanding the ethical and legal dimensions of nursing practice in Australia by referencing Australian law and reflecting the Australian clinical context and cultural norms.

This book refers to 'patients' rather than 'clients'. The question of which term is most appropriate is not easily resolved – if it can be at all – because there are many ways to interpret both terms. Consequently, we have made the decision to use the term 'patients' because it best approximates our use of the concept of vulnerability. We do not regard patients as people who are either in a contract with the nurse or merely passive and dependent on the nurse; rather, they are people who are in a relationship of power with the nurse because they are in specific situations of need. Under Australian law, this is considered a fiduciary relationship – that is, one in which the nurse is recognised as having superior knowledge and therefore more power than the patient, but the patient's authority in decision-making carries more legal and moral force. To represent patients as people who have a merely contractual or dependency relationship with a nurse would be to misrepresent their situation and to obscure the ethical and moral implications of the context of care. A patient's need and vulnerability in the context of a nurse's power constitute the source of the nurse's moral and legal obligations. Therefore, the nurse–patient relationship occupies centre stage throughout this book.

This book takes a 'relational' approach: it emphasises the centrality of relationships to nursing practice at both the theoretical and practical levels. For example, at a theoretical level the book explains personhood as a set of capacities that develop from birth and are sustained throughout life through relationships with other people. It traces the moral basis of law to our need as human beings to live together in societies, and the accompanying need to be protected from harm produced through the activities of people living in close proximity to one another. It also describes how, at a personal level, particular relationships can facilitate or erode an individual's sense of self and self-respect. This can occur, for example, through giving recognition of achievement and providing affection and encouragement, or by withholding these. The ability of relationships to impact profoundly on our lives underpins the importance of having professional boundaries and legal constraints on what nurses can do in their clinical relationships with patients.

Nurses are required to care for and protect the interests of people who are sometimes vastly different from them. How nurses respond to these differences is a measure of their humanity. In being permitted to take a role in the innermost personal lives of people, nurses have a rare opportunity to experience a relationship that can be emotionally and morally profound. Some of the most intimate experiences of life can be found in nursing: delivering a new child into the world; holding the hand of a dying man as he takes his final breath; restarting a person's heart; or consoling someone after a death in the family. In sharing these fundamentally defining experiences of human mortality, the nurse–patient relationship can deeply affirm our connections to one another.

Nurses discover that relationships work in both directions. Nurses receive far more from their patients than is often understood because when nurses honour their patients' needs – their feelings, their hopes and fears, and their bodies – they show themselves to be trustworthy, compassionate, respected and professional. By having the opportunity to act with integrity, compassion, confidentiality and competence, nurses make themselves worthy of trust and respect, and experience their lives as worthwhile and meaningful. This is why so many find nursing to be a deeply satisfying and sustaining occupation.

We begin by setting out a description and philosophy of what a person is, and endeavour to show throughout the book how that understanding of persons underpins the moral and legal obligations of nurses. Understanding persons also means understanding the different stages of life, and the different needs, concerns, aspirations and possibilities experienced at these different stages. Rather than proclaim what those needs and possibilities are, this book encourages nurses to talk to their patients, to listen to them and to learn from them. Patients teach nurses much more, and do so far more effectively, than any book ever could. To this end, case studies in this book have been taken from real life, with many of them providing a view of the clinical setting from the patient's point of view.

This book does not set out to provide a narrative of the good nurse. Rather, it provides a coherent set of conceptual resources and information to guide nurses in their relationships with vulnerable people in the clinical context. It promotes a patient-centred approach, for example, by emphasising the need for decisions about care to be informed by the patient's perspective and personal circumstances; for the patient to actively participate in decision-making; and for the patient to set their own terms for the clinical relationship and treatment wherever possible.

In focusing on the nurse–patient relationship, this book foregrounds the patient's vulnerability. Vulnerability is here used in a technical sense, and it is important for readers to understand this. Vulnerability refers to the fact that we are constantly affected by, and responsive to, other people and the world around us, in both positive and negative ways. In other words, vulnerability simply means *being affected by* people and things. We can be affected positively – for example, by the pleasure and nutrition of good food. We can be affected negatively by the pain and disability of injury or disease. This book presents the view that no person is immune to being affected and influenced by others. This view is significant because it underpins the central claim of this book: that it is our ability to be affected by another person that makes it possible for us to care for each other.

The vulnerability of people receiving nursing care is recognised in law. There are some specific pieces of legislation that relate to particular situations of vulnerability, such as the various Mental Health Acts in each state and territory, the *Disability Discrimination Act 1992*, and the *Children and Young Persons Act 2008* (ACT) (and its equivalent in the other states and territories), while other situations of vulnerability are recognised more generally in common law. Because nurses are also vulnerable, they have certain legal and moral entitlements and protections. For example, nurses have a moral entitlement to be treated with respect, and have legal protection from accusations of assault in relation to certain professional activities – for example, some involving touching or restraining patients. The connections between each clinical situation and its relevant legislation will be explained throughout the book.

Chapter 1 describes how we each *become* persons over time and through our relations with other people. This makes personhood fundamentally relational and interpersonal: we become who we are – with our tastes, talents and abilities – as a result of our interactions with the environment around us and the people in it. Moreover, this is a lifelong process. The idea that we are always in formative relations with the environment and other people is part of the concept of human vulnerability. Vulnerability can be understood as an expression of our belonging to the world with other people, and it is this belonging together in the human world that drives our capacities to care for one another. This is why skills in managing interpersonal relations and communication are central to the nursing role.

Chapter 2 provides an overview of the Australian legal system, its structure, function and philosophical underpinnings. It explains the differences between legislation, common law, criminal law and civil law, and illustrates how these are relevant to nurses and the profession.

Chapter 3 focuses more closely on the nurse–patient relationship. This relationship is called a therapeutic relationship because its function is to have a beneficial effect on the patient. In other words, the nurse–patient relationship is itself a form of therapy because nursing care is inseparable from the relationship. This chapter explores several different models of professional relationship, and explains the nature and obligations of the fiduciary relationship. It then discusses how the therapeutic relationship embodies the moral principles of non-maleficence, beneficence, autonomy and justice. Consistent with the two-way direction of relationships, it also considers some moral dangers of the relationship to both nurse and patient, and concludes with a consideration of the ways in which the therapeutic relationship can promote capacity-building in patients.

Chapter 3 also describes the regulation of nursing practice in Australia and explains why this is a necessary part of ensuring the safety and quality of clinical care. It sets out the roles of the Australian Health Practitioner Regulation Agency (AHPRA) and the Nursing and Midwifery Board of Australia (NMBA) in setting the training and practice standards for nurses and midwives, and handling complaints, investigations and disciplinary hearings.

Chapter 4 addresses the legal framework for valid consent to treatment and refusal of treatment, which is based on the right to autonomy (as discussed in Chapter 3). It considers situations where a person cannot legally consent – for example, where the person is a child or is unconscious – as well as situations where consent is not needed, such as in a medical emergency, where there is serious mental illness or where a patient needs to be restrained for their own safety. The chapter also explains the place of guardianship, advocacy and the use of advance directives in protecting a person's autonomous decision-making.

Chapter 5 takes a detailed look at the concept of negligence, and how it is tied to the nurse's duty of care towards their patients. It explains how a failure to meet that duty of care can lead to a legal finding of negligence against a nurse. It describes how a nurse's required standard of care is determined in law, and how negligence is proven (or defended). It also explains a nurse's legal liability and professional indemnity, as well as the employer's vicarious liability for the actions of nurses.

Chapter 6 looks at the cultural and ethical considerations that are relevant to nursing people from diverse cultures, with a focus on nursing Aboriginal and Torres Strait Islander people. It is important to remember that Aboriginal and Torres Strait Islander peoples are diverse groups who live a variety of lifestyles, from highly traditional to highly modern, on tropical islands, in remote deserts and in suburbia. Indigenous culture encompasses elements from ancient practices to contemporary technology. Appreciating the complexity of Indigenous Australian culture and its historical context is fundamental to providing ethical and therapeutic care.

Chapter 7 continues the focus on the nurse–patient relationship by examining legal and moral requirements around patient privacy and confidentiality, and mandatory reporting. It explains requirements in relation to the management of patient information, including reporting of child abuse, family violence and professional misconduct.

Chapter 8 takes up themes of power, autonomy and advocacy in decision-making about care. Trust is central to negotiating treatment in the nurse–patient relationship because the patient does not choose to enter into a relationship with the nurse. The chapter looks at the nature and scope of trust, and considers the extent to which nurses can be expected to accommodate patients' wishes.

Chapter 9 turns the focus more closely onto the nurse through a discussion of issues of professional self-respect, with a special focus on reporting mistakes and clinical incidents. It looks at factors that influence nurses' decisions about reporting, and explains the importance of dealing effectively and ethically with clinical errors and incidents – for the sake of both patients and nurses. Admitting to mistakes has a number of important moral and practical effects for nurses, including restoring their self-respect and putting the patient back at the centre of care.

Finding the courage and the words to admit mistakes can be facilitated in the workplace by employing specific approaches. Chapter 9 discusses an approach developed in the United States, and adopted worldwide, known as 'Giving Voice to Values' (Gentile 2010). This is a structured practical approach that helps individuals develop the skills they need to speak out when they know they should. The chapter concludes with an explanation of the open disclosure process as a means of restoring trust and justice to the clinical relationship.

Chapter 10 looks at some of the legal and ethical dimensions of two high-profile situations: abortion and euthanasia. These situations are often discussed together because they concern the limit of human vulnerability (in death) and the limit of human freedom (in determining who can legitimately kill). Our mortality matters to us; accordingly, how we die matters to us, as individuals and as a society. For these reasons, issues relating to abortion and euthanasia have tended to attract considerable public attention and invoke powerful emotions, regardless of which point of view is taken. Much of the debate around abortion and euthanasia concerns how successful the law can be in protecting the vulnerable from harm while respecting individuals' autonomy. This chapter considers some of the main ethical arguments for and against euthanasia and abortion, and sets out the relevant legal frameworks for nurses. In the previous few years, voluntary assisted dying laws have been introduced to all Australian states, but not the Australian Capital Territory and Northern Territory, which are subject to Commonwealth legislative control. While nurses often have a special interest in the morality of abortion and euthanasia, the nurse's role is clearly prescribed by law, and failure to act within the law can result in criminal charges of assault or even manslaughter.

Chapter 11 discusses ethics and aged care, with a special focus on the ways in which nurses can support the autonomy of elderly people. An older person's autonomy begins to deteriorate as the processes of biological decline begin to affect a person's mobility and mental acuity to a degree that obviously impacts their normal activities of living. One of the implications of the process of ageing is that the greatest potential for the nurse to have an impact on a person's autonomy lies within the sphere of activities of daily living. While ethical issues such as euthanasia tend to capture the public imagination, it is at the level of everyday living that the most profound ethical impact is felt. It is at this level also that the dangers (and complexities) of elder abuse typically manifest.

In any book that attempts to discuss law or ethics in relation to nursing practice, there is always much more that could be said – and so much more in a book that attempts to discuss both. This book has tried to steer a path between the need for detail and the need for economy of explanation in order to assist training nurses to orient themselves to the complex and sometimes perplexing world they will face: the world of working with fellow human beings. The world of nursing can be like the cosmos in miniature: stunningly beautiful, utterly amazing, compelling, alarming, hilarious and frightening. We hope this book is a reliable resource for navigating that world, and that it provides an opportunity for student nurses to reflect upon their own values, beliefs and attitudes as they work toward becoming the kind of people they want to be.

Online resources

Reflective questions appear throughout each chapter to help you to revise the content and draw connections with your own practice. Downloadable answer guides for these questions are provided in the online resources at www.cambridge .org/highereducation/isbn/9781009236027/resources.

Further reading

Cashin, A. (2017). Standards for practice for registered nurses in Australia. *Collegian, 24*(3), 255–66.

Gentile, M. (2010). *Giving voice to values: How to speak your mind when you know what's right*, Yale University Press.

Hewitt, J., White, B. & Del Villar, K. (2021). Voluntary assisted dying in Victoria: Why knowing the law matters to nurses. *Nursing Ethics, 28*(2), 221–9.

Ridge, R.A. (2015). Putting the I in integrity. *Nursing Management, 46*(4), 52–4.

Rushton, C. (2017). Cultivating moral resilience. *American Journal of Nursing, 117*(2), https://journals.lww.com/ajnonline/Fulltext/2017/02001/Cultivating_Moral_Resilience.3.aspx.

Snir, J., Ko, D.N., Pratt, B. & McDougall, R. (2022). Anticipated impacts of voluntary assisted dying legislation on nursing practice. *Nursing Ethics Online*. https://doi.org/10.1177/09697330211022409

1 UNDERSTANDING THE HUMAN PERSON

KIM ATKINS

LEARNING OBJECTIVES

In this chapter, you will:

→ Develop your appreciation of the complexity of the concept of 'person'

→ Develop your understanding of 'personhood' as a relation between the biological, interpersonal and social aspects of a human being

→ Develop an understanding of human vulnerability, and how this makes the capacity to care for each other possible

→ Reflect upon the ways in which your beliefs about yourself affect your capacity to care for yourself and others

In 2004, the Chief Justice of the Family Court of Australia, Alistair Nicholson, made a determination that a 13-year-old child (known as Alex) could proceed with medical treatment that would permanently change that child's gender from female to male. Justice Nicholson noted that Alex had the physical appearance of a girl and normal female chromosomes, but had a 'longstanding, unwavering and present identification as male' (*Re Alex* [2004], para. 80; see also Atkins 2005).

In coming to a coherent determination of what was in Alex's best interests, Justice Nicholson gave due consideration to Alex's personal and family history; Alex's subjective perception of his situation; the nature of Alex's relationships with family and friends; and the relevant scientific and medical information pertaining to Alex's mental, physical and sexual health.

The case of Alex has guided legal decision-making since 2005. Experiences such as Alex's raise questions about the nature of human identity:

〉〉 What is the connection between the physical body and a person's psychological outlook?

〉〉 What part do early life experiences play in shaping a personality?

〉〉 What part do social influences play in shaping a personality?

〉〉 Is there an essential defining quality that all persons share?

〉〉 What is gender, and in wat sense does it matter?

〉〉 Where do we get our ideas about persons, sex and gender, as well as what is proper or improper?

As a nurse, you will be called upon to support, care for and protect people who are vastly different from yourself. How you respond to the diversity of human beings will be a measure of your own humanity as well as your professionalism. The NMBA

7

Code of Conduct and the ICN Code of Ethics are designed to support you in this. Certainly, caring does not come as easily to some nurses as it does to others. After all, it is not always pleasant being around incapacitated, sick or grieving people. So why do people want to support the ill or incapacitated? What is it about human nature that causes people to care for each other *at all*?

This chapter will provide a response to this question through a philosophical account of being a person. This account describes being a person as a dynamic unity of personal factors (such as biology and psychology); interpersonal factors (such as relationships with immediate family and close friends); and social factors (such as type of education, or socioeconomic status). We each become an individual person with a unique identity as a result of complex processes involving all these factors (Atkins 2008; Laceulle 2018). The formation of our identity begins with the biological processes of sexual reproduction and pregnancy, followed by our early life experiences in the care of our parents. Later, we come under the influence of formative relationships of friendship, schooling and other social interactions. In addition, our personal identities are formed within our social context, which is itself the outcome of powerful historical and cultural forces. Consequently, a basic feature of being human is to be constantly affected by, and responsive to, other people and the world around us – in both positive and negative ways. This feature of human life – being affected by the people and things around us – is called vulnerability. This concept will be discussed in more detail later in the chapter, where you will see that vulnerability lies at the heart of our capacity to care for each other (Mackenzie 2020; Petherbridge 2021).

Central to this approach to the human person is the idea that we each *become* a person through a complex range of developmental processes. Becoming a person entails the acquisition of a range of physical, cognitive, emotional and interpersonal capacities, which develop over time as the human body develops, and grow through relations with other people. For example, as young children grow, they develop the ability to walk and climb, to communicate and to self-regulate emotions. These skills allow a child to understand the actions of others and to join in cooperative activity. As a result of participating in simple cooperative activities, children acquire the capacity for more sophisticated social skills, such as patience, perspective-taking and negotiation. The philosophical point here is not simply that a person has to acquire social skills to get on in life, but rather that the individual acquires the skills of personhood in a social context. Furthermore, it is from their social context that individuals develop the beliefs, attitudes and expectations that make up their personalities. Understanding individuals as (partly) the product of the society in which they grow and learn reverses the commonly held assumption that a society is the result of individuals who come together voluntarily to secure goods that an individual could not acquire alone. This book takes the approach that persons only ever emerge *from* societies. This means that a person's culture and cultural identity are highly significant because culture is a fundamental source of the meaning a person can find in their life. This is why cultural safety – having one's culture acknowledged and treated with respect – matters to us all; it therefore has a central place in the delivery of appropriate and effective nursing care. We will discuss cultural safety in Chapter 6.

In the example at the beginning of the chapter, Justice Nicholson's decision about Alex can be seen to draw upon the personal, interpersonal and social factors that have influenced Alex's personal identity. Justice Nicholson considered Alex's physical condition, and the biological and medical data related to it. He also considered Alex's early life relationships, especially his relationship with his father. Finally, he considered Alex's experiences at school and his current (as well as possible future) social situation. Justice Nicholson placed these considerations in the context of the requirements of law, including relevant legal precedents and current medical consensus. In doing so, he put together a complex picture of Alex as a young person who is both affected by and responding to his circumstances, a young person with certain physical and psychological states who is part of a circle of family and friends, who has certain social responsibilities and disadvantages, and who – like most other people – simply wants to live a life that will allow him to overcome his personal and social difficulties and thrive. In short, we understand who Alex is when we grasp the 'story' (or narrative) about his life. Every person that a nurse will come across is someone who is both affected by and responding to their circumstances. They will be someone who has physical and psychological states; who is part of a circle of family and friends; who has certain social responsibilities and disadvantages; and who is striving to live a life of their own. The person and their health issues are part and parcel of that broader context.

In setting out guidelines for nurses' and midwives' conduct when caring for persons, the Nursing and Midwifery Board of Australia's (NMBA) Code of Conduct for Nurses and the International Council of Nurses' ICN Code of Ethics for Nurses recognise the personal, interpersonal and social factors that make up a person (NMBA 2018b; ICN 2012, 2021). These have been set out in Tables 1.1 and 1.2 respectively. The most up-to-date information, standards and guidelines for nurses and midwives can be found on the NMBA website (www.nursingmidwiferyboard .gov.au).

TABLE 1.1 NMBA's Code of Conduct for Nurses

PRINCIPLE	VALUE
1 Legal compliance	Nurses respect and adhere to their professional obligations under the National Law and abide by relevant laws.
2 Person-centred practice	Nurses provide safe, person-centred and evidence-based practice for the health and wellbeing of people and, in partnership with the person, promote shared decision-making and care delivery between the person, nominated partners, family, friends and health professionals.
3 Cultural practice and respectful relationships	Nurses engage with people as individuals in a culturally safe and respectful way, foster open and honest professional relationships, and adhere to their obligations about privacy and confidentiality.
4 Professional behaviour	Nurses embody integrity, honesty, respect and compassion.
5 Teaching, supervising and assessing	Nurses commit to teaching, supervising and assessing students and other nurses to develop the nursing workforce across all contexts of practice.
6 Research in health	Nurses recognise the vital role of research to inform quality healthcare and policy development, conduct research ethically and support the decision-making of people who participate in research.
7 Health and wellbeing	Nurses promote health and wellbeing for people and their families, colleagues, the broader community and themselves and in a way that addresses health inequality.

Source: NMBA (2018b).

TABLE 1.2 The ICN Code of Ethics for Nurses

ELEMENT	STANDARD
1 Nurses and people	The nurse's primary professional responsibility is to people requiring nursing care.
	In providing care, the nurse promotes an environment in which the human rights, values, customs and spiritual beliefs of the individual, family and community are respected.
	The nurse ensures that the individual receives accurate, sufficient and timely information in a culturally appropriate manner on which to base consent for care and related treatment.
	The nurse holds personal information in confidence and uses judgement in sharing this information.
	The nurse shares with society the responsibility for initiating and supporting action to meet the health and social needs of the public, in particular those of vulnerable populations.
	The nurse advocates for equity and social justice in resource allocation, access to health care and other social and economic services.
	The nurse demonstrates professional values such as respectfulness, responsiveness, compassion, trustworthiness and integrity.
2 Nurses and practice	The nurse carries personal responsibility and accountability for nursing practice, and for maintaining competence by continual learning.
	The nurse maintains a standard of personal health such that the ability to provide care is not compromised.
	The nurse uses judgement regarding individual competence when accepting and delegating responsibility.

ELEMENT	STANDARD
	The nurse at all times maintains standards of personal conduct, which reflect well on the profession and enhance its image and public confidence.
	The nurse, in providing care, ensures that use of technology and scientific advances are compatible with the safety, dignity and rights of people.
	The nurse strives to foster and maintain a practice culture promoting ethical behaviour and open dialogue.
3 Nurses and the profession	The nurse assumes the major role in determining and implementing acceptable standards of clinical nursing practice, management, research and education.
	The nurse is active in developing a core of research-based professional knowledge that supports evidence-based practice.
	The nurse is active in developing and sustaining a core of professional values.
	The nurse, acting through the professional organisation, participates in creating a positive practice environment and maintaining safe, equitable social and economic working conditions in nursing.
	The nurse practises to sustain and protect the natural environment and is aware of its consequences on health.
	The nurse contributes to an ethical organisational environment and challenges unethical practices and settings.
4 Nurses and co-workers	The nurse sustains a collaborative and respectful relationship with co-workers in nursing and other fields.
	The nurse takes appropriate action to safeguard individuals, families and communities when their health is endangered by a co-worker or any other person.
	The nurse takes appropriate action to support and guide co-workers to advance ethical conduct.

Source: ICN (2021).

Each of the chapters in this book is informed by this picture of the human person. Chapter 2 explores how the law has an important role in stabilising society and supporting relationships of trust between people. Chapter 3 focuses on the interpersonal nature of the nurse–patient relationship, and Chapter 5 looks at the legal obligations and implications of that relationship. The understanding of the human person as embodied, social and vulnerable is central to the discussions of consent and autonomy in Chapters 4 and 6, and the role of confidentiality, trust and respect is the focus of Chapters 7 and 8.

Nursing is a profession that encompasses a huge diversity of practices and practice settings. As the population of Australia ages, the focus of health care increasingly is turning to the management of chronic disease through primary health care, self-management and disease prevention through health promotion. That means that we can expect to see more nursing practice taking place in the broader community rather than in acute-care settings, such as hospitals. This cultural shift highlights the importance of nurses having a good understanding of the nature and diversity of human beings, and of the many ways in which people live, flourish, become ill, age and die.

What is a person?

SOME BACKGROUND TO THE CONCEPT

Since the purpose of nursing is to support and promote the health and well-being of persons across the lifespan, it is important to good nursing practice that nurses have a robust understanding of the concepts of 'persons' and 'well-being'. In other words, in order to understand the needs of any individual person – as well as what constitutes a person's well-being – nurses need to have a sound understanding of what a 'person' is in general.

It is important to note that, at different times and in different places, there have been very diverse ideas about the characteristics of persons, and about who can be included in the community of persons. For example, the ancient Greeks believed that, in addition to purely human persons, there were people who were the offspring of humans and gods. Ancient Egyptian hieroglyphs depict people with a human torso and a dog's head (called 'cynocephaly'). Even today, a wide range of concepts exist pertaining to what a person is. Some people believe that ghosts are persons, or that the possession of a soul distinguishes persons from non-persons. Others – for example, the ethicist Peter Singer (1993) – believe that chimpanzees can be considered persons because they have self-awareness and a concern for their lives. Based on Singer's definition, rational, self-aware aliens from distant planets (if they were to exist) could also be considered persons.

On the other hand, at different times in history, various groups of humans have been excluded from the status of persons for a range of reasons. For example, in the past, women, Indigenous peoples and slaves were claimed to lack sufficient intellectual and moral capacity to make them full persons. Today, the concept of the person continues to be philosophically challenging. Recently, scientists in Italy successfully integrated human body tissue and artificial components to restore a man's limb function, and work has been underway for some time to repair paralysing spinal injuries with artificial nerve conductors. These kinds of medical achievements raise the question of how much of an individual's body can be replaced with artificial components while they can still be regarded as being a human being. Movies such as *Blade Runner* and *Ex Machina* play around with these ideas.

There is no *single* attribute common to all persons by which any individual can be said to be, or not to be, a person. Ideas about what constitutes personhood have varied from age to age and from culture to culture, and no doubt will be different in the future. The way philosophers express this situation is to say that personhood is 'discursive' – that is, 'personhood' is a loose concept comprising a set of attributes that hang together more or less coherently, and that are broadly agreed upon by a community. It is a flexible concept, the boundaries of which are determined differently at different times and in response to different issues. One dreadful example of this occurred in Germany and European countries under Nazi occupation during World War II. Under this regime, people of the Jewish faith, homosexuals and people with certain disabilities were excluded from the category of persons, and were imprisoned and executed on the basis of a racist ideology of Aryan supremacy (Tatz 2003). Clearly, where a society draws the line between persons and non-persons matters because, overall, the suffering of non-persons is valued less than the suffering of persons.

In Australia, the legal system and mainstream social institutions and practices presuppose three basic features of persons: first, that only members of the species *Homo sapiens* are persons; second, that persons are embodied beings; and third, that persons are socially situated.[1] These three features can be seen, for example, in the legal regulations concerning human births and deaths, and the practice of abortion. When a birth is registered, the child's name is recorded, as is the name of the mother (and father if possible) and the date and place of birth, then a birth certificate is issued. This legal process is extremely important because it marks the child's entry into the community and entitles the child to all the legal rights and protections of the laws of the community. The birth certificate is one of the first formal, legal ways in which a child is given social *recognition* as a person.[2]

REFLECTIVE QUESTION 1.1
What kind of features characterise persons?

In Australia, we do not require dogs or cats or horses to have birth certificates because those animals are not recognised as members of the community of persons. We still value and care about our animals, and they do have some legal protections, but the role and legal entitlements of animals are nothing like those of persons. Only those beings who are recognised as persons can have all the rights and responsibilities of citizenship. These rights include the right to hold a passport, own and sell property, vote and consent to medical treatment and so on. However, the birth certificate is not the only way in which legal recognition of one's membership of the human community can be bestowed. Indigenous people living in remote areas, immigrants and refugees may be unable to trace their birth records because of different cultural practices, war or social upheaval. In these cases, other means can be used to establish the person's legal status, such as sworn testimony of someone from the person's place of origin. Such testimony is simply another form of social recognition of personhood.

PERSONHOOD IS A RELATION BETWEEN THE BIOLOGICAL, INTERPERSONAL AND SOCIAL ASPECTS OF A HUMAN BEING

The practical approach to personhood on which this book is based takes as its starting point some biological and social facts about human life. In exploring these ideas, we must keep in mind that some human beings may temporarily or even permanently lose some of the capacities and attributes of persons. While the loss of all capacity does not mean that such human beings automatically lose our moral consideration or their legal standing, it can affect how they are regarded by other people. Some of these human beings will be among the most vulnerable people that you will encounter as a nurse. How you respond will be a measure of your own humanity and morality.

To begin, let's review some biological facts. We come into the world through a process of sexual reproduction that involves the bodies (or tissues, at least) of a woman and a man. As foetuses, we develop inside a person's body, and we are born physically immature and require considerable care to survive. It is now widely agreed that children's bodily experiences (sensations and perceptions) in infancy and early childhood are fundamental to their physical, psychological and moral development (or lack of development) (Anda et al. 2006; Calhoun 2008). These earliest experiences can play a crucial role in the development of emotional dispositions, intellectual capacity, the ability to understand and interact with other people, and the ability to value oneself and one's life. The reasons for this are complex and fascinating, and part of the explanation lies in the fact that human biology plays a fundamental (but not exclusive) role in the kind of *mind* that each individual develops (Gallagher & Meltzoff 1996; Hambrick et al. 2021).

Sometimes we can fail to appreciate the physical aspects of the mind. This is partly because we experience thinking differently from other bodily experiences, such as stretching, indigestion or giving birth. Thinking seems to be unconstrained by the physical limitations of time and space. For example, you can represent in your mind objects that are much bigger than your head, such as the Himalayan mountain range, and you can recall in a short period of time a series of events that took much longer in real time, such as a holiday. But other aspects of thinking can indirectly be shown to have a bodily basis. An obvious example is the effect of mind-altering chemicals, such as alcohol, narcotics and anaesthetics. Even more obvious is the effect of pain. Experiencing pain changes the way a person perceives and thinks about the world around them (Gligorov 2017).

We also know that physical factors (such as exposure to sunlight, massage, exercise and sexual activity) also have an effect upon the way a person feels, and therefore on how the person thinks and behaves. In addition, certain mental and intellectual changes are well known to accompany hormonal changes during adolescence and menopause, and large-scale changes in a person's personality are not uncommon after brain trauma following a motor vehicle accident or stroke. All this provides us with very good reasons to take seriously the idea that the human mind has a physical basis and is profoundly influenced by a range of core physical factors: sexual reproduction, experiences during infancy, developmental brain processes, developmental changes related to adolescence and ageing, and the effects of the physical environment throughout life (Keenan et al. 2016; Michel et al. 2018).

Now consider some social facts. Human life is intrinsically social because human survival requires social cooperation to ensure the provision of food, shelter, protection, companionship and sexual mates, and to pass on those skills to succeeding generations. As a result of close and prolonged interaction with carers during infancy, each individual acquires a set of skills that aid survival. These are skills in setting and achieving goals, delaying satisfaction, self-regulating emotions, communicating and forming relationships to secure personal and shared goods. It is thus clear that our basic social relations are tied directly to our biological needs. In this sense, persons are socially constructed: we acquire personhood only in a social context (Gallagher 2005, 2017). All this is a function of the simple fact that human beings have bodies – or, more specifically, are *embodied*. When you provide nursing care, you are not merely doing something to the person's body, as if it is simply a special kind of object. You are interacting with the person's *life*.

LAW AND ETHICS IN PRACTICE

In his book *The Man Who Mistook His Wife for a Hat*, Oliver Sacks describes a clinical encounter with a patient suffering from a brain injury, Mr Thompson, who had previously owned a delicatessen:

'What'll it be today?' he says, rubbing his hands. 'Half a pound of Virginia, a nice piece of Nova?'

'Oh Mr Thompson,' I exclaim, 'and who do you think I am?'

'Good heavens, the light's bad – I took you for a customer. As if it isn't my old friend Tom Pitkins … Me and Tom (he whispers in an aside to the nurse) was always going to the races together.'

'Mr Thompson, you are mistaken again.'

'So I am,' he rejoins, not put out for a moment. 'Why would you be wearing a white coat if you were Tom? You're Hymie, the kosher butcher next door.'

This banter goes on for some time, with Mr Thompson coming up with other identities for Dr Sacks, based on various visual cues, such as the stethoscope around the doctor's neck. Finally, Mr Thompson says:

'You're not my usual chest-thumping doctor. And by God, you've a beard. You look like Sigmund Freud – have I gone bonkers, round the bend?'

'No, Mr Thompson. Not round the bend, just a little trouble with your memory – difficulties remembering and recognising people.'

'My memory has been playing me some tricks,' he admitted. 'Sometimes I make mistakes – I take somebody for somebody else … What'll it be now, Nova or Virginia?'

(Sacks 1985: 103–4)

Think about how important friendships and relationships are to one's own sense of who one is. What might be the impact of being unsure if the person you are interacting with is the same person as you had interacted with previously?

PERSONHOOD AND REFLECTIVE SELF-AWARENESS

Next, briefly consider the idea that a person's sense of being someone with a life of their own – reflective self-awareness, in other words – arises from the fact that human beings are embodied (Merleau-Ponty 1961).

One of the key features that philosophers have attributed to persons is the capacity for reflective self-awareness (barring serious brain injury). This means that persons not only have awareness of their surroundings (as, say, an insect might), but they can *know* that they have this awareness. When you reflect upon your own awareness of your surroundings, you become self-aware – that is, you realise that you exist in those surroundings. For example, when you are consciously aware of hearing a piece of music, you know that it is *you* who hears the music: you are simultaneously aware of the music and of yourself. Furthermore, you may become aware that the music makes you feel a certain way, and then you may wonder why it makes you feel that way. Those further reflections may evoke a memory associated with the music, and so on.

It may sound unnecessary to say that when you know that you are aware of something, you simultaneously know that it is you who is aware, but it has important implications. If you were only ever aware of your surroundings and not of yourself, you could not, for example, intervene and change your behaviour or your personality traits. Reflective self-awareness makes it possible for us to take our own selves as objects of experience. So, just as we pass judgement on objects in the world, we can pass judgement on ourselves. For example, I may not only be aware of the colour of my hair and the size of my feet, but might also judge my haircut to be fabulous or my feet to be unshapely. In the same way, I can judge my attitudes, values and actions to be good or bad, better or worse. This awareness provides me with the opportunity to change who I am and what I do. It gives me *choice*. Being able to make considered decisions and being able to direct one's life accordingly means having autonomy. (We will consider autonomy again in Chapter 3.)

Reflective self-awareness is sometimes regarded as the function of a purely intellectual power or faculty, but it is in fact a bodily function (Atkins 2008; Gallagher 2005). Reflective self-awareness is a product of the body's ability to feel itself and to connect its feelings to bodily functions and actions through the sensorimotor system, which is coordinated in the brain. This begins in infancy. The sensorimotor system allows the infant to feel, move and coordinate its body parts in such a way that gives rise to purposeful actions without the child having to form any conscious representation or thought of what it is doing. This can be seen in various infant reflexes that precede the development of permanent fine and gross motor skills – for example, the rooting reflex, whereby if the child's cheek is stroked the baby turns their head, opens their mouth and begins sucking; and the stepping reflex, whereby when the child is held above a surface and lowered so that when their feet touch the surface, the child moves them as if to walk (Keenan et al. 2016). In these examples, the infant's body is unconsciously tracking and coordinating the movements of its body parts in relation to one another, without having to be consciously or reflectively aware of what it is doing. This ability is known as proprioception (Gallagher 2005).[3]

Proprioception is the first (and a necessary) stage in the development of a sense of self. It gives the human body the innate ability to sense itself as an integrated whole, and to regulate its movements by coordinating itself as a whole. This gives rise to a sense of unity and allows the formation of an individual perspective. Proprioception commences *in utero* and is fully developed in early childhood

(Holst-Wolf et al. 2016). It underpins both conscious and unconscious bodily movements. To illustrate proprioception in action, consider what happens during sleep. Have you ever wondered why you do not fall out of bed when you are asleep? Proprioception keeps you safely in your bed because while you are sleeping – while your usual self-awareness is inactive – your body nevertheless continues to sense where your limbs are and where the edge of your bed is, and confines your movements to the safety of the bed.

In addition to being able to sense itself (through proprioception), the child's developing body also senses the bodies of other people, notably those of its carers. This adds an interesting aspect to the development of self-awareness. In infancy, when children are bathed, they not only feel the warmth and the wetness of the water on their skin, but they also feel the size, texture and shape of the hands of the person bathing them. So the sensations that infants feel *in* their body are not simply their own inner sensations, but a mixture of perceptions of their own body and of the hands of the person bathing them. For example, an infant being bathed feels a sensation in their back as a result of the pressure from the bather's hands. The infant's body seems to treat that sensation as belonging to it, even though the hands themselves belong to someone else's body. This mixing of sensations arising from the child's own body and the body of the child's carer explains why styles of parental care, with their different rhythms of speech, types and intensity of touch, modes of play and emotional force, powerfully influence the child's developing sense of self, and make each child's self-experience complex and unique (Negayama et al. 2015). The experiences arising from the infant–carer interaction actually stimulate the growth of neural pathways in the child's developing brain that structure how the child reacts to the world around them and to other people (Gallagher & Hutto 2007; Vincini et al. 2017). This gives the child's developing sense of self an interpersonal dimension. In other words, it orients the child's brain (and behaviour) to the existence of other people – specifically, the people with whom the child has some relationship of dependency. This interpersonal orientation will later assist the child to develop their sense of being a person *in general*. Regarding oneself as a person among many other, similar persons demonstrates that selfhood has a social dimension.

Along with the development of cognitive and behavioural abilities, the infant–carer relationship is the ground for the development of moral qualities, such as self-esteem, self-trust, resilience, integrity, empathy and the ability to act from reasons of one's own. In general, children who are treated gently, have their needs met and are applauded for their endeavours will develop a positive sense of self – a strong sense of optimism, resilience and integrity, all of which are necessary for strong moral capacities. This is demonstrated by research into the effects of adverse childhood events (ACEs), including interpersonal trauma, which indicates that children who are treated roughly and are neglected have more difficulty developing a positive sense of self and empathy for both self and others (Oral et al. 2016; Perry 2013). In severe cases, they may not expect very much from life and may have reduced capacity for moral reasoning and autonomous action. Such children may instead rely heavily on strong and stable social structures (such as schooling) to provide the guidance and support necessary for healthy self-esteem and self-trust, successful relationships and social integration (Cox et al. 2020).

It is important to note that we are frequently quite unaware of our background emotional dispositions. This is because our emotional dispositions are more than mere representations in our minds upon which we can easily reflect, such as the memory of a good meal or a sad film. Rather, they function as a kind of unnoticed background against which our conscious ideas, attitudes and beliefs stand out. This is why the concept of emotional intelligence has been a focus of recent research. Emotional intelligence refers to the awareness and understanding of one's emotional dispositions and tendencies, and the ability to reason about one's emotions in order to have constructive interpersonal and professional relationships (Mestre & Barchard 2017). In fact, much of our waking life is driven by non-conscious habits and dispositions. This is why philosophers have emphasised the importance of self-reflection and self-understanding to autonomy. To genuinely understand ourselves and other people, we need to look beyond our express beliefs and attitudes to include an understanding of our background assumptions and the conditions under which those beliefs and attitudes were formed. Importantly, this includes the personal, historical and cultural context within which we each acquired our personalities and values. As a nurse, you should be aware of your own background assumptions about other people, cultures and belief systems, since they will influence how you interact with your patients and how therapeutic your relationships will be.

TO SUMMARISE SO FAR

Persons are human beings with physical, intellectual, emotional, interpersonal and social dimensions to their personalities, which develop over time and are related in complex ways. Importantly, not all our beliefs, attitudes and dispositions are conscious or intentional. It is through the interrelation of physical and psychological attributes, interpersonal relationships, social participation and reflective self-awareness that we each develop the competencies and capacities of personhood. Thus, who a person is must be understood by the story of that person's life. If we think persons can be understood simply as souls or brains or biological components, we will not be able to make sense of what people actually do, feel, think and need.

Recall Oliver Sacks' patient, Mr Thompson, who is losing his sense of self because he is losing his sense of his world and his place in it. He cannot adequately grasp his physical location (in hospital, not the delicatessen), his personal situation (being a patient with a brain disease) or the people around him (he continually misrecognises people). In a different way, a change of social context can befuddle our expectations and understandings of other people.

LAW AND ETHICS IN PRACTICE

Jenny spent a semester on a cultural exchange at a university in Greece. She was there alone over the Christmas period. One of the university lecturers who had helped her organise the exchange (a single, middle-aged man) invited her to spend Christmas Day at his home. Jenny found that she did not know how to interpret the invitation. Did he think this was expected of him as part of his role in the exchange? Was he just being polite and didn't really expect her to accept the invitation? Did he feel sorry for her? Was he making a sexual advance towards her? Or was it an innocent 'no strings attached' social invitation?

Jenny realised that her confusion arose because she couldn't construct a coherent narrative about her situation. She lacked knowledge about the Greek cultural norms around male–female interactions and student–lecturer interactions, so she lacked certainty about the kind of relationship she was in, what was expected of her, what she should expect of herself, and how she should behave.

>> **Do you think your own expectations of others' behaviour are influenced by your own culture?**

VULNERABILITY

The word 'vulnerable' has several meanings, and often conjures up the image of someone who is weak or frail, or who is being taken advantage of. However, this is a very limited and inadequate way of understanding the term. This book uses the word 'vulnerable' in a specific, technical way. *This is important.* When the word 'vulnerable' is used, it is referring to a basic condition that applies to every human being, not just individuals who are disadvantaged in some way. Vulnerability can be both good and bad. However, in its basic meaning, vulnerability is *neither* good nor bad in itself; it is just a fact of life – a necessary condition for acquiring the skills and capacities of personhood. To say that we are vulnerable to something is simply to say we can be affected by it. To say that persons are fundamentally shaped by their physical, emotional and intellectual relations to other similarly embodied individuals is to say that human beings are essentially *mutually vulnerable*. In other words, part of what it is to be a person is to be involved in a web of both voluntary and *involuntary* relationships with other persons. We fundamentally affect and influence each other, and no one is immune to being affected and influenced by others.

Some ways in which human beings affect each other are the same for every relationship. For example, all human beings can be affected physically by others by being slapped or pushed or prodded, regardless of age, gender or disability. Other ways of being affected vary from relationship to relationship, and from society to society, and vulnerabilities vary across the different stages of life and between personalities at the same stage of life. For example, teenagers tend to be more sensitive to peer pressure than middle-aged people, and some individuals are outgoing while others are more solitary. Individual relationships and characteristics are also expressed differently according to norms around friendships between men and women, public displays of emotion and styles of verbal interaction. Nevertheless, no matter how unique or solitary an individual may aspire to be, people who could *never* share the activities, ideas or emotions of other people would be incapable of really understanding either themselves or another person.

The things to which we are vulnerable are those things that can affect us physically, emotionally, psychologically, interpersonally and socially. For example, when we are affected physically, we may experience stimuli such as heat, noise, odours and textures. When we are affected emotionally, we may experience states such as joy, sadness, anxiety or relief. And when we are affected psychologically, we may experience states such as hoping, planning, remembering or imagining. We are also affected by our friendships, which may produce experiences of trust, loyalty or betrayal. Also, we may have social experiences, such as solidarity when playing in a sporting team, or national pride when visiting a historical monument. All these kinds of experiences overlap with each other: emotions are accompanied by psychological states (such as thoughts of the feared or hoped-for object); physical sensations are accompanied by emotional and psychological states; and our interpersonal and social experiences have physical, psychological and emotional aspects to them.

Vulnerability is a function of human embodiment, since it is our embodiment that determines the ways we can be affected and the kinds of experiences we can have. Our experiences may be positive or indifferent, or they may be negative. Vulnerability can give rise to negative experiences, such as contracting infections like pneumonia and influenza, because the human body is the kind of physical environment in which those bacteria and viruses can grow. If the human body were made from completely different substances – for example, plastic – those pathogens would not be able to grow in it, and so we would not be vulnerable to pneumonia or influenza; however, we would be vulnerable to melting! On the other hand, vulnerability can give rise to very positive experiences, such as the pleasure felt from listening to beautiful music, playing fun games, eating delicious food, reading scary stories, dancing and falling in love.

As we have stated, this book uses the concept of vulnerability in a technical, philosophical sense to refer to the capacity that human beings have to be affected by something. In this way, we can say that vulnerability is part of the human condition. By that we mean vulnerability is just part and parcel of being human.

Vulnerability is the capacity to be affected by something. Can you imagine what life would be like if you were not vulnerable? Can you even imagine a living creature that is not vulnerable in this sense? It seems highly likely that if a person was never affected by anything, they would never perceive or be aware of anything because nothing would affect their neurological system and brain. The biological and social characteristics of *Homo sapiens* mean that we are vulnerable creatures. Because something can happen to us, we have a reason to care about our situations. For this reason, it is important for a nurse, as a carer, to be sensitive to the different situations of people within a society. The situations of men, women, adults, adolescents and children differ in significant ways, which if they remain unnoticed can be affected adversely by what the nurse does, or fails to do.

To illustrate this idea, consider the situation of Rob, who is admitted to hospital for cosmetic surgery to reduce the size of his nose. Clearly, Rob cares about having a certain kind of physical appearance, and is vulnerable to negative feelings about his nose. A nurse who sincerely believes that a person's personality is more important than a person's physical appearance may insufficient attention to physical traits, such as the size of a person's nose. This may sound good, but the problem is that the nurse may not be sufficiently sensitive to Rob's situation. The nurse may fail to respond in a caring way to Rob's particular vulnerability, not because the nurse is cruel or stupid, but because the things the nurse cares about are so different from the things Rob cares about.

Have you ever found yourself saying to a friend that something they care about is superficial or unimportant? How do you feel when someone trivialises something you care about? From time to time, we all encounter situations that are beyond our own personal experience, and can initially make it hard for us to care appropriately about those situations. In such cases, education and imagination can be valuable tools. Nurses are often called upon to care for people from a vast range of backgrounds and lifestyles. For example, while you may not have any personal experience of cancer, you can read about its effects on the body, listen to people who have had that experience and imagine what it is like to have a diagnosis of cancer. You can also relate those experiences to your own experiences of being ill, afraid or needing help, to develop an understanding of what it might be like to have cancer. In that way, you can come to care about the situations of people with cancer, even when those situations are beyond your actual experience. In such a situation, you can see how drawing upon your own vulnerability helps you to care. Our understanding and experience of our own vulnerability can be a powerful source of empathy, understanding and support for other people.

CARING FOR OTHERS

Being affected by other people is part and parcel of being a person, and this is what makes it possible for us to care about the world and other people in it. Vulnerability gives us the capacity to care for each other because it allows us to affect each other. Because we can affect each other, we can make a difference to how each other feels. Caring for another person just is the striving to make a difference to how that person feels – both about their circumstances and themself.

However, caring – like charity – begins at home. To understand why, first consider another idea. We not only have relations with other people, through which we become capable of caring about others; we also have relations with our own selves, through which we become capable of caring for ourselves.

The idea that we have to acquire the capacity to care for ourselves may seem surprising to some. People with healthy self-esteem take that capacity for granted: it just seems obvious that we care highly for ourselves. But as psychologists and philosophers have known for a long time, this is far from straightforward. This point is important because one's capacity to understand and care for others is directly affected by one's capacity to understand and care for oneself (Ricoeur 1992). Caring – whether directed to oneself or others – entails the same basic set of skills, such as patience, tolerance, tenderness, forgiveness, trust, good judgement and the desire to do well.

To understand this, reconsider some basic features of persons. Persons have reflective self-awareness. For example, here you are, reading this book. You are not only aware of the book, you are also aware that it is you who is reading it. In other words, you have reflective self-awareness. We noted earlier that, just as we pass judgement on objects in the world, we can pass judgement on ourselves. For example, you can criticise yourself for being unfit or admire yourself for working hard. This shows that reflective self-awareness is a kind of relationship you have with yourself. You can observe your thoughts, feelings and behaviour, and you can pass judgement on yourself – even argue with yourself – rather as you might do with another person you know well.

You can, through your relationship with yourself, come to care a lot about certain aspects of yourself, or come to care very little about other aspects. When you have an experience that makes you feel good about yourself – for example, doing well in an exam – that experience tends to increase the value you attach to yourself as a learner. When you have an experience that makes you feel bad about yourself – for example, letting down a friend – that experience tends to make you decrease the value you attach to yourself as a friend (Dillon 1992). Often, mild self-criticism can motivate you to do better next time, so it can be a useful tactic to help you live up to your personal standards. The better you are able to live up to your standards in one aspect of your life, the better you will tend to feel about yourself and your life overall, so your self-esteem is likely to improve.

Although self-criticism can motivate a person to do better, prolonged and powerful self-criticism can make a person feel that they are less worthy than other people, and so reduce their self-esteem. The notion of 'self-esteem' refers to a person's sense of their inherent worthiness *as a person*. Self-esteem is not the same as pride or narcissistic self-regard. It is more than having a positive self-image: self-esteem is a very deep kind of measure of oneself and what one considers oneself to be worthy of in life. Typically, when people have high self-esteem, they set high standards for themselves, and so expect to carry out work of high quality. The person with high self-esteem cares about doing well, both for their own satisfaction and in relation to others. Conversely, people with low self-esteem can have lower expectations of themselves, and may expect to carry out work of lower quality (Dillon 2013). So how you feel about yourself may have an impact on how you treat your patients and colleagues.

Self-esteem has a very close connection with self-respect, which is related to the way a person is regarded by others. Self-respect refers to the manner in which we care about our own personal standards, beliefs, values and conduct. Self-respect is developed through being respected by others and having respectful relations with others. Much of what we each believe about ourselves is the result of 'internalising' the opinions of other people. This is a well-known psychological phenomenon. It is fine if you live in an environment where you are loved and told you are a good and clever person, but unfortunately this isn't the case for everyone. People who are subject to systematic discrimination on the basis of sex or race, for example, can come to believe that people of their sex or race really are inferior to those of other sexes or races (Dillon 1992, 2013). As in all experiences of oppression, children who are raised in situations where they are subjected to ongoing physical or psychological abuse tend to internalise the low regard their carers have for them, and come to believe that their needs are inferior to those of others (Foucault 1997; Hancock 2018). In each of these cases, the result is poor self-esteem and severe self-criticism, and the individual truly believes their life is less worthwhile than the lives of others. It is very important to people's sense of self-worth and self-esteem that they have positive experiences throughout their life that support them to value their existence. We will discuss this issue in relation to self-respect in Chapter 9.

REFLECTIVE QUESTION 1.2

Imagine an experience in the clinical setting where you fail to carry out a task to the appropriate standard – for example, you might apply a dressing that falls off soon afterwards. How are you likely to react psychologically and emotionally to this situation?

The point of this discussion has been to demonstrate that we are not just vulnerable to other things and other people; we are also vulnerable to our own selves. Each person is vulnerable to the inner psychological and emotional forces that constitute one's sense of self and identity. We have feelings and beliefs about ourselves, and we respond to these in various ways – only some of which we are consciously aware. The feelings, beliefs and attitudes we have about ourselves influence our self-esteem, and thereby affect our capacity to care both for ourselves and for other people. In short, to nurse well, nurses first and foremost need to have a good relationship with themselves.

Vulnerability and ethical life

The idea that selves are mutually vulnerable is highly significant for understanding ethics, but first we need to clarify what ethics is. *Ethics is a branch of philosophy concerned with the question of what constitutes a good life.* The concept of a 'good life' has a technical, philosophical meaning here. It does *not* refer to a life that feels good, or is 'nice', or that someone just happens to think is good. The concept of a good life refers to the kind of life in which *all* human beings can flourish physically, emotionally, psychologically, morally, interpersonally and socially. The 'goods' of human life correspond to our human, embodied capacities – things such as physical health, emotional well-being, psychological clarity and resilience, personal integrity, self-respect, friendship, collegiality, a sense of belonging and being respected, prosperity, social stability and political freedom (MacIntyre 1985; Meyers 2004).

Philosophers have attempted to develop theories of the good life by identifying the basic features of human life that allow us to value our lives. French philosopher Paul Ricoeur (1992) has provided the kind of framework that fits with the picture of embodied personhood described in this book. Ricoeur writes that the good life must satisfy three fundamental human needs: our need to value and respect our own selves through self-esteem; our need to have relationships with others in which we are mutually valued and respected (solicitude); and our need to feel part of a society in which people are treated fairly and as moral equals (justice). According to this view, an ethical life is one characterised by self-respect and self-esteem, friendship, love and cooperation, in a society free from discrimination and persecution, where there is fairness in the distribution of benefits and burdens across the whole community. Importantly, these needs are all interrelated, and together they underpin a coherent and meaningful life. Self-esteem depends upon having good relations with others (solicitude) in a just society. Solicitude is possible only between individuals with self-esteem who value fairness, and justice is only possible between individuals who consider that their own lives and the lives of others are worth living.

LAW AND ETHICS IN PRACTICE

Api is a Sudanese refugee living in the suburbs of Melbourne. He was shot and seriously injured during civil violence in Sudan. His parents died in the conflict. People occasionally remark on what a good life he has now, far from the violence and persecution he experienced in Sudan. Api replies, 'It is true that I am safe. I have a job and I am completing university studies to become an engineer. But I don't think that I can ever be free of the guilt and pain I feel for leaving my family to die. I feel that I am not a proper person for running away, even though I know it saved my life. Who could really trust me if I run away when they need help?'

Api's overwhelming suffering from the civil war has eroded his self-esteem and self-respect, and make it difficult for him to enjoy and feel deserving of the good things that life in Australia can offer him, even though he recognises their value.

>> **When you interact with a person who has a very different life experience from yours, what kind of assumptions do you make about what is 'natural' or' normal' emotional expression?**

Philosophers do not believe that the good life actually exists – there is far too much injustice and inequity in the world. The good life as a world in which all human beings flourish is an ideal; it is not real. It is a world to which we can only aspire, but it is one to which we *should* aspire.

On another level, we can consider our own, actual lives to be more or less good lives, despite the fact they are imperfect, often fragmented, plagued by ignorance and interpersonal conflict, and subject to all sorts of forces and emotions over which we have little control. We are living ethically when we try to act in ways that accord with the ideal of a good life. That is, we are ethical when we try to embody the values that would make the world a place in which everyone can flourish. That kind of a place would be one where everyone is treated fairly and without prejudice; where everyone receives good health care; where everyone enjoys the fruits of friendship and family; and where everyone works together to share the responsibilities of a good society.

In practical terms, a good life requires each of us to acquire and apply the skills, understanding, relationships and personal characteristics of a good person. The best way to do this, as Aristotle advised over 2000 years ago, is still to bring ourselves under the influence of people who have those traits we wish to acquire ourselves, and avoid those who lack them (Thomson 1966). In other words, we need to be open to being influenced and affected by the kind of people with whom we would want to live and who we want to be like (Meyers 1989). To become the kind of person we would like to be, we must become the kind of person we would like to be *with*. In addition, if we expect other people to trust us, understand us and act responsibly towards us, we have to learn to trust, understand and act responsibly towards ourselves. Only in this way will we become trustworthy, understanding and responsible people. In the context of nursing, this points to the importance of becoming skilled and professional through actively fostering relationships with other skilled and professional nurses – for example, through membership of professional organisations.

During the COVID-19 pandemic, a significant problem arose with the proliferation of misinformation about vaccines and the virus itself, especially through social media channels. This misinformation has been able to influence people in part because we are vulnerable to each other. Just as we can have our beliefs and attitudes shaped positively by other people, sometimes they can be shaped negatively – misshaped or misdirected – during times when we are unsure about what is happening, or fearful about what might happen. Under those kinds of circumstances, one can start to doubt one's knowledge or judgement, and possibly act in ways that might be unethical.

Ethics is often conflated with morals, but this is a mistake. Morals are best understood as the principles (or rules) that should guide human conduct in order for the good life to be realised (Ricoeur 1992). Moral principles are rule-like expectations or beliefs that stipulate what one ought to do in order to be 'good'. Living up to those principles places obligations on what one can do. Moral obligations, then, concern those things that each of us is required to do to create a good life.

Our moral principles have several dimensions. To illustrate, consider the life of a student nurse, Mike. Mike feels that life is good when he gains self-esteem, for example, by achieving his goals through study or sporting efforts; when he develops fulfilling friendships and professional relationships; and when he enjoys the fruits of a just society, for example, through labour laws that regulate safe work standards and levels of pay. Mike's moral obligations, then, are to act in ways that preserve and promote the conditions that make possible the life he values. Examples of such moral obligations would be respect for himself and his colleagues, trustworthiness, empathy, patience, commitment, compassion and honesty. Furthermore, justice requires that he also promotes fairness, and rejects unfairness and injustice wherever he finds it.

Moral obligations are the practical imperatives that guide our innate striving towards a coherent and meaningful life – a good life. Human persons are not isolated planets merely passing by in 'outer space'. This is why living an ethical life obliges us to respect each other. Respect requires us to refrain from deceiving and manipulating each other, and to be trustworthy and responsible. An ethical life also requires us to be empathetic, patient and fair – in short, to act in ways that preserve the conditions that make a good life possible *for anyone*.

These fundamental moral obligations are of particular relevance to the nurse because patients are especially vulnerable to the nurse's power, as a result of needing the nurse's special knowledge and skills. The issue of power and the professional relationship will be addressed in Chapter 3.

In his work on dignity therapy, Canadian psychiatrist Professor Harvey Chochinov (2013; Chochinov et al. 2022) maintains that the health professional (especially a doctor or nurse) functions like a mirror to the patient, reflecting back to the patient a view of themselves as they are regarded by the nurse or doctor. If the nurse regards the patient as a lost cause, the patient can come to regard themself in the same way, becoming depressed and feeling worthless. Alternatively, if the nurse regards a patient as a valuable individual whose feelings, thoughts and recovery are important, the patient will find it easier to maintain their self-esteem and motivation to do well. All these experiences are tied to mutual vulnerability. The nurse can support the suffering person by being open to the person's need to be regarded as a worthy member of humanity. That means regarding the patient as the

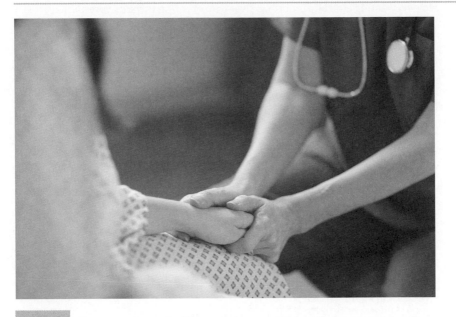

FIGURE 1.1	The nurse plays a significant role in supporting a suffering person's trust in their own capacity to recover and live well again.

subject of a web of rich, complex and moving experiences and relationships that matter, and not merely a bundle of worn-out tissue or a pit stop in a nurse's busy day (Chochinov 2013; Chochinov et al. 2022). Chochinov maintains that health professionals must embrace humanity as central to their practice and as a source of compassion. In other words, he argues that medical and nursing education must inculcate in doctors and nurses an appreciation of the significance and value of literature, music, art and history – those disciplines in which the rich tapestry of human lives, loves and sufferings is described and explained.

Perhaps this sounds like an onerous view of ethics. However, for a nurse to have a good relationship with their patients – a therapeutic relationship – they are going to need to use more than science; they will require ethics. That means utilising a skillset that acknowledges our mutual vulnerability and promotes self-esteem through solicitude and justice. The nurse will need to use empathy, recognition, tolerance, trust and imagination. They will also need to exercise humility, openness and an appreciation of human diversity – a sense of humour comes in handy, too. Finally, the nurse will need to appreciate not only the person's social situation and their cultural background, but the ways in which social forces and interpersonal relations mould and influence that person's outlook, values and responses.

However, acting ethically is not merely a way of acting towards your patient: it is a way of acting towards yourself – *a way of life.*

Conclusion

Being a person does not consist in something simplistic like having a soul or a brain. It is a complex, dynamic and social process across the lifespan. Personhood in general, and our personalities in particular, are the combined effects of our biology, our relationships, our life experiences, the social and cultural institutions within which we live, and our self-reflections and self-conceptions. Our vulnerability – our capacity to be affected – makes us the kind of beings who can grow, change and respond to circumstances and other people in reflective, rational, emotional and imaginative ways. The dynamic and interpersonal features of personhood give the nurse–patient relationship its therapeutic power. It places the nurse in a special position to promote and restore health and well-being. How the nurse uses that power will affect not only the patient's well-being, but the nurse's personal and professional identity as well.

REFLECTIVE QUESTIONS 1.3

1 If you had to nurse a person who had been convicted of a serious crime, what kind of principles might guide how you treat the person?
2 What are the three key elements of personhood?
3 What is human 'vulnerability' in the sense that it is being used in this book?
4 What is 'mutual vulnerability'?
5 What is self-respect? How does a person develop self-respect? Why does a nurse's self-esteem matter?
6 How does our vulnerability make it possible for us to care for each other?
7 What are the three basic needs that a good life must strive to meet?
8 How does your conception of the good life inform what you do and think?

Further reading

Bolt, J. (2019). The concept of vulnerability in medical ethics and philosophy. *Philosophy, Ethics and Humanities in Medicine, 14*(6), https://doi.org/10.1186/s13010-019-0075-6

Brison, S. (2002). *Aftermath: Violence and the remaking of a self.* Princeton University Press.

De Chesnay, M. (ed.) (2011). *Caring for the vulnerable: Perspectives in nursing theory, practice, and research,* 3rd ed. Jones & Bartlett.

Dillon, R. (2013). Self-respect and self-esteem. In H. LaFollette (ed.), *International encyclopedia of ethics.* Wiley Blackwell.

Emerging Minds. *Website*. Especially information on adverse childhood events (ACEs): https://emergingminds.com.au/resources/background-to-aces-and-impacts

Heaslip, V. & Ryden, J. (2013). *Understanding vulnerability: A nursing and healthcare approach*. Wiley & Sons.

Nussbaum, M. & Sen, A. (1993). *The quality of life*. Clarendon Press.

Sacks, O. (1985). *The man who mistook his wife for a hat*. Picador.

Sinclair, S., Hack, T.F., Raffin-Bouchal, S. et al. (2018). What are healthcare providers' understandings and experiences of compassion? The healthcare compassion model – a grounded theory study of healthcare providers in Canada. *BMJ Open*, *8*(3), e019701.

Case cited

Re Alex [2004] Fam CA 297

Notes

1   Australian law recognises 'artificial persons', but these are corporations, constituted by actual human persons, with specific legal obligations and responsibilities that are shared among the board of directors.

2   It is important to note that even babies whose birth is not registered are entitled to legal protections; however, if the formal social processes of legal recognition are not followed, the child effectively is excluded from all subsequent rights and opportunities. For example, a Medicare card cannot be issued and regular medical care cannot be given; enrolment at school cannot be undertaken; a passport cannot be issued; a bank account cannot be opened; legal employment or even marriage cannot be undertaken, and so forth.

3   See Gallagher's (2005) discussion of the case of Ian Waterman, who lost all ability to detect sensations in his body below his neck as the result of a head injury. He cannot sense where his limbs are, or how they are behaving, without looking at them. He has no feeling in his body and no proprioceptive awareness of his body other than of his head. He manages to control and coordinate his movements only by visually monitoring and coordinating the parts of his body as he executes the movement. For example, he cannot walk by simply putting one foot in front of the other. He has to watch his feet in order to walk, and he has to both see and imagine the route he is walking, then consciously coordinate it all. If he stops visually monitoring his body parts, he stops walking.

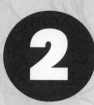

2 THE LEGAL SYSTEM

BERNHARD RIPPERGER

LEARNING OBJECTIVES

In this chapter, you will:

→ Gain a basic understanding of the law and its role in everyday life

→ Learn about the major institutions that make up the Australian legal system

→ Be able to identify the sources of law

→ Develop an awareness of key features of some areas of the law that are relevant to nurses

→ Gain an appreciation of the role of law in defining a nurse's 'scope of practice'

Although nursing is a health-care profession, and nurses are required to have clinical skills in order to practise, the law establishes expectations that must be met. When a health-care professional such as a nurse fails to meet these standards, the law can intervene in a number of ways that can have very significant consequences.

For example, in 2011 a six-year-old boy named Jack was admitted to the Children's Assessment Unit at Leicester Hospital in England around 10.30 a.m. Jack had Down syndrome and a known heart condition. He had been suffering from vomiting and diarrhoea, and had difficulty breathing. He was cared for by a trainee paediatrician, Dr Hadiza Bawa-Garba, and nursing staff, including Ms Isabel Amaro. Jack died that evening from an infection. His death was immediately reported to the Coroner.

During the coronial inquest, expert evidence was given that suggested the death was preventable. The Coroner adjourned the hearing and the matter was referred to the police. Both Dr Bawa-Garba and Ms Amaro were charged with 'manslaughter by gross negligence', which carries a maximum penalty of life imprisonment. Both were convicted and each received a two-year suspended prison sentence.

It was found that Dr Bawa-Garba had failed to adequately assess the patient, respond to findings from laboratory tests that showed the boy was deteriorating, keep proper notes and refer to a consultant for further advice.

The nurse, Isabel Amaro, had failed to undertake and record regular readings of the boy's vital signs and oxygen saturation levels, and she had also failed to keep a proper fluid balance record, even though he was on intravenous fluids. Ms Amaro had also turned off the oxygen saturation-monitoring equipment without telling Dr Bawa-Garba and it was alleged that she had failed to escalate her concerns about the deteriorating condition of the boy to senior nursing and medical staff, which delayed his reassessment. These failures were said to have contributed significantly to the boy's death.

Following their convictions, Dr Bawa-Garba and Ms Amaro faced professional disciplinary hearings and were 'struck off' their respective registers, although Dr Bawa-Garba later appealed and had the penalty reduced to a suspension.

Source: *Bawa-Garba v General Medical Council* [2018] EWCA Civ 1879; Findings of the Conduct and Competence Committee, Nursing and Midwifery Council (UK), 4 August 2016.

Other chapters of this book will look in some detail at what *the law* is as it applies to different aspects of nursing practice in Australia. However, in this chapter we will focus more on what *law* is in general, and on some of the basic philosophical and legal principles that make up the Australian legal system.

Accordingly, this chapter will briefly introduce the main features of the Australian legal system, including:

→ the different parts or 'arms' of the government
→ the sources of law
→ some key features of different branches of law relevant to nursing.

A basic knowledge of the legal system is fundamental to understanding the law as it applies to nursing practice. As we will see, both later in this chapter and elsewhere in this book, the whole concept of a 'profession of nursing' is in part a product of the law. Indeed, the very first principle of the Code of Conduct for Nurses requires that 'Nurses respect and adhere to their professional obligations under the National Law and abide by relevant laws' (NMBA 2018b). This chapter will look at this aspect of the role of law in nursing through a discussion of a nurse's 'scope of practice'.

The law and its role in everyday life

Before looking at the specific features of the Australian legal system, it is worth reflecting on some more fundamental questions, such as 'What is law?' and 'What is the role of law in everyday life?'

Law is a complex system of rules, processes and values that are publicly shared and exist to help people decide how to behave. Law plays an important role in stabilising society (Habermas 1996). It is a feature of modern societies that in our everyday lives we are surrounded by and interact with many people who we do not personally know. These people may be from different backgrounds to ours and they may have different world-views and values. This unfamiliarity can make the task of coordinating our day-to-day activities challenging, as we cannot know for sure how people will respond in various situations. In the absence of well-established or specific social bonds (like the relationships we may have with family, friends or other 'neighbours'), there can be a degree of uncertainty involved when we have to interact with other people. Put simply, the question can easily arise: Why should I trust this stranger? The law plays an important part in answering this question. This is because most people obey the law most of the time. This phenomenon is known as 'general compliance'. It is this feature of law that has a powerful effect in stabilising society because it means we can generally know how other people will respond in everyday situations.

In addition to this stabilising effect of the law, there is also a 'disburdening' effect. That is, the law makes it easier for us to move around and interact in everyday life. Imagine that every time we met a new person or found ourselves in a new situation we had to worry about or negotiate what rules were going to apply or what behaviours were expected. That would be a difficult, time-consuming and risky process (and there is a good chance that no agreement would be reached). The law, however, allows us to enter into interactions both with new people and in new contexts without the effort that would be involved in establishing a relationship with these people. This is because the law has already defined a lot of the rules and behaviours that are relevant to the new interaction or situation. For example, when I enter a shop for the first time, the law has already established the rules around how I can buy something, my rights and obligations as a purchaser and the rights and obligations of the shopkeeper as a seller. The law enables us to adopt legally defined and protected roles that we know will be recognised and respected.

The role of law in stabilising our expectations and behaviours, and in disburdening us in our everyday interactions, is especially important in situations where there is an inequality of power or specific vulnerability. For example, when I am unwell and go to a hospital, I know that the people who present themselves as nurses are properly trained and have a legal responsibility to provide me with care. I also know that the medicine and equipment that will be used to treat me have been tested to make sure they are safe and reliable. In short, part of the reason why I am able to enter into a nurse–patient relationship is because the law provides me with a baseline level of trust and confidence – this is what it means for nursing to be a profession.

The social effectiveness of the law is one criterion of whether a particular law can be said to be 'legitimate'. A legitimate law is one that is regarded by society as having authority, as being a rule that should be followed. If a law cannot guarantee general compliance, it fails as a law and is unlikely to have a strong enough claim to affect people's behaviour. This can happen when the law does not keep up with social change, which can lead to many contentious issues, including in relation to abortion and euthanasia (which will be discussed in Chapter 10). However, the law does not simply claim to be effective at organising social interaction. When we say a law is legitimate, we are also saying that it deserves to be followed – that we respect it. General compliance is not enough to justify a law as legitimate. It also has to be capable of being followed out of *respect* for the law.

The philosophical underpinnings of why the law must also make this moral claim on us are varied and complicated, and are beyond the scope of this chapter. However, it is generally accepted that we respect the law because of its basis in the value we attach to autonomy and democracy. In short, a law is legitimate if it is one that I as a citizen could choose to obey (by choosing I exercise my autonomy) and one that I have agreed to myself (through the democratic process).

The law is a public expression of the general will of the citizens of a political community reached through a deliberative democratic process – for example, where the people elect representatives who make laws on their behalf. Legitimate laws are those that, in a sense, we have freely chosen to impose on ourselves. This is why the law can simultaneously both command obedience and expect compliance out of respect for the law.

REFLECTIVE QUESTION 2.1
What are the two criteria of a legitimate law?

The major institutions of the Australian legal system

In order to understand how the law works, it is necessary to have a basic understanding of both the major institutions of the legal system and the key principles and institutions of the system of government that exists in Australia.

PRINCIPLES AND STRUCTURE OF GOVERNMENT

Australia is a democracy, which means that the political community in Australia is organised according to the principle that the source of legitimate power is the 'will of the people'. The specific form of democracy that is in place in Australia is known as 'representative government'. This means that members of the political community periodically choose representatives who are responsible for deciding how society should be organised. These representatives make decisions on behalf of everyone about what policies and values should be given priority, what laws should be in place and how those laws are to be enforced.

Australia inherited its system of government from England and, despite some changes, the fundamental principles of that system remain in place. Certain principles and conventions exist in the Australian democratic system, which limit the direct involvement of the people in decisions about the way government operates. The most obvious example is that Australia's head of state is the King, who is represented in Australia by the Governor-General and the Governors of the various states. This is very different from other democratic countries that elect their head of state, such as France or the United States.

Another principle that is regarded as fundamental is the doctrine of the 'separation of powers'. In order to avoid the abuse of power by the head of state, the responsibilities of government have, over time, been divided up among different 'arms of government': the executive, the legislature and the judiciary. Each of these will be discussed in detail below; however, in brief the three arms are responsible for:

→ developing policy and administering the law
→ making the law
→ giving effect to the law (Sanson & Anthony 2018).

Despite some limitations on the separation of powers and other peculiarities of the system of government, the key principle of any modern, democratic society, such as Australia, is that it is governed in accordance with the 'rule of law'. This means that the Australia Government exercises its power through the law, and is accountable to the law. That is, every action and every part of government are subject to the law.

LAW AND ETHICS IN PRACTICE

Before colonisation, Aboriginal and Torres Strait Islander peoples, living in what is now called Australia, had their own systems of law. When the British colonised Australia, they decided that English law would apply, including in relation to Aboriginal and Torres Strait Islander peoples. This decision was justified on the basis of a principle of international law that where foreign land was simply occupied, rather than conquered, the law of the occupying power was to apply. This required a finding that the land was empty when it was colonised. This was not literal because it was clear that there were many people living here when the British arrived, but instead it was argued that as Aboriginal people did not cultivate the land; it was not their property. This was a doctrine known as *terra nullius*.

Terra nullius applied in Australia until the High Court decision of *Mabo v Queensland (No 2)* handed down in 1992. The *Mabo* decision allowed some legal recognition of certain rights of Aboriginal and Torres Strait Islander peoples in relation to land. However, these rights can be modified by Australian law, and there remains very little recognition of customary law in the Australian legal system (Sanson & Anthony 2018).

》》 Thinking about what makes a law 'legitimate', what do you think are some of the ongoing consequences for Aboriginal and Torres Strait Islander peoples of the doctrine of *terra nullius?*

THE FEDERATION OF AUSTRALIA

Australia's has a federal system of government. This means that Australia is made up of a number of distinct political communities, namely, the states and territories. Australia used to be made up of several self-governing colonies. These colonies agreed to unite and form a government that could rule the nation as a whole, and in 1901 the Commonwealth of Australia was created through federation.

The key feature of federation was the enactment of the Australian Constitution, the legal document that creates the Commonwealth of Australia and establishes its key legal institutions. Constitutional law is a very complex area well beyond the scope of this chapter; however, it is important to know a few of the important features of the Constitution because it sets out the most important rules for how the political and legal system in Australia works. For example, the Constitution includes:

➔ a formal separation of powers at the Commonwealth level
➔ a limitation on the Commonwealth's legislative powers (in terms of subject matter, or the areas in which the Commonwealth parliament is able to make laws)
➔ a rule stating that where a Commonwealth law is inconsistent with a state law, the Commonwealth law will prevail.

The federal structure of Australia adds a level of complexity to both the political and legal systems because, in addition to the rules and conventions that govern each political community, there are rules and conventions that govern the relationship the Commonwealth government has with each state and territory government.

LAW AND ETHICS IN PRACTICE

When is a national law not a national law? Section 51 of the Constitution gives the Commonwealth parliament power to legislate in respect of certain subject matter, such as taxation, currency and military defence. The Commonwealth can also legislate with respect to matters referred to it by the states or in relation to matters incidental to the subject matter in section 51.

Section 51 does not include health as one of the areas on which the Commonwealth can legislate. At the time of federation, it was thought that issues relating to health services would be managed more appropriately at a state level.

Since that time, changes to the ways health-care services are funded and provided made a national scheme to regulate the various health-care professions both important and desirable. However, the Commonwealth had no power to pass a law to govern the professions. The Health Practitioner Regulation National Law is not a law of the Commonwealth; rather, following a period of negotiation, each state and territory agreed to pass a law in its own jurisdiction that was the same, or at least largely the same (there are some differences between states in the 'national law') as the law of the other jurisdictions.

>> **Why is it useful to have a national law regulating the health-care professions?**

The arms of government

As noted above, the government is made up of the executive, legislative and the judicial branches, each with its own distinct legal structure and responsibilities in the exercise of power. We will now examine each of these in turn.

THE EXECUTIVE

The executive is the branch of government that most people associate with the term 'the government'. The executive includes the prime minister (or premier at the state level) and the various other ministers who are appointed to assist them.

Ministers are responsible for the administration of the government on a day-to-day basis. They are allocated 'portfolios', which are generally based on subject matter such as 'finance', 'health', 'law and justice' and so on. The ministers are identified by a title that reflects these responsibilities – for example, the minister for health is responsible for all the laws relating to health services.

In order to assist ministers in carrying out these duties, there is the bureaucracy, or 'public service'. This includes large departments, which are structured hierarchically and are responsible directly to the minister, and smaller bodies, which may have a degree of independence from the minister's direct control.

One reason why people associate the executive branch with the government as a whole is that it is very powerful in Australia. This is because it usually controls the legislative branch (because the political party that wins the most seats in parliament forms the government) and so can directly affect how law is made. Further, in addition to being able to have law made the way it wants, the executive can use its control over government finances to influence how law is created and enforced.

For example, one of the largest parts of the bureaucracy of each state in Australia is in relation to the health portfolio. All states and territories have a minister for health, who is responsible for administering the law relating to health and for the delivery of publicly owned or funded health services. In addition, the health portfolio usually involves control over spending very large amounts of money. In New South Wales, the total health budget in 2021–22 was over $30 billion (New South Wales

Health 2021), while in Tasmania it was over $10 billion (Tasmanian Government 2021). The ability to decide how this money is spent means the executive has a lot of power.

THE LEGISLATURE

Following the Westminster system of government (named after the location of the UK parliament) the legislature is responsible for making law. In Australia, the legislature of each state and territory, as well as the Commonwealth, is known as a parliament. The parliaments of the Commonwealth and most of the states (other than Queensland, which only has a lower house) are made up of two 'houses' – a lower house, made up of representatives of particular geographical areas or 'electorates', and an upper house, which acts as a house of review. As the legislature is made up of those who are elected by the people, it is the central part of the democratic system. One of its roles is to hold the executive accountable for its actions.

However, the legislature's most important role is to create laws. The process of creating a law starts with the introduction of a Bill into the parliament. This is most often done by a minister; however, any member of parliament can introduce a Bill. The process by which a Bill becomes law is set out in Figure 2.1.

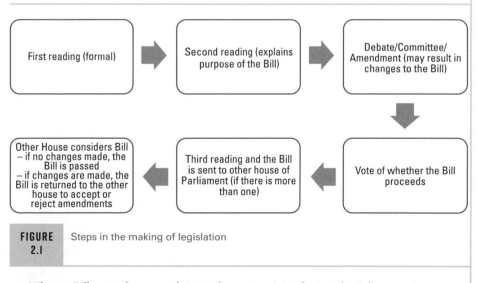

FIGURE 2.1 Steps in the making of legislation

When a Bill is read a second time, the person introducing the Bill presents a speech (either orally or in writing), which is called the 'second reading speech'. This provides an explanation of what the Bill is trying to achieve and why. This speech can be referred to later when a court is trying to interpret what the law means.

Once a Bill has passed through the parliament, it is sent to the Governor (or Governor-General at the federal level) for approval – this is a formal process called 'assent'. This makes the Bill an Act. There is one further step before the Act becomes law, which is known as commencement. Some Acts commence on the day of assent; others will commence at a later time, when the Governor issues a proclamation that states when the Act commences. The Act itself will state whether it commences on assent or on proclamation.

Many Bills that are passed are 'amendment' Bills. This means that they make changes to existing Acts. This is required when certain problems with the existing law are identified by the courts or when a change in policy means the law needs to be changed. When an amending commences, it makes changes to the principal Act – it is now common for the amending Act to then be repealed. This can be confusing when you are looking for an important change that has been made by an amending Act: a search for the amending Act will reveal it has been repealed; however, the changes that were made will be in force as part of the principal Act.

THE JUDICIARY

The third arm of government is the judiciary. This is made up of the judges and the courts. An independent judiciary is regarded as fundamental to the rule of law.

The function of the judiciary is to give effect to the law. It does this primarily by resolving disputes between people according to law. This requires a judge to determine the facts of the dispute, identify the relevant law and then apply the law to the facts. This will sometimes involve the judge having to interpret what the law means in the specific circumstances of the case.

The judiciary is bound by the law; it must act in accordance with the power and responsibilities given to it by the law. This includes a requirement that judges act in accordance with fundamental principles of fairness. This idea of fairness requires judges to act impartially, ensure that the parties to a dispute are given an opportunity to participate in the proceedings and give detailed reasons for their decisions.

Judicial proceedings that take place in courts are generally very formal. There are strict procedures that have to be followed by the parties to the proceedings, and usually hearings are conducted in accordance with special sets of rules. For example, in hearings before courts, the 'rules of evidence' apply. These are a set of legal rules and principles that decide what type of evidence a court can take into account and what information it must not consider. For example, the rules of evidence usually do not allow someone to give evidence that is an opinion about whether something is true unless that person is an expert.

A key principle in the operation of the judiciary is 'jurisdiction'. This refers to the power of a court to hear and determine a matter. A court must have the necessary jurisdiction, otherwise its decision will not be valid. A court's jurisdiction can be defined in a number of ways. The first relates to whether the court is dealing with an issue under federal or state law. In the case of the former, it will be exercising 'federal jurisdiction'. (Note that the *Judiciary Act 1903*, which is a Commonwealth law, allows a court of a state to exercise federal jurisdiction.)

Jurisdiction can also be defined by what outcomes a court can decide in relation to a dispute. For example, some courts can only hear matters involving an amount of money below a specified total, and some courts can only impose a limited punishment in a criminal matter. There are also courts that have a specialised jurisdiction, such as those dealing with children. Jurisdiction is also used to describe the type of law or legal issue a court can determine. For example, the same court may at different times exercise either its civil or its criminal jurisdiction.

Finally, there is an important difference between two types of jurisdiction: 'original' and 'appellate'. 'Original' jurisdiction means the court has power to first hear and decide the dispute. 'Appellate' jurisdiction is when a court reviews an earlier decision by a court in relation to the same dispute. It is important to note that although a right to appeal is an important feature of the judicial system, in many cases appeals are not the same as a new or second hearing of the dispute. For example, an appeal may often only be heard if one of the parties can show that the original court made an 'error of law'.

The hierarchy of courts is a very important part of the judicial system. There are different hierarchies in the federal and the state and territory judicial systems. However, the court that sits above them all is the High Court of Australia. It is the highest appeal court in the country in relation to both federal and state jurisdiction. It also has some original jurisdiction, including where the Commonwealth is a party to a dispute.

Table 2.1 sets out the system of Courts in Australia.

TABLE 2.1 Outline of Australian judicial system

	HIGH COURT	
	Federal system	States and territories
Superior courts	Federal Court Family Court	Supreme Court (including Court of Appeal; Court of Criminal Appeal in NSW)
Intermediate courts	Federal Circuit Court	District Court (NSW, Qld, SA, WA)/County Court (Vic)
Inferior courts		Magistrates Court (ACT, Qld, SA, Tas, Vic, WA) Local Court (NSW, NT)

In the federal system, the superior courts are the Federal Court and the Family Court. The Federal Court has original jurisdiction in relation to a range of disputes under Commonwealth law, such as bankruptcy and corporations law. It also hears appeals from the Federal Circuit Court. The Federal Circuit Court has similar jurisdiction to the Federal Court (and Family Court), but was created to deal with less complex cases. It also hears some appeals from certain Commonwealth tribunals (tribunals will be discussed later in this chapter). The Family Court is a specialised jurisdiction that deals with family disputes, including with regard to parenting.

In most states and territories, there are three levels in the court hierarchy. At the lowest level is the Magistrates Court (in New South Wales, this is the Local Court). These courts hear most civil and criminal matters in each state, but have limited jurisdictions. They can generally only hear disputes involving small amounts of money and can only deal with less serious criminal matters. A nurse facing a criminal charge involving misuse of a small quantity of drugs would most likely be dealt with in the Local Court.

Most states also have an 'intermediate' court known as a District Court (in Victoria, this is the County Court). These courts generally deal with more serious criminal matters and civil claims that involve larger sums of money. They also have an appellate jurisdiction in relation to the Local or Magistrates Courts. Finally, each state and territory has a Supreme Court (these are the only courts a state is required to have under the Constitution). These courts generally have unlimited jurisdiction in relation to civil claims and will deal with the most serious criminal matters. A nurse facing a charge such as murder or negligent manslaughter would usually be dealt with in the Supreme Court. As medical negligence claims often involve significant damages and large amounts of money claimed in compensation, they are also usually dealt with by the Supreme Court.

Supreme Courts also have appellate jurisdiction in relation to the lower courts. In addition, they have the power to undertake 'judicial review'. This is a special form of review whereby the court determines whether a decision-maker has properly exercised their power. This jurisdiction is often used to review decisions made by the executive branch of government.

It is important to be aware of the hierarchy of the courts in order to understand the doctrine of 'precedent'. This will be examined in more detail below; in brief, this doctrine means that a decision of a higher court on a question of law is binding on lower courts within the same hierarchy in relation to the same kind of case.

TRIBUNALS AND OTHER BODIES

Tribunals and other bodies have become an increasingly important part of the legal system in Australia. Tribunals have some of the characteristics of a court in that they:

→ are established to resolve disputes

→ are independent

→ must act fairly

→ are usually required to give reasons for their decisions

→ often involve hearings between parties

→ can make orders that can end a dispute.

However, technically, tribunals are not courts but are administrative alternatives (Sanson & Anthony 2018). This means that tribunals are required to decide disputes in accordance with specific rules that are set out in legislation. Because tribunals are administrative alternatives, the people who sit on them are usually not judges, and in many cases do not even need to be lawyers; rather, they are people who are skilled and experienced in the subject area over which the tribunal has jurisdiction. For example, when dealing with a complaint under the National Law, the relevant tribunal will generally include a legally trained person, a community representative and a member of the same profession as the health practitioner whose behaviour is under review.

Tribunals were created to be faster, cheaper and more flexible than courts. Often hearings are less formal and many of the rules that apply in a court may not be applied in a tribunal (such as the rules of evidence). As simpler and less formal forums, it was originally intended that parties could at tribunals appear without lawyers; however, it is now often the case that lawyers will be used. In part this is because some of the powers a tribunal can exercise may have significant consequence for the parties. For example, a tribunal can decide whether a nurse is guilty of professional misconduct and can order that they be suspended or disqualified from registration.

Other bodies have been established to exercise certain functions that are independent from direct control by the executive. Most states have an ombudsman who can investigate complaints about poor government administration and can make recommendations or report to parliament if they find the complaints are justified. Some states have special bodies to investigate public corruption, such as the Crime and Corruption Commission in Queensland. These can have quite extensive powers. Moreover, some states have specialised bodies to examine and investigate complaints about professionals, such as the Health Care Complaints Commission in New South Wales.

COVID-19: An insight into the rule of law in Australia during a pandemic

Since early 2020, one of the defining features of life in Australia – and in most other places around the world – has been the COVID-19 pandemic. The front line of the response to the pandemic has been the health system and the people who work within it. However, it is also the case that the law is 'an integral part of the public health framework that protects the community during a pandemic' (Bennett & Freckleton 2021).

A major part of Australia's response to COVID-19 has involved state and territory governments using a range of legal tools to help manage the crisis. The daily experience of press conferences during the pandemic regularly involved updates about the health system's response to the disease, but also included announcements about restrictions being imposed on individuals' rights and liberties. Typically, ministers and health officials stood alongside law enforcement officers to explain what and why certain measures were being imposed by the government. These public health orders were often very wide-ranging, including the imposition of quarantine, border closures, lockdowns, curfews, wearing of face masks, and the use of QR codes when entering shops or businesses. (Bennett & Freckleton 2021). The restrictions also impacted the way the community interacted with the health-care system: visits to hospitals were banned or significantly limited. Later in the pandemic, the issue of vaccinations, and in particular the debate over whether vaccinations could or should be mandatory, became a prominent issue.

Although, in the Australian context, the community response to the legal measures that were imposed demonstrated a significant level of compliance (remembering the importance of general compliance to the question of legitimacy), these measures have often been contested in both the medical (or more broadly scientific) and legal professions, as well as in the general community (Bennett & Freckleton 2021). It is well beyond the scope of this chapter to discuss these issues in detail; however, it is useful to think about the justification for these types of legal measures. As noted by the Australian Human Rights Commission, all human rights come with responsibilities – Article 29 of the Universal Declaration of Human Rights (United Nations 1948) says 'everyone has duties to the community'. This means we all have a responsibility to respect each other's rights and not do things that endanger the rights of others. This principle can help explain why certain measures taken by the government to limit the usual exercise of individual rights in the interests of everyone are justifiable (the second limb of the test of legitimacy discussed earlier) (Australian Human Rights Commission 2022a).

The legal response to the pandemic also provides an insight into the federal system of government. As discussed above, the Commonwealth has the power to legislate only with respect to certain matters, with health not included. However, because COVID-19 posed a threat to the nation as a whole, the Commonwealth was required to provide national leadership, which it did by providing economic support through financial subsidies to the unemployed and to affected businesses. It also exercised its power by making or using laws with respect to many matters, such as quarantine, external affairs and the movement of people in and out of Australia. The states, however, have responsibility for public health and (generally speaking) police and the enforcement of law, and many of the measures taken that impacted society on a day-to-day basis were the result of public health measures imposed by state governments under public health legislation (Twomey 2020).

As the pandemic saw both levels of government use their powers to implement new legal measures, this gave rise to the need for a significant degree of coordination and cooperation. For example, while the Commonwealth could impose requirements for people arriving in Australia to be quarantined, the administration of these measures – from implementing COVID-19 testing to policing compliance – was left up to the states. The Commonwealth also provided some assistance – for example, by arranging for the Army to assist in monitoring quarantine arrangements. At times, however, the different levels of government did not agree on what measures should be taken, which created a degree of complexity. For example, some states decided to move schooling to an online environment (in line with their responsibility for education); however, at one point the Commonwealth offered funding to private schools to return to face-to-face teaching, thus undermining the position of the states (Twomey 2020). However, it was in the area of aged care that the complexity of the Commonwealth–state relationship created the most difficulty. In its Special Report on Aged Care and COVID-19, the Royal Commission into Aged Care Quality and Safety (2020) examined how a lack of clarity about roles, including a dispute between the Commonwealth, the NSW state government and the aged care provider about whether infected residents should be transferred to hospital, may have contributed to the tragic loss of life at the Newmarch House aged care facility in Sydney.

Generally speaking, although there have been failures and controversies, and some high-profile voices of dissent, arguably the legal response to COVID-19 has demonstrated both the commitment of the people and governments of Australia to the rule of law, and the effectiveness of this model of social coordination in maintaining a free and secure way of life.

The sources of law

The sources of law can be categorised as primary and secondary (Sanson & Anthony 2018). Primary sources of law are those that directly create law or give immediate effect to law. These include legislation, delegated legislation (or Regulations) and court judgments. In this context, court judgments give effect to both legislation (including delegated legislation) and also to the 'common law'. What is meant by the common law will be explained below.

Secondary sources of law are those that do not have direct legal effect in the Australian legal system but may have some influence on how primary law is made or interpreted. These sources include international law, especially any treaties to which Australia is a signatory, and reports of bodies such as the Australian Law Reform Commission. Included in this category are also such things as codes of practice, guidelines and some policies.

LEGISLATION

As discussed above, legislation is created when a Bill is made into an Act of Parliament. Because legislation is created by the representative part of government, it is considered the paramount source of law in Australia. This idea is sometimes called 'parliamentary sovereignty'. It means that if the legislature disagrees with an act of the executive or a decision of the judiciary, it can (with some exceptions) overrule it by passing legislation.

The general structure or layout of all Australian legislation is the same. Each Act will have a name and year, and often a number, to identify it. An Act usually has both a long title and a short title. The long title includes the subject matter and purpose of the Act. Usually, Acts are referred to by their short title (which will be specified in the Act itself). Very large Acts may have a number of chapters, each containing several parts. Parts may be further broken up into divisions. The body of the Act is set out in numbered sections. At the end of the Act there may also be schedules, which have numbered clauses. Schedules are usually used to add details or to include prescribed forms. Often, there is also a schedule explaining how any changes that are made to the Act are to apply in different circumstances.

Reading legislation is often trickier than it looks. Sometimes a reference to a specific section of the Act seems to be enough to describe what the law is on a given issue. However, it can be misleading or not very helpful to only consider one section. It is important to look at the broader context of the Act, and it is often necessary to refer to other parts of the legislation, particularly where a section uses a term that is defined in the Act. For example, section 17A of the *Poisons and Therapeutic Goods Act 1966* (NSW) sets out the circumstances in which a nurse can possess, use or supply a poison, restricted substance or drug of addiction. Section 4 of the Act defines the terms 'poison', 'restricted substance' and 'drug of addiction' as things appearing in various schedules of the 'Poisons List'. In turn, the 'Poisons List' is a list created under section 8 of the Act. The Poisons List itself is not part of the legislation, but is found in a separate legal document called a 'proclamation' (in this case, the Poisons and Therapeutic Goods (Poisons List) Proclamation 2016). As this example shows, it may be necessary to look at several different areas of an Act, and indeed sometimes at things other than the Act, to understand how legislation applies to any particular situation.

In addition to legislation often being complex to read and understand, the law has specific rules about how legislation is to be interpreted. In fact, the Commonwealth and most states and territories have a separate piece of legislation that sets out rules about how to interpret legislation – for example, the *Acts Interpretation Act 1901* of the Commonwealth (see the Appendix for a table of relevant legislation). Over the years, the courts have argued over various principles and rules about how a piece of legislation should be understood. Some argue that the literal meaning of the words should be used. Others say that the words should be interpreted in light of the context, or the purpose of the legislation – what it was intended to achieve. This is why it is usually necessary for a lawyer to assist in explaining what a piece of legislation means.

DELEGATED LEGISLATION

Legislation, even very detailed legislation, is often not able to set out what should happen in every situation that it is designed to cover. New circumstances may arise or different ways of implementing the law may become preferable to others. In order to enable the executive to carry out its function of administering the law on a day-to-day basis, many Acts delegate some authority to the government to make rules with the force of law. This is known as delegated legislation.

The most common form of delegated legislation is known as Regulations. Although Regulations are made by the executive, not the legislature, the power to make a Regulation must first be given to the executive by a specific section of an Act. For example, section 45C(1) of the *Poisons and Therapeutic Goods Act 1966* (NSW) says that 'the Governor may make Regulations, not inconsistent with this Act, for or with respect to any matter that by this Act is required or permitted to be prescribed or that is necessary or convenient to be prescribed for carrying out or giving effect to this Act'. It is very common for an Act to include a Regulation-making power in this way. This is a method for the parliament to, at the same time, enable and limit the power of the executive to make Regulations.

Regulations have the same legal effect as Acts. They also look a lot like Acts and are set out in a similar style. The main difference is that instead of 'sections' each numbered provision is often called a 'clause'. Because they do not go through the parliamentary process, Regulations are easier to make and to amend and so are often used to deal with matters of detail. For example, clause 122 of the Poisons and Therapeutic Goods Regulation 2008 (NSW) lists the current prescribed type A drugs of addiction. This list can be changed and updated more easily as new drugs are registered for use – there is no need to go through the process of the legislature having to pass an amending Act.

During the COVID-19 pandemic, another form of delegated legislation was commonly used. Many of the restrictions that were imposed by the various governments around Australia were through 'public health orders' (for example, in New South Wales) or 'emergency management directions' (for example, in South Australia). As with regulations, the power to make a public health order or emergency management directions must be given to the executive in legislation: in New South Wales, section 7 of the *Public Health Act 2010* allows the minister, if they consider on reasonable grounds that a situation has arisen that is, or is likely to be, a risk to public health, to take such action, and by order give such directions as they consider necessary to deal with the risk and its possible consequences; in South Australia, section 25 of the *Emergency Management Act 2004* allows the state coordinator, if they are of the opinion it is necessary to do so, to do various things including issuing directions. The value of these legal instruments lay in their ability to be highly detailed and specific in terms of their operation and to be changed very quickly as circumstances required.

CASE LAW

Case law is the law that is created by decisions made by the courts. This is often known as the common law. The High Court of Australia in *Lipohar v The Queen* (1999: 44) said:

> The common law has its source in the reasons for decisions of the courts which
> are reasons arrived at according to well recognised and long established judicial
> methods. It is a body of law created and defined by the courts.

For many centuries, in the tradition of English law, it was the common law and not
legislation that was the most important source of law. The legislature was much
less active and less concerned with passing legislation. Common law was made
by judges and applied to all people, rather than to particular classes (such as the
clergy) or in particular places – this is why it is called the 'common' law.

Central to the development of the common law is the doctrine of precedent.
As discussed above, the purpose of law is to provide social stability, which requires
laws that are general and consistent. However, a judge only decides the case they
are hearing. The direct effect of a judgment is only binding on the parties to the
proceedings. It is the doctrine of precedent that allows the common law to develop
general principles, so the decision in one case can have a broader application. The
doctrine of precedent works on the basis that similar cases should be decided in
the same way. The principles that can be drawn from earlier cases become the body
of the common law.

The doctrine of precedent is another reason why the publication of written
judgments (an explanation of the judge's reasons for their decision) is important
in the Australian legal system. Written judgments do not just provide transparency
for the parties to the proceedings; they also enable the reasoning used in one case
to be applied in other similar cases.

An important part of the doctrine of precedent relates to the hierarchy of courts
described above. Generally speaking, a court is only required to follow a decision
made by a higher court. There is no strict requirement that a judge must follow a
decision made by a judge of the same court; however, it is usual that a judge will do
so, unless they fundamentally disagree with the principle established by that case.
This means decisions of the High Court have the effect of settling the common law
in Australia, and those decisions will bind all courts:

> This Court is the final appellate court for the nation. When an appeal is dealt with
> in this Court, and its reasons are published, those reasons will form part of the
> common law of Australia and will bind *all* courts in the country. (*Lipohar v The
> Queen*: 50)

As noted above, the legislature can override or change the common law. However,
it is also possible for the common law to evolve without any involvement by the
legislature. In *Breen v Williams* (1996: 47), the High Court said:

> In a democratic society, changes in the law that cannot logically or analogically
> be related to existing common law rules and principles are the province of the
> legislature. From time to time it is necessary for the common law courts to

re-formulate existing legal rules and principles to take account of changing social conditions. Less frequently, the courts may even reject the continuing operation of an established rule or principle. But such steps can be taken only when it can be seen that the 'new' rule or principle that has been created has been derived logically or analogically from other legal principles, rules and institutions.

Even though legislation is an increasingly prominent part of the legal system, the common law remains very important. The law relating to negligence is a good example of this, and will be discussed in some detail in Chapter 5.

SECONDARY SOURCES

Secondary sources of law have no direct legal effect, but can influence the way the law is applied or interpreted, or can have other indirect legal consequences. For example, official reports by bodies such as the Australian Law Reform Commission and research by academics can influence the way the executive and the legislature design legislation. In certain circumstances, such material can also be used by a court in interpreting the law. Another secondary source is international law. Courts will sometimes take into account principles from international law, such as treaties and other instruments to which Australia has agreed, when interpreting the law.

Other secondary sources of law include 'codes' and 'guidelines'. These include documents that set out standards and rules of behaviour and competency that are specific to an industry or profession. Strictly speaking, these do not have direct legal effect – a code is not the same as an Act or Regulation. However, in certain circumstances codes can have a significant impact on the law. For example, the Code of Conduct for Nurses is issued by the Nursing and Midwifery Board of Australia (NMBA), which is a National Board established under Part 5 of the Health Practitioner Regulation National Law. A National Board is given power under the Act to develop and approve codes and guidelines. The Code of Conduct for Nurses has been approved by the NMBA, and it is very important as it sets out the legal requirements and expectations of the profession. Under section 41 of the Act, the code is stated to be 'evidence of what constitutes appropriate professional conduct or practice' for nurses. Accordingly, if a nurse's conduct varies significantly from the code, this could have significant legal implications – it may be a basis for criminal proceedings (if the variation was extreme), a claim of negligence (see Chapter 5) or result in disciplinary proceedings (see Chapter 3).

It is necessary to remember, though, that no matter how important the code is, it is not a law. This means that if there is ever a situation where the code requires something that is contrary to an Act, Regulation or the common law, those laws prevail. Indeed, the Introduction to the code notes:

The code is not a substitute for requirements outlined in the National Law [*Health Practitioner Regulation National Law Act 2009*], other relevant legislation, or case law. Where there is any actual or perceived conflict between the code and any law, the law takes precedence. Nurses also need to understand and comply with all other NMBA standards, codes and guidelines. (NMBA 2018b: 3)

REFLECTIVE QUESTION 2.3

How can the law be changed?

Areas of the law of particular relevance to nurses

This section will shift focus from the structure of the legal system to examine some substantive areas of the law. It will set out the most basic division within the law: that between criminal and civil law. There will then be a brief outline of two areas of law that are relevant for nurses: the coronial system and disciplinary proceedings.

CRIMINAL LAW

The most fundamental division in law is between criminal and civil law. The criminal law is probably the area of law best known to most people from news and popular culture. The criminal law establishes various offences – these are rules that describe conduct regarded as so socially unacceptable that it deserves punishment. Criminal proceedings involve one party (the prosecution) attempting to prove that the other party (the defendant) has committed an offence. In addition, criminal law also covers matters such as the powers of police to investigate alleged crimes and the procedures that apply to hearing matters before the court. The criminal law also includes the penalties that can be imposed if a court finds a person guilty of an offence.

The fact that nurses work with patients who are vulnerable means there are opportunities for criminal behaviour. These can include physical acts that cause harm, such as assault and sexual assault, and even murder. For example, Niels Hoegel, who was a nurse in Germany, has been convicted of the murder of six patients but has confessed to murdering many more (perhaps over a hundred more). According to news reports, prosecutors alleged he would give patients various drugs in order to show off his skills at resuscitation and to 'fight off boredom' (The Guardian Australia 2018). More commonly, nurses may be accused of offences relating to property theft or abuse of drugs. It is important to appreciate that these possibilities exist because nurses have a professional responsibility to report suspected crimes (see Chapter 7). Also, in some circumstances it is itself a crime for a nurse not to provide information to the police if they believe a serious crime has been committed.

Although the criminal law is a combination of both legislation (laws created by the parliament) and common law, most criminal offences are found in legislation. All jurisdictions in Australia, including the Commonwealth, have a principal piece of legislation, such as the *Crimes Act 1958* (Vic) or the *Criminal Code Act 1899* (Qld), that sets out the major criminal offences such as murder, sexual assault and robbery. However, criminal offences can be found in a wide range of legislation. For example, section 113 of the Health Practitioner Regulation National Law (NSW) creates an offence of someone using the title 'nurse' if they are not registered as a nurse.

In most (but not all) cases, a criminal offence involves a physical component (an act) and a mental component (an intention). For example, the offence of murder involves a person deliberately doing something that causes the death of another person (the act) with the intention to either kill or inflict grievous bodily harm, or with a reckless indifference to human life (see, for example, section 302 of the *Criminal Code Act 1899* [Qld]). In some less serious offences, it may not be necessary to have a criminal intention. These are offences of 'strict' or 'absolute' liability. For example, an offence of exceeding the speed limit can be committed without having an intention to drive too fast. It is also important to remember that the criminal law does not require an accused person to have a criminal *motive* in order to be guilty. This means that an intentional act done out of kindness or a sense of moral responsibility could still be a criminal offence (see the discussion of euthanasia in Chapter 10).

Another feature of the criminal law with which many people are familiar is the 'burden of proof'. This is the requirement that the prosecution must prove that all the elements of the offence – the necessary acts and intentions – existed. The standard the prosecution has to meet is very high – 'beyond a reasonable doubt'. The burden always rests with the prosecution. There is no obligation on the accused person to prove any fact or issue that is in dispute, or to prove their innocence. This is known as the presumption of innocence. Even if an accused person gives evidence, they do not have to prove that their account is true: the prosecution has to prove that it could not reasonably be true.

If a person is found guilty of a crime, a court will have a range of options when it comes to sentencing (the punishment). In certain circumstances, the court may decide not to proceed to a conviction even though the person is found guilty. This is usually done if the offence is not very serious and the person has no previous criminal history. The courts also have a number of non-custodial sentences (sentences that do not involve a person going to prison) that they can apply, including fines or orders requiring a person to perform community service. For more serious matters, a person can be sentenced to imprisonment.

The vast majority of criminal matters in Australia are dealt with in the lower courts before a magistrate sitting alone. As noted earlier, there are limits to the penalties a magistrate can impose, even if the maximum penalty for an offence is quite high. More serious offences are dealt with in the higher courts, and can involve a number of preliminary stages before the case is finally heard. In these more serious matters, there will usually be a jury as well as a judge.

A person who is convicted and sentenced will have a right of appeal to a higher court against their conviction, and sometimes just their sentence if they think it is too severe. Usually the prosecution can only appeal against a sentence if they think it is inadequate. There is no right for the prosecution to appeal against a decision not to convict a person. This is part of the principle of 'double jeopardy', which prevents a person being prosecuted more than once for the same conduct or event. That is, if a person is found not guilty at a criminal trial, they cannot later be found guilty of an offence that relates to the same set of facts.

It should be noted that although 'double jeopardy' prevents a person being punished twice for the same conduct, this principle does not extend to professional disciplinary action. That is, a person may be subject to both criminal and disciplinary proceedings arising from the same incident. The NSW Court of Appeal in *Health Care Complaints Commission v Litchfield* (1997: lines 18–22) said:

> Disciplinary proceedings consequent upon a conviction in criminal proceedings are not barred by … any wider principle of double jeopardy … The converse is also true and adverse disciplinary action does not bar later criminal proceedings arising out of the same facts.

This is why, in the case of Jack at the beginning of the chapter, the health-care professionals were dealt with under both the criminal law and the relevant disciplinary regime.

CIVIL LAW

There are many ways in which a nurse can become involved in matters involving the civil law. The easiest way to define the civil law is that it is any area of law that is not criminal. However, this covers a very diverse range of law, including torts (civil wrongs), family law, contracts, corporations law, property law and employment law.

Civil law is important for nurses because it governs the nature of their employment (for example, whether they are employees or contractors) and their various rights in the workplace, but it is also relevant for a wide range of issues discussed elsewhere in this book, including consent, confidentiality, discrimination, guardianship and negligence. Indeed, it is far more likely that a nurse will be involved in a civil law issue than a criminal law issue.

While civil law involves rules that govern behaviour, it focuses more on how people should conduct themselves within specific relationships – for example, where there is a duty of care, within a family, in business and so on. Civil law typically involves regulating and resolving disputes between people (though here a person can be a 'legal person', which includes a company or the government) rather than the state enforcing rules of behaviour, which is what happens in criminal law. Usually the burden of proof lies with the person bringing a claim against another person. The standard of proof in most civil proceedings is the 'balance of probabilities', which is a lower standard than the criminal standard. One of the most important areas of civil law for nursing practice is the law of negligence. This will be discussed in more detail in Chapter 5.

Unlike in criminal cases, where a court will impose a punishment, in a civil case the court will order a particular remedy that is designed to resolve the dispute. For example, in relation to negligence, the usual remedy is an award of monetary compensation; in a contract dispute, it might be payment of money or an order requiring that the person fulfil their obligation under the contract; in family law there are orders about parenting responsibilities and division of property; in corporations law it may be a civil penalty (a bit like a fine) or orders restricting people acting as directors of a corporation. Most cases are dealt with in the lower courts unless there are serious issues or large amounts of money in dispute. Some matters can only be heard in courts with a special jurisdiction.

CORONERS AND INQUESTS

Very occasionally in a nurse's career, they may find themselves involved in a matter concerning the Coroner. Coroners investigate certain kinds of deaths in order to determine:

→ the identity of the deceased
→ the date, place and circumstances of the death
→ the cause of death (Coroner's Court of New South Wales 2020b).

The difference between the circumstances and cause of death can be explained as follows:

> If one is inquiring into a death following a fall from a height, the cause of death would be the injuries sustained in the fall. The manner of death would be how that fall came about. Did the deceased jump, was he pushed or did he or she fall accidentally? (Waller 1994: 67)

Certain deaths have to be reported to the Coroner, such as if the death was violent or unnatural – for example, homicide, suicide or drug, alcohol or poison-related deaths. 'Reportable deaths' are discussed in more detail in Chapter 7.

In some cases, the Coroner will decide to hold an inquest. An inquest is 'a court hearing where the Coroner considers evidence and submissions in order to make the determinations noted above' (Coroner's Court of New South Wales 2020a). The Coroner can require people to produce documents, and can call witnesses to give evidence of their knowledge of the circumstances of the case under investigation. It is also common for the Coroner to obtain expert reports, including from a post-mortem examination of the deceased.

An inquest is quite different from a normal court hearing. There are no parties to the proceedings, although interested persons may be allowed to question witnesses and make a submission to the Coroner. The Coroner will be assisted, either by police or by a lawyer (or both), who will prepare a brief of evidence for the Coroner and will examine witnesses and make submissions. The rules of evidence that apply in other courts do not apply in an inquest.

When a case is before them, the Coroner has special powers over the body of a deceased person. This includes the right to the remains of the deceased, and to retain organs even after the other remains are released, if it is considered necessary for investigating the cause of death. In some cases, the Coroner can order the exhumation of a body for further testing.

The Coroner's role is to find out what happened, not to hold someone responsible for causing the death. The Coroner cannot find someone guilty of a crime relating to the death. If at any time during the course of an inquest or inquiry the Coroner forms an opinion that someone may have committed a serious offence in connection with the death, the Coroner is required to suspend the inquest or inquiry and refer the matter to the police or other authorities to consider whether someone should be prosecuted for a crime (Coroner's Court of New South Wales 2020a). If the prosecution decides not to prosecute, or the prosecution is unsuccessful, the Coroner may decide to continue the inquest.

The Coroner may also refer concerns about the professional conduct of a health-care professional to a relevant disciplinary body. Similarly, although the Coroner cannot decide that someone should be held liable for the death because they were negligent, the Coroner's finding may be relied upon 'in subsequent civil proceedings or insurance claims' (Coroner's Court of New South Wales 2020a).

Following an inquest, the Coroner may make recommendations to governments and other agencies with a view to improving public health and safety. However, the Coroner has no power to enforce compliance with such recommendations (Coroner's Court of New South Wales 2020a). For example, in the matter of Ahlia Raftery, the Coroner found that

> [She] died on 19 March 2015 whilst she was a patient in the Psychiatric Intensive Care Unit of the Mater Mental Health Centre … The cause of Ahlia's death was neck compression due to hanging. Ahlia died as a consequence of actions taken by her with the intention of ending life. (Coroner's Court of New South Wales 2017)

The coronial inquest had heard that there were a number of procedural problems that contributed to Ahlia's death, including in relation to the way nursing staff took observations of their patients, particularly at handover times. Accordingly, the Coroner made a number of recommendations that these procedures be modified. Another important recommendation made by the Coroner was that the NSW Minister for Health should consider increasing nursing-to-patient ratios at the facility (Coroner's Court of New South Wales 2017). The Minister for Mental Health advised the Attorney-General that all the recommendations were accepted and arrangements were being made for their implementation (New South Wales Communities and Justice 2022).

A list of the Coroners Acts is included in the Appendix.

DISCIPLINARY HEARINGS

Serious complaints against nurses will often result in formal disciplinary proceedings. In this section, we will examine a few of the legal principles that apply in disciplinary hearings, making them different from other types of civil proceedings. Chapter 3 will outline the system for the regulation of nursing practice in Australia and some of the underlying ethical and legal principles involved.

Serious disciplinary proceedings will usually be heard in a tribunal. Because of their nature, these are generally more formal than many other types of proceedings heard in a tribunal. The tribunal will usually be made up of a lawyer (sometimes a judicial officer), professional representatives and community representatives. A nurse who is appearing before the tribunal in a disciplinary hearing will usually be allowed to have legal representation.

The NMBA (or the Health Care Complaints Commission [HCCC] in New South Wales or Health Ombudsman in Queensland) will refer a complaint that has been made about a nurse that is considered sufficiently serious to the tribunal and will appear at the hearing of the complaint. The complaint will set out the alleged facts of the case and assert that they support a finding that the nurse is guilty of either 'unprofessional conduct' (called 'unsatisfactory professional conduct' in New South Wales) or the more serious finding of 'professional misconduct'.

Unprofessional conduct and professional misconduct are defined in the various state and territory Health Practitioner Regulation National Laws. For example, section 5 of the *Health Practitioner Regulation National Law Act 2009* (Qld) defines 'Unprofessional conduct' of a registered health practitioner to mean:

> professional conduct that is of a lesser standard than that which might reasonably be expected of the health practitioner by the public or the practitioner's professional peers, and includes:
>
> **(a)** a contravention by the practitioner of this Law, whether or not the practitioner has been prosecuted for, or convicted of, an offence in relation to the contravention; and
> **(b)** a contravention by the practitioner of
> > **(i)** a condition to which the practitioner's registration was subject; or
> > **(ii)** an undertaking given by the practitioner to the National Board that registers the practitioner; and
> **(c)** the conviction of the practitioner for an offence under another Act, the nature of which may affect the practitioner's suitability to continue to practise the profession; and
> **(d)** providing a person with health services of a kind that are excessive, unnecessary or otherwise not reasonably required for the person's well-being.

In the same Act, 'professional misconduct' of a registered health practitioner is defined as:

> **(a)** unprofessional conduct by the practitioner that amounts to conduct that is substantially below the standard reasonably expected of a registered health practitioner of an equivalent level of training or experience; and
> **(b)** more than one instance of unprofessional conduct that, when considered together, amounts to conduct that is substantially below the standard reasonably expected of a registered health practitioner of an equivalent level of training or experience; and
> **(c)** conduct of the practitioner, whether occurring in connection with the practice of the health practitioner's profession or not, that is inconsistent with the practitioner being a fit and proper person to hold registration in the profession. (at section 5)

The Australian Health Practitioner Regulation Agency (AHPRA) has published a Regulatory Guide that gives examples of what constitutes unprofessional conduct and professional misconduct.

In proceedings in the Tribunal, the onus of proof is on the NMBA (or HCCC in New South Wales or Health Ombudsman in Queensland) and the civil standard of proof applies. If the tribunal is satisfied that the facts of a complaint are proven it can caution or reprimand the practitioner, impose conditions on the practitioner's registration or order the practitioner to seek and undergo medical or psychiatric treatment or counselling or to complete an educational course. If the tribunal considers that those facts support a finding of unprofessional conduct or professional misconduct, it can impose stronger sanctions, including a fine, or suspend or cancel the practitioner's registration (AHPRA 2020b).

As discussed above, the law does not consider there to be any principle of 'double jeopardy' that prevents disciplinary action being taken against a nurse for conduct that has also been the subject of criminal or civil proceedings. This is because the regulation of nurses, including the complaint-handling and disciplinary process, is designed to protect the community and the integrity of the profession from the harm caused by unsatisfactory professional conduct or professional misconduct. Action taken against a nurse in a disciplinary setting is protective in nature, not a punishment. In *Health Care Complaints Commission v Do*, the NSW Court of Appeal stated (at 35):

> The objective of protecting the health and safety of the public is not confined to protecting the patients or potential patients of a particular practitioner from the continuing risk of his or her malpractice or incompetence. It includes protecting the public from the similar misconduct or incompetence of other practitioners and upholding public confidence in the standards of the profession. That objective is achieved by setting and maintaining those standards and, where appropriate, by cancelling the registration of practitioners who are not competent or otherwise not fit to practise, including those who have been guilty of serious misconduct. Denouncing such misconduct operates both as a deterrent to the individual concerned, as well as to the general body of practitioners. It also maintains public confidence by signalling that those whose conduct does not meet the required standards will not be permitted to practise.

This is also why ethical values such as honesty and integrity, as much as technical clinical skills, are relevant to a person's suitability for registration as a nurse.

LAW AND ETHICS IN PRACTICE

In 2019, a nurse was alleged to have stolen and used a dying patient's credit card. She was charged by police; however, the charges were dropped because the police could not prove that the patient had not consented to the nurse using the card. However, disciplinary action was taken against the nurse. The tribunal hearing the matter found that the nurse had acted dishonestly in using the patient's credit card. She had also failed to give a truthful account to her manager. Further, she had failed to notify the National Board that the police had charged her with a criminal offence. The tribunal held that each finding amounted to unsatisfactory professional conduct and, taken together, they amounted to professional misconduct (*Health Care Complaints Commission v Shrimpton*).

≫ **Why is it that a nurse's honesty in reporting matters is considered so important?**

REFLECTIVE QUESTION 2.4

What might be the legal consequences if a nurse who is employed in a community health-care clinic is found to have substituted a drug that was prescribed for a patient with a non-prescription drug and then taken the patient's prescribed medicine for their own use?

The role of law in defining a nurse's scope of practice

The idea of 'scope of practice' is a very important one for all health-care practitioners. It is also conceptually quite complex. For example, the Registered Nurse Standards for Practice define 'scope of practice' as 'that in which nurses are educated, competent to perform and permitted by law' (NMBA 2016). It notes that the 'actual scope of practice is influenced by the context in which the nurse practises, the health needs of people, the level of competence and confidence of the nurse and the policy requirements of the service provider' (NMBA 2016). Accordingly, scope of practice is an idea that brings together professional skills, knowledge and training, ethical standards and legal responsibilities to inform the day-to-day decision-making of a nurse when engaged in their profession.

In recognition of the importance and complexity of 'scope of practice', the NMBA has published a number of tools to assist nurses to identify their scope of practice and make informed decisions about what they should do in their everyday practice in a consistent way – these can be found at the following link: www .nursingmidwiferyboard.gov.au/codes-guidelines-statements/frameworks.aspx. It is the nurse's responsibility to know what their scope of practice is and act within it.

LEVEL OF TRAINING

Nurses can only deliver treatment appropriate to their level of training. For example, a nurse without neonatal training would be practising outside their scope of practice if they were to give advice or treatment in relation to a premature baby.

Even within a group of similarly qualified nurses, there can be differences in the level of training where specific procedures are concerned. For example, nurses employed in a coronary care unit may be trained to insert an intravenous cannula. However, unless a nurse has undergone the specific training for that unit and has been assessed for competency, they would be practising outside their scope of practice if they inserted an intravenous cannula while working in the coronary care unit. This could lead to disciplinary action being taken. For example, in April 2022, a Nursing and Midwifery Professional Standards Committee made a finding of unsatisfactory professional conduct against nurse Thamsanqa Ndiweni. Nurse Ndiweni, while working a shift in an aged care facility, caused an injury to a patient when attempting to replace a catheter. Although he was first registered in Australia in 2012, he had practised almost exclusively as a mental health nurse and had only inserted a catheter twice before, the last time being about three or four years previously. Part of the reason for the finding of unsatisfactory professional conduct was that in accepting the shift, he knew that he had not refreshed his clinical skills generally and the work involved clinical experience outside his scope of practice.

CONTEXT OF PRACTICE

The NMBA decision-making tools noted above include a useful one-page summary guide and a flowchart that sets out how nurses should approach decision-making in relation to their scope of practice.

The first step is to start with an assessment of the patient's needs. The nurse next has to consider whether the activity falls within contemporary nursing practice. This includes considering whether any necessary regulatory authority has been or can be obtained, whether the activity complies with nursing standards of practice and whether any other necessary health-care practitioners are available to assist. Even if these criteria are met, the nurse then has to consider the organisational context. Is this an activity that is permitted by the organisation employing the nurse? Does the organisation have the skill mix to enable the provision of the required care? Finally, a decision must be made about the most appropriate person at that organisation to deliver the care required. This includes the nurse considering whether they have the confidence to provide the care.

Nurses should only deliver treatment appropriate to their level of appointment in an organisation. What a nurse is permitted to do will be informed by the statement of duties or position description under which the nurse is employed, irrespective of their level of skill and training. For example, consider a nurse who has many years' experience in an emergency department (ED) and is employed in a community health centre to provide health-promotion activities. They should not perform the kind of procedures they may have undertaken in the ED in their role at the community health centre. For example, even if the nurse was trained and experienced in venepuncture or suturing, they would not be permitted to carry out these procedures at the community health centre unless they were described in their statement of duties.

Similarly, a registered nurse employed by a nursing agency to fill casual vacancies at different hospitals in a city would not normally be permitted to undertake the range of procedures that permanent staff at one of those hospitals would carry out. It is essential that nurses understand the positions they occupy and the responsibilities *and constraints* of those roles.

STATE AND COMMONWEALTH LEGISLATION

Legislation governing what nurses are permitted to do varies from one state or territory to another (as can be seen in the tables of legislation included in the Appendix). For example, the *Poisons Act* in Victoria has slightly different provisions for registered nurses to administer medications in the absence of a medical officer than does the *Poisons Act* in Tasmania. There are also different mandatory reporting requirements and different requirements around detention under the Mental Health Acts of each state and territory. Practising registered nurses need to be aware of and understand the legislative frameworks within which they practise, and any relevant differences when they move between the states and territories for employment.

THE EMPLOYER'S POLICY FRAMEWORK

Each place of employment will have its own set of policies concerning what registered nurses are permitted to do. Employers' policies provide guidance to staff about how they are to act in order to meet specific legislative requirements and national safety and quality standards. For example, each hospital in Australia is developing its own policy to implement the Open Disclosure Framework, which deals with clinical incidents (see Chapter 9 for discussion), and health-care services usually have guidelines for the management of patient information in order to meet their requirements under various privacy legislation.

Employers will usually have policies that relate to specific activities of registered nurses, such as what to do with patients' belongings, how to manage complaints and what to do about blood spills. Some policies spell out the processes by which a registered nurse can formally be recognised as clinically competent to carry out certain procedures, such as venepuncture or intravenous cannulation. The process for establishing clinical competence is sometimes called 'credentialling'. This usually involves completion of a specified training program plus an examination of the practical and theoretical components. Credentialling is one of the ways in which a nurse's scope of practice can clearly be determined. A registered nurse who previously had been taught to cannulate – and had even cannulated many times – would nevertheless be acting outside their scope of practice if they inserted a cannula at their place of employment without being credentialled *at that place of employment.*

Each of the above requirements functions to ensure that nursing practice is safe for the patient, the nurse and the employer. When nurses practise outside their scope of practice, they place patients at risk of harm. Nurses who work alone – for example, as agency staff in under-resourced facilities or in remote locations – are particularly at risk of overstepping their scope of practice. This is because they are surrounded by fewer reminders and role models than are nurses in larger organisations – especially teaching hospitals – and may feel under pressure from other staff or the local community to provide extended care.

In addition to any concerns about impact on the patient, if they act outside their scope of practice, a nurse may face a number of legal consequences. These could include criminal charges if, for example, they do something they know they are not qualified to do or not capable of doing properly, causing serious harm to a patient. Criminal charges could also arise if they fail to do something or even take the necessary steps to ensure an appropriate level of care is given to a patient. For example, thinking back to the case of Jack at the start of the chapter, the nurse Isabel Amaro was found guilty of manslaughter for contributing to the death of the patient by, in part, not properly advocating for his care when his condition was deteriorating (Findings of the Conduct and Competence Committee, Nursing and Midwifery Council (UK), 4 August 2016).

A nurse who fails to act within their scope of practice may not provide a reasonable standard of care and so may be found negligent. As will be discussed in Chapter 5, the reasonable standard of care is an objective one, and the level of the individual nurse's training and experience will not necessarily be relevant.

Failing to act within scope of practice may involve conduct that could lead to disciplinary measures. That is, it may constitute unprofessional conduct or even professional misconduct. Another consequence may be that the employer terminates the nurse's employment.

REFLECTIVE QUESTION 2.5

Think about Jack's case at the start of this chapter. How is the idea of a practitioner's 'scope of practice' relevant to the issues raised by the boy's death?

Conclusion

The law is a fundamental part of modern society. It plays an important role in giving people confidence in their day-to-day interactions with other people, whether they are thinking about it or not. Thankfully, the law operates in the background of our lives most of the time. The law is more prominent, however, when it comes to regulating certain types of relationships, such as those between nurses and patients. The vulnerability of patients and the relative power of nurses mean the law has a greater role in providing protection and security to better stabilise that relationship. It does this in a number of ways: in addition to the usual application of the criminal and civil law, the law also regulates the profession of nursing in accordance with the clinical and ethical standards defined by the profession itself.

Generally speaking, if nurses abide by the standards of the profession and approach their day-to-day practice in accordance with those standards (including an understanding of their scope of practice), the law will remain in the background. However, even if a nurse acts completely professionally, given the environment in which they are employed, there will be circumstances where they will come into contact with the law – either because of a death that has to be reported to the Coroner or because they are a witness to the wrongful acts of another person, including a colleague. For this reason alone, it is important that nurses have a familiarity with the legal system and some key principles of Australian law.

REFLECTIVE QUESTIONS 2.6

1 What is the rule of law and why is it important?
2 What could a nurse do if they were convicted of a crime or found guilty of unprofessional conduct but they do not agree with the decision?
3 Why is it important to know that there is a difference between a state or territory law and a Commonwealth law?
4 Is it a crime for a nurse to make a mistake?
5 Can a nurse be deregistered for conduct that does not relate to their skill as a nurse?

Further reading

Australian Health Practitioner Regulation Agency (2020). *Regulatory guide*. www.ahpra.gov.au/Publications/Corporate-publications.aspx

Australian Human Rights Commission (2022). COVID19 and human rights. https://humanrights.gov.au/about/covid19-and-human-rights

Bennett, B. & Freckleton, I. (eds.) (2021). *Pandemics, public health emergencies and government powers: Perspectives on Australian law*. Federation Press.

Coroner's Court of New South Wales: www.coroners.justice.nsw.gov.au

Habermas, J. (1996). *Between facts and norms*. MIT Press.

Nursing and Midwifery Board of Australia (2019). DMF A3 nursing flowchart and DMF A4 nursing summary guide. www.nursingmidwiferyboard.gov.au/Codes-Guidelines-Statements/Frameworks.aspx

Redfern Legal Centre (2016). *The law handbook*, 14th ed. Thomson Reuters.

Royal Commission into Aged Care Quality and Safety (2020). *Aged care and COVID-19: A special report*. https://agedcare.royalcommission.gov.au/publications/aged-care-and-covid-19-special-report

Sanson, M. & Anthony, A. (2018). *Connecting with law*, 4th ed. Oxford University Press.

Starr, L. (2018). Negligent care leads to manslaughter convictions. *Australian Nursing & Midwifery Journal*, 20 May.

Twomey, A. (2020). *Multi-level government and COVID-19: Australia as a case study*. Melbourne Forum on Constitution Building. https://law.unimelb.edu.au/__data/assets/pdf_file/0003/3473832/MF20-Web3-Aust-ATwomey-FINAL.pdf

Waller, K. (1994). *Coronial law and practice in New South Wales*, 3rd ed. Butterworths.

Cases cited

Bawa-Garba v General Medical Council [2018] EWCA Civ 1879

Breen v Williams [1996] HCA 57; (1996) 186 CLR 71

Health Care Complaints Commission v Do [2014] NSWCA 307

Health Care Complaints Commission v Litchfield [1997] NSWCA 264

Health Care Complaints Commission v Ndiweni, Professional Standards Committee Inquiry, 23368/22, 29 March 2022

Health Care Complaints Commission v Shrimpton [2019] NSWCATOD 25

Inquest into the death of Ahlia Raftery, State Coroner's Court (NSW), 9 June 2017

Lipohar v The Queen [1999] HCA 65; (1999) 200 CLR 485

Mabo v Queensland (No 2) (1992) 175 CLR 1

Re Isabel Amaro; Findings of the Conduct and Competence Committee, Nursing and Midwifery Council (UK), 4 August 2016

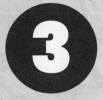

3 THE NURSE–PATIENT RELATIONSHIP AND THE REGULATION OF NURSING PRACTICE[1]

KIM ATKINS

LEARNING OBJECTIVES

In this chapter, you will:

→ Be able to explain the concept of a 'therapeutic relationship' and how it differs from friendship or paternalism

→ Describe the power that characterises the nurse–patient relationship

→ Develop your ability to identify risks in the nurse–patient relationship

→ Be able to explain the key legal and moral responsibilities of the nurse–patient relationship

→ Describe the four principles of bioethics

→ Explain why nursing is a 'regulated' practice

Christine is a patient in the medical ward where you are working. She is anxiously awaiting some test results. You notice that she asks your fellow nurse, Carole, to call the resident doctor for her because she wants to ask the doctor some questions about things that are bothering her. Carole agrees, but then goes to morning tea.

When you ask Carole why she hasn't called the doctor, Carole replies, 'I could call the doctor but I know that she won't come until her regular round at 11.30 a.m. Christine will just have to wait. If she asks me again, I'll just say that the doctor is busy but will be here at 11.30. She isn't going to complain. She knows how busy these doctors are.'

The focus of this chapter is the moral aspects of the nurse–patient relationship. Some people might think Carole is treating Christine with disrespect by misleading and then avoiding her. Others might think Carole is just being realistic. After all, the doctor really is busy and will not be free until 11.30 a.m. In order to work out whether or not this is an appropriate way to treat a patient, the nurse will need to have a good understanding of their responsibilities to their patients and the moral basis of those responsibilities.

Rights and obligations are like two sides of the same coin. A legal right comes with a corresponding obligation, or duty. A right is a legal *entitlement* to do something, and an obligation is the *constraint* upon individuals' behaviour that comes with that entitlement. However, the nurse–patient relationship involves more than legalities. As discussed in Chapter 1, interpersonal relationships involve moral values, such as respect, beneficence and compassion.

The therapeutic relationship: Power and vulnerability

The nurse's relationship with a patient is called a *therapeutic* relationship. Such a relationship exists to have a healing or beneficial effect on the patient. In a very real sense, the relationship is part of the nursing care because the care is inseparable from the relationship. For this reason, the Nursing and Midwifery Board of Australia (NMBA) has set down guidelines for professional boundaries for nurses and midwives in its Code of Conduct for Nurses (NMBA 2018b).

The nurse–patient relationship is complex, but it has some basic features that are important for nurses to understand. First, it is a relationship of power. The nurse is in a position of power over the patient because patients have needs that they cannot meet themselves, and that require the assistance of the nurse. Nurses' power lies in their capacity to influence treatment, and thereby influence a patient's recovery. The NMBA's Code of Conduct for Nurses recognises the significance of the nurse's power (NMBA 2018b). Principle 4: Professional behaviour (point 4.1) states:

> Adhering to professional boundaries promotes person-centred practice and protects both parties. To maintain professional boundaries, nurses must:
>
> **a.** recognise the inherent power imbalance that exists between nurses, people in their care and significant others and establish and maintain professional boundaries

The term 'power' can be used to express several meanings, such as agency, authority, control, influence and dominance. In a relationship of power, one of the parties has more control, influence and authority *in the particular situation* than the other. It is important to note that the power is to be understood in relation to a particular situation. In a situation where you need expert health care, it is of limited use to be physically strong, well educated and aware of your rights if you do not understand the physiological facts about your illness, what options for treatment are open to you or how the health-care system functions. A person in this situation will be unable to determine the best course of action simply because they lack the necessary know-how. In contrast, nurses typically know much of this, and have a relationship with their health-care colleagues through which they can influence the ways in which care is delivered.

Nurses' professional power lies in the fact that they have a great deal of knowledge that patients typically do not possess – for example:

→ expert theoretical knowledge about the human body and pathophysiology
→ clinical experience of a range of conditions and treatments
→ a general understanding of human psychology
→ professional training in dealing with people – especially sick people
→ knowledge about the side-effects and rates of success of particular treatments
→ knowledge about the structure and function of the health-care system
→ knowledge about the particular health-care organisation – for example, the hospital or clinic
→ particular knowledge and understanding of the patient's condition and what can be expected of it.

The patient's lack of knowledge requires trust in the nurse. This trust gives the nurse power over the patient because the patient has to take the nurse at their word, and cannot know (or at least cannot know initially) whether or not a nurse is acting honestly. Normally, the people we trust are those we know well personally, but in the clinical setting the patient is required to trust complete strangers. This can be very difficult to do, even though nurses are generally highly trusted. Patients' dependence on the trustworthiness of nurses can make them vulnerable to being harmed if a nurse fails to live up to that trust. This places an important moral obligation on the nurse to be honest and trustworthy, and to respect confidentiality. Confidentiality and trust will be discussed in more detail in Chapters 7 and 8.

In addition to expert knowledge, the nurse has a network of collegial relations upon which to call at any time in order to assist or advise in planning and delivering care – for example, fellow nurses, doctors, dieticians or technicians. The patient often has no such network of interpersonal, practical and professional support, and consequently may feel lonely, isolated and anxious.

In a clinical setting, nurses have freedom of movement, so can come and go from the clinic or hospital as they please. In contrast, patients may be required to wait to see a doctor, to have observations taken, to receive medication, to have tests or receive results, to have a referral written and so forth – all in order to have their health needs met. In this way, patients' freedom and control over their personal circumstances are significantly reduced, making them dependent upon others.

The nurse is also free of the anxiety that comes with being ill. The mere fact of requiring investigation or treatment of a condition creates anxiety in the minds of most people. Even the most experienced health-care practitioners feel some anxiety when their own health is called into question. This is a psychological pressure that can put patients at a disadvantage by making it more difficult for them to articulate their needs and negotiate their treatment options in a confident way.

Such conditions create a certain kind of vulnerability for individuals who find themselves dependent upon a nurse. These individuals are vulnerable simply by virtue of needing to rely on the nurse for something that is fundamental to their well-being and peace of mind. Being vulnerable in this sense does not mean that patients have no power at all in their lives, or are incapable of defending themselves; rather, it means that, *in this particular situation* – their illness – their capacity to maintain their own well-being is compromised because they depend upon the professional abilities of the nurse. The more complex a person's health-care needs, the greater their vulnerability, because the more they will need to rely upon health-care professionals to meet those needs. While this increases the power of the health-care professional, it also increases that provider's duties, and their moral and legal responsibilities to the patient.

REFLECTIVE QUESTIONS 3.1

1 Think of a patient you have nursed or read about. Make a list of the ways in which the patient is vulnerable to the nurse's power.
2 What cues does a patient give you to show they trust you?
3 How do you think a patient would feel and behave if they did not trust their nurse?

Models of the professional–patient relationship

As discussed briefly in the Introduction, the relationship between the nurse and the patient can be understood broadly as a 'fiduciary relationship'. In law, 'fiduciary' refers to a situation where 'one person justifiably places confidence and trust in someone else and seeks that person's help or advice in some matter' (Merriam-Webster Dictionary). This type of relationship has a particular set of features that make it significantly different from other types of professional relationship (Frankel 2011). Before considering the character of the fiduciary relationship more closely, we will next consider four common models for the professional–patient relationship, and look at their moral aspects (Bayles 1989; Coady & Bloch 1996; Stein-Parbury 2009). These models are not the only kinds of models that are credible, but they do express some very common understandings (and misunderstandings) of the professional–patient relationship.

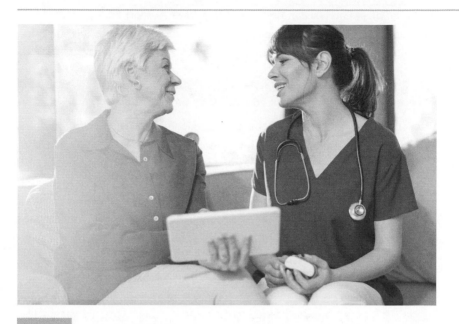

| FIGURE 3.1 | An ethical relationship is one where the patient's authority in decision-making takes priority over the nurse's knowledge and power. |

THE AGENCY MODEL

In the agency model of a professional relationship, the professional acts as an agent of the patient – that is, the professional does exactly the things that the patient would do, were the patient able (Bayles 1989: 71). In this model, the professional's actions are directed solely by the wishes and inclinations of the patient, regardless of the professional's own judgement about the wisdom of those actions. For example, Karen has a seven-year-old son with protruding front teeth. Karen tells the school nurse that she does not want her child to attend the school dental clinic because he will feel embarrassed about his teeth. On the agency model, the nurse would be morally obliged to respect Karen's wishes, even if the nurse believed that the child needed to be seen by a dental therapist. Here, the patient (Karen, as the guardian of her son) has all the authority and all the responsibility.

A serious problem with the agency model is that it sometimes asks professionals to act against the values and standards to which they are committed, and which comprise good professional practice. In this way, the patient can compromise the professional's self-respect. For example, by insisting that the nurse slavishly obey her, Karen makes no place in the relationship for the expert knowledge, training and skills that are part of the nursing role. Karen thus fails to give the nurse due professional recognition, and fails to treat her with appropriate respect.

THE CONTRACT MODEL

Another way of characterising the professional–patient relationship is as a contract – that is, an agreement freely negotiated between two equal parties (Bayles 1989: 72). Here, both parties agree to the conditions of the contract, and both parties are equally bound by the contract. The contract imposes clear mutual rights and obligations upon the parties. For example, if I enter into a contract with a builder to build my house, the contract sets out what the builder is required to do and what I am required to do, and it also sets out the penalties for each of us should we fail to uphold our ends of the agreement.

Although a contract assumes that the parties to it are equal, it is clear that such equality is impossible in many situations, and this is almost always the case in health care. In a health-care situation, the patient typically has far less knowledge about their situation than the professional, and consequently has less choice about alternative courses of action. Medical, nursing and allied health knowledge is difficult to acquire – usually requiring formal university training – and its application to particular situations requires careful judgement informed by knowledge of similar cases. In addition, the professional typically has more freedom to enter the contract than the patient. For example, a general practitioner has many more patients to select from than individuals have general practitioners to choose from. This is especially the case in rural and remote Australia, where there are fewer doctors and nurses per capita than in urban areas, and the costs and inconvenience of travel to attend a clinic may be significant.

In contrast with a contractual model, an approach that has been gaining popularity in recent times has been to promote the 'expert patient'. On this approach, patients (and the public in general) are encouraged to learn about the latest health research and evidence base for treatments so that they can understand how alternative treatments will impact upon their particular lives, and therefore be equipped to make more fully informed choices about health care. Programs such as Self Management UK in the United Kingdom (www.selfmanagementuk.org) exemplify this approach.

THE FRIENDSHIP MODEL

The friendship model (Bayles 1989: 74) acknowledges the personal nature of the professional–patient relationship. This model is characterised by mutual trust, affection, cooperation and a shared interest. This may seem like a good model from the patient's perspective, because one characteristic of friendship is that friends accord each other's interests more weight than they do non-friends' interests. In the friendship model, the patient may expect the professional to show them special favour by 'pulling some strings' – for example, by putting the patient ahead of more needy people on a clinic waiting list.

However, there are a number of morally significant differences between friendship and a professional relationship. Most notably, the mutuality of the professional–patient relationship is quite limited, unlike normal friendships. Remember, a professional acts in the patient's interests; the patient does not act in the professional's interests. We see health professionals only when we need them to do something for us. Coupled with this need is an inequality of knowledge and the personal motivation for entering the relationship. Importantly, the affection characteristic of a friendship is inappropriate in a professional relationship.

The defining feature of friendship is the willingness to be influenced by the friend's interests, simply for the friend's sake (Kennett & Cocking 1998). For example, if my friend Linda asked me to go to a golf tournament with her when her favourite player visited town, I would agree to go – not because I like golf (I have no interest), but because I am open to being influenced by her interests on account of the affection we feel for each other. This dynamic is dangerous in a professional relationship because it may result in a patient adjusting their views about what they need in order to keep things comfortable between themself and the professional (and vice versa). Rather than probing problems critically, the relationship would be driven by maintaining mutual affection. In reality, health-care judgements need to be based on expert knowledge, experience and objective evidence.

PATERNALISM

The paternalist model (Bayles 1989: 74) describes a relationship where someone (Person X) makes a decision about what happens to someone else (Person Y) on the basis that X knows better than Y what is in Y's best interests. The word 'paternalism' comes from the Latin word *pater*, meaning father. Parents, for example, exercise paternalism over their children by making decisions on their behalf when their children lack the knowledge and capacity to make appropriate decisions about their own actions. As a model for professional–patient relationships, paternalism has some benefits – for example, it recognises the inequalities and power imbalance in the relationship, and allows the professional to use their superior knowledge to further the patient's interests more effectively than the patient could. So paternalism is not *necessarily* incompatible with respect for the patient's autonomy.

However, paternalism has a very limited scope within health care. Where patients lack knowledge, the professional should be able to provide that knowledge in a form sufficient to allow patients to exercise their own responsible decision-making. This is also known as 'supported decision-making', and is the preferred contemporary approach to shared decision-making. Much information that professionals have is irrelevant to the patient's decision-making process, in any case. For example, if I require treatment for a leg ulcer, I do not need to know detailed pathophysiology about the interaction of antibiotics with cell membranes; I just need to know enough to understand how various courses of action will affect me. I need to know what will happen if I do not have regular dressings, if I do not take antibiotics or if I continue to play with the neighbour's dog or smoke cigarettes. I also need to know the likelihood that the ulcer will get better with rest alone.

Often patients begin a relationship with a professional when they have little knowledge, but that changes over time as the patient understands more about the process in which they are involved. Paternalism can easily be taken too far if the professional, having made a judgement that the patient is incompetent, does not adjust that attitude in response to the patient's increased knowledge over time. Patients may become unsatisfied with a treatment if they feel they have been excluded from the decision-making process, and this can result in a loss of trust, and consequently loss of compliance with needed treatment.

As noted earlier, strategies such as the 'expert patient' approach attempt to build the capacity of patients to make decisions that best suit their own lives. Another strategy with this aim is the 'Ask Share Know' project (https://askshareknow.com .au). It encourages patients to ask health professionals the following three key questions:

1   What are my options?
2   What are the possible benefits and harms of those options?
3   How likely is each of those benefits and harms to happen to me?

Paternalism in health care can take the form of a 'deficit' model, where the health and well-being of a particular community are judged by comparing it to what another 'mainstream' community has, rather than by understanding the strengths and resources of the supposedly 'deficient' community. This approach has tended to characterise the delivery of Aboriginal health care in Australia (Verbunt et al. 2021). A serious problem with this approach is that it presents poor health outcomes of Aboriginal communities as the fault of those communities insofar as they fail to meet the standards and norms of mainstream Australian communities. Consequently, this approach 'misses important structural, political, and cultural contexts, that present and enable opportunities to improve health' (Verbunt et al. 2021).

An example of a health care service that has actively addressed paternalism in health care delivered to Aboriginal Australians is the Dalarinji model at St Vincents Hospital in Sydney (Presz et al. 2022). This service was jointly developed by the Emergency Department and the Aboriginal Health Unit to improve health outcomes for Aboriginal people. In another setting, success in lifting COVID-19 vaccination rates among Aboriginal communities has been shown to the result of leadership and management by Aboriginal health practitioners (Naren et al. 2021).

THE FIDUCIARY MODEL

While the fiduciary model of relationship (Bayles 1989: 78; Bayles 2009) does not exhaust the nurse's legal responsibilities to the patient, it provides a sound way to understand the nurse's professional and legal obligations to the patient. The fiduciary model recognises the nurse's superior knowledge and power, but gives priority to the patient's authority in decision-making. According to this model, both parties are responsible for their actions, and the judgements of both should be taken into consideration when coming to a decision about care. However, as long as the patient is mentally competent, the patient is the final authority in decision-making. At the same time, health-care professionals have special obligations to the patient arising from their superior clinical knowledge, by virtue of which the patient is required to *trust* the professional.

In a fiduciary relationship, the patient has an active role to play in decision-making. The use of the word 'consent' rather than 'decide' to express the patient's role in determining treatment is meant to indicate the cooperative nature of the decision-making process. For example, it is standard practice in obstetrics for the woman and the obstetrician to share the decision about the mode of delivering the baby. They may agree to trial a normal delivery where there is a likelihood of needing a caesarean section, even though it is likely to make the birthing process longer and more tiring for the woman.

The decision-making process needs to be cooperative because the nurse has technical knowledge but does not necessarily have knowledge of the patient's personal situation, and how treatment will impact the patient's life. This is especially so when the patient's lifestyle and circumstances are very different from the nurse's. Because nurses typically lack both sufficient knowledge of and authority over a person's life, their expertise does not entitle them to make decisions that have significant effects on the patient's lifestyle or plans without the patient's consent. The role of the nurse within the fiduciary relationship is to provide expert advice in such a way that maximises the patient's capacity to further their own (reasonable) values and interests. Because the fiduciary relationship is based in justifiable trust in the nurse's expertise, the nurse has an obligation to provide information that is up to date, relevant and evidence based, and to do so in such a way that patients can understand its significance for their personal situation.

REFLECTIVE QUESTIONS 3.2

Think of a patient for whom you have cared.
1 What model best describes that relationship?
2 What would you change about that relationship if you could? Why?

Legal responsibilities of the professional relationship

The legal responsibilities of the nurse that arise from the nature of the therapeutic relationship with the patient are regulated by several Acts and also by common law.

The nurse is legally obliged to be truthful, trustworthy and confidential (although only up to a point – see Chapter 7), and to fully inform the patient of the nature of proposed treatments *and* alternatives. These obligations arise from the patient's vulnerability to the nurse's power – the possibility that the patient can be harmed by the nurse's acts or omissions.

The nurse has a legal responsibility called a 'duty of care' (Forrester & Griffiths 2014: 102). A duty of care refers to the legal obligation on a nurse to exercise reasonable care and skill in the provision of professional treatment. A reasonable standard is that which could be expected of other similarly trained and experienced nurses. To determine what is 'reasonable', a nurse's actions would be compared with the actions of other nurses with a similar level of training and clinical experience, employed in a similar role. So it would be reasonable to expect that a first-year graduate registered nurse would deliver a lower standard of care than a very senior nurse with many years' clinical experience. In determining the practical scope of a nurse's duty of care, one must determine the nurse's actual scope of practice, which gives consideration to the complexity of a patient's illness, the degree of the patient's dependence on the nurse and the nurse's level of knowledge, training and practical competency, and the employer's policies and organisational culture (APNA 2019).

The maintenance of a reasonable standard of care in order to meet a legal duty of care is the central reason why nurses are reminded continually that they must work within their 'scope of practice'. A nurse's scope of practice is determined by four main factors:

1   the nurse's level of training
2   the nurse's level of appointment (the position the nurse is employed to fill)
3   state and Commonwealth legislation
4   the employer's policy framework.

REFLECTIVE QUESTION 3.3

You are working with a registered nurse who has not had any training in intravenous cannulation, although she has seen many cannulations performed by other clinicians. She decides to insert an intravenous cannula into a patient and she does a good job. Is she acting outside her scope of practice?

Nurses who act outside their scope of practice fail in their duty of care. If a nurse acts outside her scope of practice and the patient is harmed by her actions, the nurse is liable for a charge of negligence. Duty of care and negligence will be discussed in detail in Chapter 5.

Moral responsibilities of the professional relationship: The four principles of bioethics

In recent times, the moral principles underpinning the nurse's duty of care and standard of care have become known as the 'four principles of bioethics'. These are non-maleficence, beneficence, respect for autonomy and justice (Beauchamp & Childress 2019). While these concepts are philosophically and practically quite complex, for our purposes this book will adopt the following general meanings:

➜ *Non-maleficence* means refraining from deliberately inflicting harm on a person, including oneself.

➜ *Beneficence* means actively bringing about a benefit for a person, including oneself.

➜ *Respect for autonomy* means acting in a way that protects and promotes the capacity for self-determination.

➜ *Justice* means acting fairly.

These principles are generally considered to be the main moral justifications for the professional activities of all health-care professionals, and this approach sits comfortably with the concept of mutual vulnerability that frames this book. Arguably, the four principles do not exhaust the moral features of a nurse's actions; nevertheless, they provide a useful guide to moral decision-making and action in nursing practice.

PRINCIPLE I: NON-MALEFICENCE – DO NO HARM

Non-maleficence is the principle that one should not deliberately inflict harm on a person, including oneself. Sometimes, when considering how to treat a person, this idea is expressed as 'first, do no harm'. In other words, the nurse should not provide treatment to a person if the treatment is more likely to harm than to help the patient. For example, nurses caring for the aged – whether in the home or an aged-care facility – should not automatically take the view that people should shower every day. While it is clearly a good idea to shower daily, a wet bathroom can pose a real danger to an unsteady or frail person. Wet surfaces, poor lighting and hard edges can lead to a fall and a fractured femur, which in the frail elderly may result in a lengthy and painful hospital stay, and possibly premature death. From the point of view of non-maleficence, when you are planning care for a patient, you need to consider carefully whether carrying out the care will pose a significant risk of harm. If providing that particular item of care will likely harm the patient, then you should not do it.

There is a further consideration here, which leads to the principle of beneficence (discussed below). Where *not* providing the care will *not* harm the patient, you should not provide it. In the above example, if it will not harm the patient to not shower every day, then the nurse should not, as a general rule, shower the frail elderly person on a daily basis.

For the principle of non-maleficence to guide your actions in avoiding harm, you need to have a sense of what harms are possible for your patients. In order to know whether a course of action will harm your patient, you will need to have knowledge of your patient's health as well as their needs and personal preferences. You will also need to know what the goals of care are – for example, is care aiming at a complete recovery (curative) or simply managing symptoms to make the patient as comfortable as possible (palliative)? If you do not know where potential harms lie, you may not be able to avoid them. In your daily nursing practice, you will need to have up-to-date, practical knowledge of the harms that pose risks for your patients, as well as the likelihood of any harms eventuating. For example, if you are dispensing medication, you will need to know:

→ the clinical indications for the drug
→ the correct dosage
→ side-effects and interactions with other drugs.

In addition, you will need to know:

→ the patient's medical condition
→ their other medications
→ any allergies
→ whether the patient is showing signs of being adversely affected by the drug
→ where to find authoritative information about the drug
→ what to do in the event of a reaction or adverse effect.

If you do not have this knowledge, then you will not know how to avoid medication-related harms to your patient. In short, in the clinical setting non-maleficence requires that nurses observe a reasonable standard of care. In order to act on the principle of non-maleficence, you must be able to implicitly or explicitly recognise the kind of care that falls below a reasonable standard for a nurse of your level of training. When your actions are guided by the principle of non-maleficence, you are living up to a minimum standard of care and meeting your legal responsibility of a duty of care.

Interestingly, non-maleficence requires quality-of-life decisions. A judgement about what counts as a harm for a person implies a judgement about what constitutes a good for that person. Judgements about harms and goods are judgements about what constitutes a good or bad quality of life. However, something considered a harm by one person may not be considered in the same way by another. For example, some people want to have a private room when they are admitted to hospital because they are anxious that a shared ward will deprive them of privacy and rest. Others are anxious about being put in a single room because they fear being lonely or neglected.

PRINCIPLE 2: BENEFICENCE – FOR THE BENEFIT OF A PERSON

Sometimes we are morally obliged not merely to refrain from harming someone, but to actively contribute to the person's welfare. This is the principle of beneficence. An act is beneficent when it is done with the intent of benefiting another (Beauchamp & Childress 2019). Nursing care entails the principle of beneficence because a defining characteristic of the therapeutic relationship is that the nurse provides the patient with a benefit. It is not enough that the nurse merely refrains from harming the patient. For example, a child health nurse at a primary school is required to provide parents and children with evidence-based information about such things as healthy diet, developmental milestones and hygiene. A nurse who sat in the school office all day reading research articles would not be exercising a standard of care that satisfied the principle of beneficence.

Like non-maleficence, acting on beneficence implies a standard of care. In order to act in ways that benefit a patient, the nurse must have sufficient knowledge of such things as the patient's condition and possible complications, treatment options and consequences, and the risks present in the environment where treatment will take place. Beneficence also requires judgements about quality of life. In order to know what will be of benefit to the patient, the nurse needs to know what the patient considers to be a good or poor quality of life. For example, a nurse in a hospital or aged-care facility might think it is good for a long-stay female patient to wear lipstick to 'brighten' her up. However, the patient might resent such an activity and regard it as an attempt to make her conform to a stereotype of femininity that she finds inappropriate.

The principle of beneficence also entails judgements of utility (or usefulness). In deciding whether the nurse is obliged to carry out a certain action in order to benefit a patient, the nurse must balance the benefits against the risks of any particular procedure. For example, the nurse may have to balance the need to get a post-operative patient up and moving about to prevent a venous thrombosis, against the risk of increasing the patient's pain and having to administer painkillers, which may decrease the patient's level of consciousness and respiration.

PRINCIPLE 3: RESPECT FOR AUTONOMY – ALLOWING PEOPLE TO MAKE THEIR OWN CHOICES

Autonomy is a form of self-governance that is sometimes called 'self-determination'. Respect for autonomy means allowing people to make their own decisions about how they live. If being autonomous means doing what you really want to do, then people are able to do what they really want to only when they are able to make decisions that are informed by facts and grounded in their conception of the life they want to live. Another way to express this is to say that we do what we want when our actions are the result of our own motives, reasoning and decision-making, rather than those of someone else. The extent of misinformation associated with the COVID-19 pandemic has been identified as a factor undermining both patients' and health professionals' desire to do what they really want to do.

Autonomy refers to the capacity to make informed decisions about one's life in order to determine for oneself whether or not a course of action is in one's best interests. Autonomy does not mean being able to do whatever you happen to feel like doing. In theorising autonomy, moral philosophers typically distinguish between decisions that genuinely reflect a person's interests and commitments, and decisions that are merely impulsive, transitory or formed as a result of some kind of coercion. Only those decisions that genuinely reflect a person's interests and commitments can be said to be autonomous (Korsgaard 1996).

A person's beliefs, knowledge, values and commitments are the basis of autonomy because they constitute the person's *reasons* for the decisions and actions they undertake. In this way, autonomy entails reasons-responsiveness. People are reasons-responsive when their choices and actions are driven by their own considered reflections and reasoning and when, if asked, they can explain their actions by appealing to their own beliefs, knowledge and values (and not those of someone else).

By contrast, a non-autonomous person is someone who acts without stable or deeply held reasons, or due to reasons that are incoherent and/or contradictory in themselves. For example, a person who chooses a course of action solely on the basis of what someone else thinks (a family member or friend, perhaps) is not autonomous because that person is not acting from reasons of their own. In a different way, a person who acts differently from one day to the next, depending on mood, cannot be said to be acting autonomously either, since their conduct is not driven by a firmly held belief, value or commitment. When asked to explain how their behaviours express their firmly held beliefs, values or commitments, these people cannot provide *reasons* of their own – in the first example because their reasons are borrowed from someone else, and in the second example because the behaviour is not motivated by any belief or value that abides from one day to the next. Respect for autonomy, then, is the recognition and valuing of a person's capacity to act from reasons of their own. So when we say that we should respect autonomy, we mean that we should take seriously a person's *considered* choices and the reasons for what they do.

Respect for autonomy has both a passive and an active form. In its passive form, it requires us to *refrain* from unduly interfering with another person's decisions and actions – for example, by not trying to convince a person to undertake a course of treatment. In its active form, respect for autonomy requires us to *act* in such a way that enables a person to exercise autonomous choice – for example, by giving the person options for their care, or adjusting the timing of some aspects of the care to allow the person to observe a spiritual obligation.

Respect for autonomy is a basic obligation within the nurse–patient relationship. It means allowing the patient to make decisions about what happens to them as part of their care. For the nurse, this involves providing patients with all the information they need, in a form they can understand, so they are able to make an informed decision that is in their best interests. Furthermore, this obligation requires the nurse to actively promote patients' control over their own situation, and assist them to avoid becoming dependent upon the nurse (Beauchamp & Childress 2019; Dunn et al. 2008). Here, encouraging the 'expert patient' can empower persons to competently choose between treatment alternatives on the basis of their own reasons.

Some people will genuinely be unable to understand the implications of their behaviour, perhaps as a result of a brain injury or dementia, so may not be fully autonomous (unless they have an advance care directive – see Chapter 4). Others may experience temporary impairment as a result of medication or an accident. In such situations, respect for autonomy will involve promoting independence as far as possible (for example, through supported decision-making), but may be morally less significant than beneficence. Consider the following situation.

LAW AND ETHICS IN PRACTICE

Linda is transferred from the emergency department to your unit for an urgent angioplasty (repair of a blocked artery in the heart) later that day. Without this surgery, her likelihood of having a life-threatening heart attack is high. She becomes increasingly anxious. Suddenly she says that she is going home.

》 How might you try to get Linda to stay while still respecting her autonomy?

PRINCIPLE 4: JUSTICE – BEING FAIR

The concept of justice is very complex, especially when it comes to dealing with the vast array of issues arising from the provision of health services. However, it is broadly understood as fairness, or the idea of giving and receiving what is due to someone. Of course, what is due to a person will vary depending upon the circumstances. For example, in the game of basketball I am treated justly when my team receives a penalty for a foul by the opposition – in other words, when the rules of the game are applied consistently to all of the players and no one is given any special favours. When I rent a house, I am treated justly when the terms of the lease are adhered to by my landlord, and I am not asked to undertake maintenance or repairs that arise from reasonable wear and tear. As a person, I am treated justly when I am seen as being capable of determining for myself what is in my best interests, and when I am afforded the same basic rights and obligations as everybody else. What is due to a person, then, is treatment that recognises the person's moral and legal equality among all other persons.

In the nurse–patient relationship, the principle of justice gives rise to the obligation to treat patients with respect for their humanity, and to give patients their due. For example, patients should not be moved up the waiting list because they happen to have a friendship with the person who compiles the waiting list. Older patients should not be charged a higher fee than younger patients for an identical service, nor should patients be given preferential treatment because they may be a celebrity, a politician or a colleague. Justice requires that the professional does not 'play favourites'.

Justice may require that certain patients who appear to be very similar receive different treatments. For example, two women who have each recently delivered their first baby may require different levels of support and care, depending upon their psychological and family circumstances. It may appear to one new mother that another is the nurses' favourite because the nurses feed her baby during the night, whereas the first mother has to get up several times during the night and receives little assistance. However, it may be that the apparent favourite has an illness that isn't obvious and that can be triggered by sleep deprivation, especially if accompanied by pain after a traumatic birth or acute anxiety, which can accompany a birth. In such a case, there is a clinical indication for special care, because it is required to assist the woman in acquiring the capacity to adequately care for both her child and herself. In other words, any apparent disparities in the kind of care given to different patients must be justified by clinical need, and appropriate according to the four principles of bioethics.

In summary, the characteristics of the nurse–patient relationship require the recognition of certain moral rights and obligations. These oblige the nurse to minimise harms to patients; to act for patients' benefit; to facilitate patients' self-determination; and to treat patients fairly. The source of these moral obligations lies in the human condition of mutual vulnerability and our common humanity.

TABLE 3.1 Overview of moral rights and duties of the nurse–patient relationship

	RIGHT	DUTY
NON-MALEFICENCE	That any possible harms arising from treatment will be kept to a minimum	To minimise any possible harm arising from treatment
RESPECT FOR AUTONOMY	To self-governance; to determine for oneself whether a treatment is in one's interests	To support a person in making their own informed decisions as far as possible, and to refrain from inappropriate paternalism
BENEFICENCE	To have one's welfare actively promoted	To act in such a way that actively contributes to the welfare of others
JUSTICE	To be treated fairly and as an equal with other persons in relevant respects	To treat people fairly and as equal with other persons in relevant respects

Risks of the nurse–patient relationship

So far, we have examined the key moral principles that underpin good nursing practice and promote the therapeutic relationship. It is important to remember that the therapeutic relationship is just that: a *relationship*. That means it works in two directions, and can be driven by both the nurse and the patient. Sometimes the relationship can have a detrimental effect on nurses, especially if they are not careful to take a professional, moral approach towards patients and their role.

Nurses need to empathise with their patients, but if empathy becomes sympathy it can lead the nurse to over-identify with the patient's suffering and thus lose professional distance. Empathy involves a kind of distance; it is an understanding of how things are for the patient without actually experiencing the feelings of the patient. Sympathy loses that distance; it is an understanding of how it is for the patient by closely and imaginatively experiencing the patient's feelings (Burton 2015). The presence of these emotions in the nurse's relationship with the patient can adversely affect the nurse's judgement about what is best for the patient. For example, sympathy can give rise to the temptation to protect the patient from bad news, perhaps by withholding information about possible side-effects of treatment. This can deprive the patient of relevant information needed to exercise autonomy.

When a nurse loses professional distance and closely identifies with the emotions of a patient, they can mistake their own emotions and emotional needs for those of the patient. When this happens (called 'projection'), the nurse may misinterpret the patient's behaviour and regard it as an attempt to meet needs that the patient does not have (Freud 1991: 241). For example, a nurse may interpret a patient's reluctance to talk as a symptom of shyness or sadness when in fact it may be that the patient finds the nurse's behaviour overbearing, and is trying to avoid interacting with the nurse (Coon & Mitterer 2010; Lilienfeld et al. 2010).

It is not only nurses who can endanger the therapeutic relationship. Patients are human too, and they bring their own character flaws to the relationship, just like anybody else. Patients – and their relatives and friends – have been known to be emotionally manipulative to obtain favourable treatment, information or drugs. When under stress, some people act in ways even they do not fully understand, or of which they may not be fully aware. For most people, the clinical situation is very different from everyday life. It can be a strange and curious situation to navigate, and a place where our everyday responses and coping mechanisms may not work as well as they normally do. For this reason, patients can become dependent upon their nurses, and this can lead to a range of problems. Being cared for can create a feeling of intimacy with one's nurse. Even when the nurse remains professionally detached, the patient can mistakenly interpret the nurse's care as an indication of friendship or romantic interest, and this can lead to unwelcome behaviour, such as flirting, inappropriate sharing of personal information, touching or gift-giving.

Patients can also mistake their own feelings of gratitude for feelings of friendship or romantic interest in the nurse. Patients and their family members can also become emotionally involved with the nurse, and feelings such as gratitude, anxiety or grief can become confused. Misunderstandings fuelled by strong emotions can become explosive in the context of grief or serious complications. Patients or family members can feel let down, and blame the nurse if their seriously ill relative deteriorates, even when they have received medical advice that deterioration is inevitable.

Living in small communities, where the nurse and patient may know each other outside of the clinical setting, can give rise to particular problems – especially as residents age and become more vulnerable.

LAW AND ETHICS IN PRACTICE

Elizabeth was a nurse working in the health centre of a small remote island community. The centre had a number of aged-care residents. Elizabeth became close to a resident elderly couple, Jean and Alan. After Alan died, Elizabeth took on some of Alan's roles, such as maintaining the family property on the island and doing Jean's banking. After the funeral, Jean's daughter – who lived interstate – became concerned when she could not locate the title deeds to the family property; this alarm grew when she discovered that Alan had written a large cheque to Elizabeth shortly before he died. Elizabeth left the island suddenly and the police were called to investigate. Meanwhile, management of Jean's finances was placed with the Public Trustee.

>> **Has Elizabeth done anything wrong?**

In small communities, both nurses and patients can feel uncomfortable about – and even resentful of – the closeness of the clinical relationship. Patients can worry about their privacy and their reputations in the community, and nurses can worry about being expected to give continued advice or support long after the patient has left the clinical setting.

It is important for the health and well-being of both the patient and the nurse that nurses understand the special nature of the therapeutic relationship, especially the greater power held by the nurse in that relationship. The close nature of the nurse–patient relationship requires emotional and intellectual maturity and discipline from the nurse to ensure that the relationship is both a healing one for the patient and a source of self-respect for the nurse. The NMBA provides a Code of Conduct for Nurses (NMBA 2018b) to guide nurses in making decisions with patients and their families.

Regulation of professional nursing practice

WHAT IS REGULATION?

Nursing is a regulated practice. Regulation is a means of ensuring that only practitioners who are suitably trained and qualified can practise, and that they do so in a manner that is both competent and ethical. It consists of rules and standards that must be observed by nurses and midwives, and by the organisations that educate nurses.

The regulation of nursing encompasses:

→ standards for registration
→ the development of codes and guidelines for practice
→ management of complaints and notifications of practice issues
→ accreditation of educational curricula (Chiarella & White 2013).

In Australia, a number of key health professions, including nursing, are subject to regulation by the Australian Health Practitioner Regulation Agency (AHPRA). Although AHPRA combines the regulation of nursing and midwifery professions, in this chapter we will focus on the impact of regulation for nurses. Under a coordinated national scheme, AHPRA regulates nurses and midwives in collaboration with the Nursing and Midwifery Board of Australia (NMBA). The NMBA states its function as:

→ registering nursing and midwifery practitioners and students
→ developing standards, codes and guidelines for the nursing and midwifery profession
→ handling notifications, complaints, investigations and disciplinary hearings
→ assessing overseas trained practitioners who wish to practise in Australia
→ approving accreditation standards and accredited courses of study. (NMBA 2021b)

The NMBA comprises nursing and midwifery boards in each Australian state and territory. While the National Board sets policy and professional standards, the state and territory boards manage notifications against practitioners and decisions for the registration of individual nurses. Each individual board across Australia, including their membership, is publicly available on the NMBA website.

WHY DO NURSES NEED TO BE REGULATED?

As we have discussed previously, the role of a registered nurse entails that the nurse has a high degree of responsibility and power. This means nurses are in a position to cause harm and suffering to patients (and their families) if care is unsafe or of a poor quality. The safety and quality of patient care depends on the competent performance of the nurse's responsibilities. The systematic training and personal commitment of nurses to high standards of practice is part of what makes nursing a profession. The Australian Council of Professions (2003) defines a profession as follows:

> A Profession is a disciplined group of individuals who adhere to ethical standards and who hold themselves out as, and are accepted by the public as possessing special knowledge and skills in a widely recognised body of learning derived from research, education and training at a high level, and who are prepared to apply this knowledge and exercise these skills in the interest of others.
>
> It is inherent in the definition of a Profession that a code of ethics governs the activities of each Profession. Such codes require behaviour and practice beyond the personal moral obligations of an individual. They define and demand high standards of behaviour in respect to the services provided to the public and in dealing with professional colleagues. Often these codes are enforced by the Profession and are acknowledged and accepted by the community.

As professionals, registered nurses are expected to self-regulate – that is, maintain an appropriate level of knowledge, practical competency and ethical standards. In addition, government also plays a significant role in the regulation of nursing and midwifery practice. State and federal governments each have a role in setting practice standards, employment standards and training requirements for educational institutions such as universities and the workforce (Chiarella & Staunton 2020). For example, the Australian Commission on Safety and Quality in Health Care (ACSQHC) is a national body that, in consultation with health professionals, sets standards for patient care in hospitals. In addition, each public hospital network in Australia has a credentialling process by which individual clinicians are determined to meet standards required for employment in those health services.

HOW ARE NURSES REGULATED?

The regulation of nursing and midwifery by AHPRA is underpinned by the *Health Practitioner Regulation National Law Act 2009* (AHPRA 2018). Although AHPRA is a national scheme, when it came into effect, each state and territory passed its own specific *Health Practitioner Regulation National Law Act.*

REFLECTIVE QUESTION 3.4

During morning tea break, your colleagues are discussing the need for registration as a nurse and one of them claims that the national scheme is unnecessary. How would you respond to this claim?

AHPRA plays a role in facilitating a health workforce that is mobile and flexible, providing high-quality education and training, and assessing overseas qualified practitioners for their suitability to practise in Australia. Read about the national scheme on AHPRA's website: www.ahpra.gov.au.

ACCREDITATION

While the NMBA is responsible for the regulation of nurses and midwives, it is the Australian Nursing and Midwifery Accreditation Council (ANMAC) that is responsible for accrediting education providers and programs of study for the nursing and midwifery professions (see www.anmac.org.au) according to accreditation standards (ANMAC 2021).

REGISTRATION AS A NURSE OR MIDWIFE

The regulation of nursing and midwifery aims to ensure that only appropriately qualified, endorsed and approved individuals can enter the profession and earn the right to use the protected title of 'nurse' or 'midwife' (see the section on 'Protected titles' below). Although not yet registered as qualified professionals, nursing students are also registered with AHPRA by the relevant educational institution where they are enrolled to study.

Once qualified, nurses and midwives must apply to AHPRA for registration. Once approved, registration must be renewed each year. In order to be registered, nurses must demonstrate that they:

→ are of good character (through a criminal conviction check)
→ have the appropriate level of English language skills
→ have recent practical experience
→ have undertaken regular, continuing professional development
→ have appropriate professional indemnity insurance (NMBA 2021a).

Each nurse or midwife must demonstrate that they meet these professional standards. If, for example, a nurse has not undertaken continuing professional development in a year, registration will not be renewed automatically; rather, the nurse may be asked to explain their circumstances.

REFLECTIVE QUESTION 3.5

Xin Xiou successfully completed his Bachelor of Nursing in 2013 and is applying for registration in 2019. He did not register with AHPRA immediately after being awarded a Bachelor of Nursing as he was active in his parents' business. He now wants to begin practising as a registered nurse, and makes an application for registration to AHPRA. Will Xin automatically receive registration and be able to apply for a nursing role?

Registration as a nurse does not automatically follow completion of a nursing qualification. The Nursing and Midwifery Board of Australia sets standards for registration that must be met before registration is granted. This is important because registration with the board confers a protected title and a position of responsibility in the community.

PROTECTED TITLES

According to the Health Practitioner Regulation National Law (see section 113: 141), it is an offence to call oneself 'nurse' or 'midwife' unless registered with AHPRA, *even if you have been awarded a Bachelor of Nursing or a Bachelor of Midwifery.* The title 'nurse' and 'midwife' are 'protected titles' – that is, it is unlawful for someone to 'knowingly or recklessly take or use a title' and/or make a member of the public or other health professional believe they are registered as a nurse or midwife when they are not. This is referred to as 'holding out', and is an offence that carries a maximum penalty of $30 000.

Holding out as a nurse or midwife has serious implications for the public and places them at serious risk of harm. Here are some examples of cases involving the use of protected titles that were investigated and resolved by AHPRA:

> In 2017 a woman in Victoria pleaded guilty to claiming to be a registered midwife. In the Frankston Magistrates court on 19 June she was found guilty of using the title 'Midwife' so as to reasonably indicate that she was both qualified and authorised to practice as a midwife when no longer registered as such. The court imposed a two year good behaviour bond and ordered her to pay the legal costs of AHPRA (who had brought the charges against her) of $17,000. (NMBA 2017)

> In 2019, a South Australian woman who continued to work as a nurse in aged care after her registration was suspended was convicted of 66 charges laid by AHPRA. The woman was ordered to pay AHPRA's prosecution costs of $1100 and imposed the Victims of Crime Levy of $10 560. (NMBA 2020)

'Nurse', 'registered nurse', 'nurse practitioner', 'enrolled nurse', 'midwife' and 'midwife practitioner' are protected titles under Australian law. Employers can check whether a person is registered or endorsed by consulting the National Register.

REFLECTIVE QUESTIONS 3.6

You become aware that a person practising homeopathy calls themselves Nurse Simona Brady.

1 Is Simona unlawfully using a protected title?
2 How would you find out whether Simona is a registered nurse?
3 What should you do if she is not?

THE NATIONAL REGISTER

The National, or Public, Register is a register of all health practitioners who are approved to practise within the scope of their registration. Anyone, including members of the general public, can access information held on this register. If a person's name appears on the register against a certain profession, this means the person is legally registered to practise. Employers regularly check this register when considering an application for employment or reviewing longer-term employees.

There is also a register available to the public of practitioners who:

➜ have had their registration cancelled

➜ have signed an undertaking not to practise, either permanently or for a defined period of time

➜ have had certain conditions imposed upon their practice.

These categories and their meaning are explained below. This register has recently been expanded to include former registered health practitioners who have been prohibited from providing health services or using a title. When the agency believes it is in the public's best interests, the register may also include a list of practitioners who have agreed not to practise (AHPRA 2021b).

PROFESSIONAL STANDARDS

Nurses and midwives must meet the professional standards laid out by the NMBA. Earlier in this book, we referred to the various codes that are endorsed by the Australian College of Nursing (ACN), the Australian Nursing Federation (ANF) and the NMBA. These include codes of conduct, standards for practice, and codes of ethics for both nurses and midwives. It should be noted that these are regularly reviewed and revised. For example, following a review by representatives of the NMBA, ACM, ACN and ANMF, the NMBA recently adopted the International Council of Nurses' ICN Code of Ethics for Nurses (ICN 2012, 2021) and the International Confederation of Midwives' Code of Ethics for Midwives (ICM 2014).

COMPLAINTS

Anyone, be it a fellow professional or a member of the public such as a patient, a patient's family or even a neighbour, can make a complaint to AHPRA about a nurse's or midwife's performance or conduct. With the exception of Queensland, this is termed a 'notification'. In Queensland, this is simply termed a 'complaint'.

A breach of any of a nurse's professional standards may be the result of impairment such as physical or mental illness, drug or alcohol addiction or serious disability. However, it may be due to incompetent practice or a result of professional misconduct.

NOTIFICATIONS MADE TO AHPRA

When AHPRA receives a complaint or notification about a nurse, it is evaluated to determine whether the complaint falls within AHPRA's scope of regulation. If it does, AHPRA refers the complaint to the relevant state nursing and midwifery board for consideration of whether there is a serious risk to the public that requires immediate action. If the board determines that there is a risk, an immediate action will be taken. For example, the nurse's or midwife's right to practise may be suspended immediately and remain in force until the complaint has been fully investigated. During this time, the nurse or midwife will have the opportunity to respond to the notification. In this way the regulatory authority acts to protect the public first and foremost, while treating the nurse or midwife justly.

A board receiving a notification has several options. It may:

→ decide to take no further action
→ refer the notification to a health complaints authority, or
→ initiate an investigation of the nurse or midwife.

An investigation may take the form of interviewing the practitioner and relevant witnesses to an event or conduct, accessing patient notes and/or speaking with an employer. Depending on the circumstances of the notification, a health or performance assessment may be required. Following receipt of all relevant information, a board may then decide to caution the nurse or midwife, or to accept an undertaking from the nurse or midwife. Alternatively, a board may decide to impose conditions on the nurse's or midwife's registration or in severe cases of professional misconduct refer the matter to a panel or a tribunal. For example, in 2021 a nurse was suspended for 18 months after he 'published "disgraceful" content about women on social media' (AHPRA 2021e). The Tribunal observed that the nurse had published material on his Facebook page that 'encouraged manipulative, coercive and misogynistic behaviour' and 'described attempts to overcome explicit non-consent of women to sexual activity' (AHPRA 2021e).

The most recent information about how notifications are managed can be found on the APHRA website (www.ahpra.gov.au/notifications/how-we-manage-concerns.aspx).

MANDATORY REPORTING REQUIREMENTS

A mandatory notification to AHPRA is required when any registered health practitioner or their employer has a reasonable belief that a practitioner has engaged in 'notifiable conduct' – that is, if the practitioner has:

→ practised the profession while intoxicated by alcohol or drugs
→ engaged in sexual misconduct in connection with the practice of the practitioner's profession

→ placed the public at risk of substantial harm in the practitioner's practice of the profession because the practitioner has an impairment

→ placed the public at risk of harm because the practitioner has practised in a way that constitutes a significant departure from accepted professional standards (AHPRA 2021g).

LAW AND ETHICS IN PRACTICE

In the mental health unit where Shana is working the afternoon shift, a recently admitted patient requires an injection. Shana and Brian, a nursing colleague, enter the room to ensure the medication is able to be administered since the patient is suffering a psychosis episode and has been aggressive. Following the injection the patient is verbally abusive and tries to punch Brian as he leaves the room. He responds by restraining the patient using a choking hold on the patient's neck with his arm and pushing his finger into the patient's eye. Shana calls another nursing colleague and together they break up the altercation. Shana is very concerned for the patient's welfare as the choking hold lasted more than a few seconds and the patient's eye is bruised. Shana is concerned about the way Brian restrained the patient.

>> **What should she do?**

Mandatory reporting and the requirements you should be aware of are discussed in more detail in Chapter 7.

Conclusion

The nurse–patient relationship can be described as therapeutic when it has the effect of promoting the healing and well-being of the patient. A therapeutic nurse–patient relationship requires professional skills and values from the nurse, supported by the legal regulation of the nursing profession in general. Nurses' skills and values include:

→ recognising and responding appropriately to the duty of care to the patient

→ understanding and responding appropriately to the various ways in which the patient is vulnerable in the clinical setting

→ understanding and responding appropriately to the issues of power in the relationship

→ understanding and responding appropriately to moral and legal responsibilities

→ understanding and working within one's scope of practice

→ identifying and managing risks effectively.

The regulation of the nursing profession as a whole aims to protect the safety and quality of nursing practice by ensuring that:

→ only properly qualified and credentialled individuals can call themselves 'nurses'
→ nurses have the necessary skills and values to undertake patient care.

This occurs primarily through AHPRA, which has set standards and processes for:

→ nurse registration
→ training and ongoing education
→ safety and quality in clinical practice
→ professional conduct
→ managing complaints about a nurse's conduct.

The overall expectations of professional nurses are also set out in the Code of Conduct for Nurses (NMBA 2018b) and the ICN Code of Ethics for Nurses (ICN 2012, 2021).

REFLECTIVE QUESTIONS 3.7

1 What does it mean to say that the nurse has a relationship of power with the patient?
2 What are some of the key moral responsibilities that the nurse has to the patient?
3 What are the key legal responsibilities that the nurse has to the patient?

Further reading

Banks, S. & Gallagher, A. (2009). *Ethics in professional life: Virtues for health and social care*. Palgrave Macmillan.

Beauchamp, T., Walters, L.R., Kahn, J.P. & Mastroianni, A.C. (2013). *Contemporary issues in bioethics*, 8th ed. Cengage Learning.

Frankel, T. (2011). *Fiduciary law*. Oxford University Press.

Kennedy Sheldon, L. (2005). *Communication for nurses: Talking with patients*. Jones and Bartlett.

Martins, V., Santos, C. & Duarte, I. (2020). Bioethics education and the development of nursing students' moral competence. *Nurse Education Today*, 95, 104601.

Nibblelink, C. & Brewer, B. (2018). Decision-making in nursing practice: An integrative literature review. *Journal of Clinical Nursing*, 7(5–6), 917–28.

Unruh, K.T. & Pratt, W. (2007). Patients as actors: The patient's role in detecting, preventing, and recovering from medical errors. *International Journal of Medical Informatics*, 76(Supp. 1), S236–44.

Note

1 Previous editions of this chapter were co-authored by Sheryl de Lacey.

4 CONSENT

KIM ATKINS

Ping Le is admitted to the surgical ward for an operation to relieve severe pain in her right hand arising from carpal tunnel syndrome. Ping Le will be asked to sign a consent form for the operation. As part of preparing her to give consent, you ask her whether the surgeon has explained the operation and its risks. Ping Le replies, 'The surgeon can just give me the form to sign. You can do what you like as long as it makes the pain stop.'

The focus of this chapter is consent. Consent concerns the granting or withholding of permission to receive care. It may seem surprising that Ping Le would let a surgeon operate on her without wanting to know exactly what is going to happen to her, but some people do occasionally respond in this way – for example, when they can no longer tolerate a painful condition. But is this acceptable from a legal point of view? What if Ping Le had a mental health condition that affected her ability to understand the surgery being proposed? Who could consent for her in that case? This chapter addresses the legal requirements of consent for adults and children, and looks at the place of guardianship and advocacy in decision-making. It also considers the situation of people who are not mentally competent and may require emergency care or need to be restrained against their will. Consent is fundamental to the moral and professional principle that health care should be geared to the patient's interests as the *patient* understands them. This is sometimes referred to as 'patient-centred care' or, more precisely, 'person-centred care' (Santana et al. 2017).

Consent in the context of person-centred care

The concept of person-centred care refers to the idea that patients (or health-care consumers) are regarded as partners in the process of planning and delivering health care. This is required in order to ensure that health-care services meet the actual needs of patients, from the perspective of the patients themselves. The Australian Commission on Safety and Quality in Health Care (ACSQHC) National Safety and Quality Standard 2 is 'Partnering with Consumers' (ACSQHC 2018). Standard 2 requires the involvement of consumers in the planning, design, delivery and evaluation of health services (ACSQHC 2018).

It is not acceptable to regard patients or consumers of health services as passive recipients of treatment that has been decided by experts. This principle is particularly relevant to consent because in health care people may be asked to agree to treatment that carries very real risks, and the ultimate significance and impact of those risks must be determined from the perspective of the person who will have to bear the impact.

The requirements for consent

Consent can be verbal, written or implied. The fiduciary nature of the nurse–patient relationship requires that the nurse respect patients' authority to make decisions concerning their lives. In a practical sense, that means the nurse is required to do whatever is reasonably possible to facilitate the patient's autonomy. This involves the nurse doing what they can to optimise the patient's ability to make thoughtful, reasoned decisions that are in accord with the patient's values, commitments, aspirations and personal circumstances. This is the philosophical and moral framework that informs legal requirements of valid consent to treatment.

It should be noted that a person who has the capacity to consent also has a legal right to withhold consent. In *Brightwater Care Group (Inc) v Rossiter* (2009: 229), Justice Martin of the Western Australia Supreme Court stated:

> an individual of full capacity is not obliged to give consent to medical treatment, nor is a medical practitioner or other service provider under any obligation to provide such treatment without consent, even if the failure to treat will result in the loss of the patient's life.

The capacity to consent to (or refuse) treatment is assumed by common law. In addition, it is specified in some state and territory legislation (in the Australian Capital Territory, the Northern Territory, South Australia and Victoria). Consent to treatment is legally binding ('valid') only when three conditions are satisfied:

→ The person giving consent is *competent* to make a decision about their health care.

→ The person has been *fully informed* of the treatment and its alternatives.

→ the consent is given freely and *voluntarily* – that is, there has been no coercion (Willmot et al. 2013).

If one or more of these requirements is not met, the consent is not valid, and if the treatment is given, the treatment may constitute a trespass against the person, for which the administering staff may be liable for disciplinary action, or for charges of assault and/or battery (McIlwraith & Madden 2014). In the clinical setting, an assault may occur without any intention on the part of the clinician to harm the person, and by means of actions that are actually intended to benefit the patient. For example, technically a nurse may occasion assault by something as seemingly straightforward as going to a patient's bedside and saying, 'I'm going to look at your dressing', then proceeding to pull back the blankets and expose the patient's body without waiting for the patient's response. While it is highly unlikely that a patient would instigate legal action for an event like this, every nurse must understand the legal requirements of consent. Where a nurse has actioned an assault, the patient can sue for compensation for any damages (recall the discussion of criminal law and civil law in Chapter 2). Assault will be considered in more detail in Chapter 5. Table 4.1 sets out the requirements for consent.

TABLE 4.I Consent requirements

SITUATION	REQUIREMENTS OF CONSENT	WHO CAN CONSENT
Life-threatening emergency	Consent is not generally required, but in the case of people of the Jehovah's Witness faith, life-saving blood transfusions cannot be given without the person's consent.	Consent is not required
Routine, minor medical and nursing care	Consent is required.	The patient A young person A legal guardian A 'substitute decision-maker' if the person is a child or is over 18 years old but lacks capacity*
Complex invasive treatment, such as dental extraction or minor surgery	Consent is required and must specify the treatment agreed to.	The patient A young person may consent if they can demonstrate full comprehension of the nature, risks and implications of the proposed treatment. A legal guardian A 'substitute decision-maker' if the person is a child or is over 18 years old but lacks capacity

>>

»

SITUATION	REQUIREMENTS OF CONSENT	WHO CAN CONSENT
'Special procedures', such as sterilisation, participation in certain research or sexual reassignment surgery	Consent is required and must specify the treatment agreed to. Greater comprehension is required for consent to special procedures.	The patient A legal guardian if a child or young person The Guardianship Tribunal if the patient is subject to guardianship The Family Court if the procedure is considered to be beyond the capacity of the parents or legal guardian to fully comprehend If the person is over 18 years old and lacks capacity, consent can only be provided by the Guardianship Tribunal or, in Northern Territory, the Magistrates Court or the Supreme Court.
Not for resuscitation	Consent is required if the patient is mentally competent.	The patient, or if the patient is not mentally competent, the patient's representative
Involuntary detention of a person with a serious mental health condition that represents a significant and imminent risk to the person or to other people	Consent is not required. Police can detain a person with a serious mental health condition for medical assessment. The detention must be supported by an assessment by an independent doctor. Detention is for a specific and short period of time, and must be reviewed by a magistrate.	Consent is not required
Community treatment order or community counselling order	Consent is not required.	A magistrate makes a community treatment order; however, the patient can appeal an order through the Mental Health Tribunal or Guardianship Tribunal.

* The guardianship legislation of each state and territory sets out a hierarchy of 'persons responsible' or 'automatic substitute decision-makers' with respect to medical and dental treatment. This hierarchy can be consulted by health-care professionals when determining from whom they should seek substitute consent if a patient is incapable of providing consent to treatment. However, only once all steps taken to support the person to make decision/s informally are exhausted, and the person is unable to make the decision, should substitute decision-making be considered.

COMPETENCE TO CONSENT

Competence in making a decision about one's health care involves the ability to comprehend and analyse information about any proposed treatment, and to apply it meaningfully to one's own situation in weighing up treatment options. In one of the most-cited Australian legal cases concerning consent, the judge noted that legal consent to treatment requires that a person understand 'in broad terms, the nature of any procedure proposed to be performed upon them' (*Rogers v Whitaker* 1992).

It is common for doctors and nurses to assess a person's competence to consent; however, where there is any doubt about competency, a proper assessment needs to be carried out carefully and without prejudice by an appropriately qualified person, such as a psychologist or psychiatrist. A judgement that a person is not competent must be supported by appropriate evidence, such as the patient's youth, level of consciousness or presence of a mental health problem that is affecting their ability to comprehend.

The following factors should be considered when forming a judgement about a person's competence (Berglund 2012: 116):

→ the person's language skills (for example, is English a second or additional language?)
→ the extent of the person's cognitive abilities (for example, does the person have dementia or a brain injury?)
→ the stability of the person's cognitive abilities (for example, does the person become disoriented at times?)
→ environmental factors affecting the person's cognitive abilities (for example, does the person have pain, anxiety, fear or sleep deprivation, or are they being affected by medication?).

REFLECTIVE QUESTIONS 4.1

1 What kind of questions would you ask a person if you were concerned that they might not understand a procedure that has been scheduled for them?
2 What kind of responses might indicate that the person does not fully understand the implications of the procedure?
3 What would you do if you identified concerns about lack of competency?

In assessing a patient's competence to consent fairly and without prejudice, the nurse (or doctor) should consider whether the patient has views with which the practitioner strongly disagrees or that they mistrust. In some cases, if the nurse disagrees strongly with a patient's world-view, the nurse may regard the patient as mentally incompetent or incapable of appreciating the clinical information, and therefore unable to consent to or refuse treatment. However, it is important to understand that while a person's decision-making in one area might appear to be less than ideal, their decision-making in another context might be excellent. Decision-making, like cognition in general, can be content-dependent. Consider the following case.

Deirdre is an 84-year-old woman who is having dressings for a leg ulcer and antibiotic treatment. She is forgetful and exhibits behaviour that the nurse considers eccentric: Deirdre enjoys singing during the day, scratches herself a lot and frequently talks to herself. At times, she speaks about characters she likes from books she has read.

One morning, Deirdre refuses to have her dressing done, and swears at the nurse. The nurse attempts, unsuccessfully, to coax her into cooperating. Deirdre tells the nurse to 'go and dance in a sunny field', and can be heard talking to herself about 'Parrot', and what he would think and do. Parrot is a character in a novel.

>> Do you think there is anything about Deirdre's behaviour that indicates whether or not she is competent to refuse treatment? What are you basing your judgement on?

BEING INFORMED

Being fully informed requires that the patient be provided with sufficient information that is relevant and in a form that they will comprehend, and that no relevant information is withheld. Furthermore, consent is legally valid only for *specified* treatment. In other words, a person consents to a specific, named treatment – not treatment in general. When a person with diabetes consents to a blood sugar test, they are not consenting to have *any* blood test. Similarly, when a person consents to a wound dressing, they are *not* also consenting to having a bed bath, or back care, or any other kind of treatment or care. The reason for this requirement is to provide a patient with protection from unnecessary interventions by the clinician. For example, if in the course of an operation to remove a person's appendix it was discovered that the patient had gallstones, the surgeon could not operate to remove the gallstones because the person had not consented to that specific treatment. Treatment for which a patient has *not* consented can be given only in extreme circumstances where the patient would die or be gravely injured if treatment were delayed. For example, if during an appendectomy it was discovered that the patient had a leaking aortic aneurysm, a surgeon would be justified in operating on the aneurysm because, if left, this condition would likely result in grave injury or death.

The manner in which information about treatment options is presented can have a significant impact on how well the person can comprehend that information and its relevance to them. For example, recent scholarship and practice in trauma-informed care explains how stress and trauma can interfere with a person's ability to comprehend complex information and undertake reflective decision-making (Blue Knot Foundation 2021). Following these guidelines can enhance patient understanding:

→ As far as possible, first establish what the patient knows already, then build on that.

→ Speak slowly, clearly and at the required volume, and pause regularly.

→ Avoid technical terms, and use language that is simple and direct.

→ Demonstrate procedures by using the relevant body part, a model or a drawing/ photograph.

→ Use analogies with situations with which the patient is familiar – for example, car engines or plumbing are often used to explain cardiovascular function.

→ Encourage the patient to ask questions and to paraphrase what you have said.

→ Give the patient time to think the information through, then have a follow-up session where possible.

→ Be careful about using examples from your personal experience – this may influence the patient unduly.

→ Resist the urge to protect the patient from harsh reality by playing down risks.

→ Do not withhold relevant information.

→ Refer the patient to further useful sources of good information.

VOLUNTARINESS

Voluntariness is a key component of consent. Consent must be given freely and without coercion. This requires the person consenting to have a clear mind and to make their decision by reference to their own needs and values. A range of factors can interfere with voluntariness, such as:

→ being under the influence of alcohol, analgesics or other drugs – such as sedatives or narcotics – that can affect cognition. If a patient was given a sedative and asked to sign a consent form shortly afterwards, the consent may not be legally valid

→ sustaining a brain injury or having a pathology that decreases cognitive ability – for example, severe concussion, psychosis or dementia

→ being unduly influenced by the needs of someone else – for example, having plastic surgery or reproductive sterilisation (vasectomy or tubal ligation) in order to please a partner

→ feeling threatened or intimidated (see the example below).

A police officer apprehended a man after receiving a call that the man was behaving strangely. The man was asked by the police officer to accompany him to a psychiatric hospital. The man cooperated, believing that unless he complied with this request – that is, unless he went voluntarily – he would forcibly be taken to the psychiatric hospital.

The High Court of Australia found that the man did not give valid consent because he was coerced by the fact of having a reasonable belief that he had no choice but to comply. (*Watson v Marshall* 1971)

>> **Nurses often expect the people they are nursing to be 'compliant' – that is, to go along with what the nurse asks or expects of them. How might you determine whether a patient is genuinely consenting or just being compliant?**

Coercion can be exercised in quite subtle ways. For example, it is a normal part of socialisation to learn to obey authority – be that police officers, teachers or parents – so it is not surprising that in a clinical setting people tend to comply with what they think doctors or nurses expect them to do without considering whether or not those expectations are reasonable. An uncritical attitude towards the judgement of nurses and doctors is reinforced by the widespread belief that nurses and doctors will always do the right thing. Clinicians must be aware of this tendency and ensure that they do not use it – intentionally or otherwise – to pressure patients into doing what the clinician wants. Clinicians can be coercive without saying anything directly but instead acting as if they expect the patient to simply agree with them. This is a particular risk for people who are normally dependent upon other people in their everyday lives, such as children, those with limited physical or intellectual capacity, or people who have experienced long-term abuse or dependency, because they may not be confident, experienced or skilled in resisting power. The fiduciary responsibilities of the clinician require the patient's (or a representative's) *active* involvement in the decision-making process, and not merely their passive compliance with whatever the clinician proposes.

In the clinical setting, obvious coercion is rare. It is more likely to occur in relation to individuals who the nurse considers to be demanding or 'difficult' – for example, people with mental health conditions (who historically have been stereotyped and subject to excessive control measures). For example, a person presenting at an emergency department may be told that the doctor will not see them unless they agree to some initial treatment process first; or that the hospital will not treat them if they do not comply with expected 'normal' behaviour. It may be otherwise conveyed to the person via words or actions that they can expect unfavourable treatment if they do not comply with the clinician's directions. Certain kinds of behaviour can also be coercive, such as standing over the person, acting impatiently towards them or treating them as if their questions are unnecessary, unreasonable or foolish.

REFLECTIVE QUESTIONS 4.2

1 How would you be able to tell whether a patient is feeling intimidated by or fearful of you?
2 Do you think feelings of fear or anxiety might affect a patient's decision in relation to consent?
3 Can a patient withhold consent for treatment that is clinically indicated – that is, if they need the treatment that is being proposed?

It is important to be aware that consent does not need to be in writing. It may be inferred from a person's behaviour. For example, if a patient holds out their arm when a nurse approaches with a sphygmomanometer, it is reasonable to infer that they are consenting to having their blood pressure taken. Similarly, if a patient pulls back the bedclothes and presents a wound when a nurse comes to do the patient's dressing, consent can be inferred. It is reasonable to infer that a person presenting at an emergency department complaining of illness is consenting to be seen by a doctor. However, this does not mean that the person is consenting to any further treatment, such as blood tests, electrocardiograms or x-rays. Failure to obtain valid consent for further treatment is a trespass of the person.

Sometimes it may not be clear whether consent can safely be inferred, so it is advisable to always ask the person for permission to provide a treatment. Consider the following example.

LAW AND ETHICS IN PRACTICE

On your first afternoon on the orthopaedic ward, you are asked to look after Steve, who has had a surgical repair of a fractured femur and tibia in his left leg following a motorcycle accident. You approach Steve and say that you are going to do his pressure area care. Steve turns away from you.

>> Is he consenting?

Consent and children

When someone reaches the age of 18 years, they are regarded as an adult in the eyes of the law and are assumed to be competent to give consent unless there is reason to believe otherwise. Until then, a young person or a child is considered a 'minor', and usually requires a parent or legal guardian to consent on their behalf. However, children between the ages of 14 and 17 can consent under certain conditions.

Parents can only consent to, or refuse, treatment that is in the interests of the child. A parent's right to consent to treatment for their child is not based on the idea that the child is the property of the parent. Rather, it is based on the fact that the parent is normally (though not always) in the best position to exercise the interests of the child. The High Court of Australia has stated:

> Once it is accepted that the power of parents to give a valid consent to the medical treatment of their children does not arise from a duty or from a natural right of almost absolute control over the person of the child, it follows that the common law gives this power to parents simply because it perceives them to be the most appropriate repository of such a power. (*Dept Health and Community Services v JWB and SMB* [*Marion's* case] 1992)

The Supreme Court of Australia has the power to overrule decisions by parents to consent to or refuse treatment:

> Historically, the common law has conferred on the State Supreme Court the overriding power to ensure that parents, and others, act in a young person's best interests. This power derives from what is known as the '*parens patriae*' jurisdiction of the Supreme Court and originates from the ancient power of the English king to care for those subjects who could not care for themselves. The *parens patriae* jurisdiction of the Supreme Court allows it to act as the final decision-maker in relation to the medical treatment of a child, even if its orders go against the parents' decision. (New South Wales Law Reform Commission 2002)

One area of potential conflict between doctors and parents is the administration of blood products to children. This mainly concerns families of the Jehovah's Witnesses faith. Each state and territory has legislation that permits the administration of blood products to children without the parents' consent under certain conditions. The administration of blood products must be an appropriate form of treatment for the child's condition, and the blood products must be administered in order to save the child's life. If required to serve the child's best interests, a child can be removed from parental care and detained in hospital for medical treatment (see the Appendix for a table of relevant legislation). In September 2013, the NSW Supreme Court dismissed an appeal by the lawyers of a male youth of Jehovah's Witnesses faith, aged 17 years and eight months, who was refusing a life-saving blood transfusion. The court determined that the state had an interest not only in keeping the youth alive until his 18th birthday, but also in ensuring he received treatment that would allow the continuation of his life thereafter (see *X v The Sydney Children's Hospitals Network* 2013).

Sometimes young people aged between 14 and 17 years seek medical treatment independently of their parents. In some cases, the young persons do not wish their parents to know about the treatment sought – for example, contraception. In Australia, both common law and the statute law of some states and territories recognise that young people between the ages of 14 and 17 years can be capable of understanding the nature and implications of some medical treatments, and for that reason can consent to such treatment without requiring the consent of their parents or legal guardians. As long as a young person can be shown to have sufficient understanding of the nature, risks and implications of the proposed treatment, they can legally consent. For example, in South Australia the *Consent to Medical and Dental Procedures Act 1985* makes provision for a child to consent under two conditions: (1) the doctor is of the opinion that the child is capable of understanding the nature, risks and implications of the proposed treatment, and the treatment is in the child's best interests; and (2) that opinion is supported in writing by at least one other medical practitioner. However, whereas adults are required only to understand the nature and implications of medical treatment in broad terms, young persons are required to demonstrate a much more comprehensive understanding (Staunton & Chiarella 2013).

In determining the status of a young person's consent, Australian common law has drawn upon the UK case of *Gillick v West Norfolk AHA* (1986). This case was brought before the House of Lords to determine whether a young person could consent to medical treatment. It arose after an objection was made against the government health service providing contraception to sexually active young people. The majority of the House of Lords judged that a minor could consent under certain circumstances. Furthermore, in those circumstances a parent had no right to prevent treatment.

In Australia, when there is conflict between what a young person wants and what the young person's parents want, the conflict can be resolved in one of two ways. The most common is by a medical officer making a decision about the young person's capacity based on professional judgement in conjunction with the consent of either the parent or the young person. The second way to resolve a conflict is to apply to the Supreme Court or the Family Court for a judicial determination of whether the treatment is in the person's best interests.

LAW AND ETHICS IN PRACTICE

A 15-year-old girl disclosed to her GP that she had a 16-year-old boyfriend and was sexually active. She requested the oral contraceptive pill, but insisted that her parents were not to be told (Bird 2018).

>> Think about your own expectations or beliefs about the significance of a person's age on their decision-making. How would you know whether your beliefs were getting in the way of a patient's autonomous decision-making?

The court will also hear applications for determinations related to sterilisation, hormonal therapy for long-term contraception, participation in medical research, administration of drugs of addiction or psychotropic drugs, or organ donation.

In addition, sometimes medical treatment is so complex and its implications so profound that parents or legal guardians find themselves unable to provide informed consent. This was the situation in the case of *Re Alex* (discussed at the beginning of Chapter 1), where a young person, Alex, requested sexual reassignment surgery. Alex's legal representative made an application to the Family Court to determine consent, which the court did (see Atkins 2005).

It is essential for nurses to understand that if a young person has a right to consent, they also have the right to confidentiality. The same principles that apply to adults apply to young people receiving medical and nursing care (see Chapter 7). The nurse is not at liberty to disclose information about the person's treatment or condition to the person's parents (or other family members) without consent.

Advocacy

Consent is an expression of autonomy, but autonomy is not an all-or-nothing affair. Individuals differ in their degree of autonomy at different times in their lives, and any individual may be more or less autonomous in the different spheres of life. Sometimes the nurse will need to advocate for people who are unable to exercise autonomy for a range of reasons – perhaps because they are very young, are unconscious, have a serious mental health condition or brain injury affecting their cognition, cannot understand English or for some other reason cannot understand the nature of their illness or treatment. Advocacy is part of the fiduciary relationship, and can be understood as a positive offshoot of paternalism (recall the discussion of paternalism in Chapter 3). When you act as an advocate, you act in the person's best interests; you take the patient's interests and values as the goal of your actions. Advocacy is something akin to taking sides with the patient. You try to respect the patient's autonomy by seeking to further the interests of the patient as the *patient* understands them.

The skills needed for advocacy are the same ones that are important for both caring and autonomy – for example, good listening and comprehension, an appreciation of different perspectives, empathy, trust, the confidence to speak out and a commitment to both the patient's good and the nurse's professional good. A nurse is often thought to be an appropriate advocate because the nurse is the clinician who often spends the most time with the patient, and so may come to understand the patient's clinical and personal needs. Understanding those beliefs and values that are relevant to the patient's nursing care is part and parcel of the fiduciary relationship, and so is central to the nursing role.

Advocacy organisations can be called in to help support a person in making decisions about their care. This may be particularly helpful in the case of a person living with a disability or someone who is a refugee.

LAW AND ETHICS IN PRACTICE

Beela is an Aboriginal woman from a remote community, admitted to the coronary care unit of a major hospital. The coronary care unit is a mixed-sex unit. When taken to her bed, Beela retreats to the bathroom, where she huddles in the corner crying and will not come out.

>> **How might a nurse advocate for Beela?**

Advocacy can be difficult when the nurse and patient have very different cultural backgrounds (see Chapter 6 for more discussion of culturally safe nursing practices). Unless Beela's nurse understands her cultural context, the nurse will not be able to advocate effectively. Beela is facing a number of personal, social and cultural challenges. First, in her mind she is sharing a room with a man. In her kinship group, this is highly improper and would normally have implications for her kinship relations in the future. Second, she is alone, far from her family and community in a strange and intimidating setting: a high-tech Western hospital. To compound her difficulties, Beela may not speak English, and nurses in Australia's acute hospitals are highly unlikely to speak her language. Beela may feel that she is subject to mystifying decisions from people who are quite unlike the people to whom she can relate or who understand her. She is confined inside a complex building when she normally spends a lot of time outdoors, and there are no sacred places that can offer her a sense of repose and safety. Beela feels that she has lost control of her life. She needs someone to advocate for her.

Beela's case is complex, and advocacy would entail seeking advice and involvement from a number of other people, including Aboriginal health liaison officers, social workers, and Beela's relatives and friends. In other cases, advocacy can be as simple as being present during the doctor's consultation to provide psychological and moral support. Understanding a patient as a unique person with their own particular needs will help the nurse to understand what is needed for effective advocacy in each patient's situation.

Although nurses often need to advocate for their patients, the nurse cannot always side with the patient. Nurses' commitments to nursing practice, to the institution in which they work and to their personal values may all be sources of conflict with a patient's point of view. There is a limit to how much support one person can give to another's interests without undermining their own. This is particularly the case in multicultural settings. For example, some cultures believe that only certain family members can make decisions about the health care of other family members, and all cultures have a variety of rules about how women and men should interact, which can sometimes become a problem if the nurse and patient are not of the same gender. The patient or their family may rate such considerations as the nurse's gender more highly than clinical considerations, such as professional expertise and speediness of recovery.

Nurses' responsibilities towards patients need to be understood directly in relation to their fiduciary obligations and the legal requirements for valid consent. The nurse must provide information, advocate for the patient's interests and, as far as reasonably possible, eliminate unwarranted influences on the patient's deliberations. Consent is more than a signature on a form: it is the patient's considered agreement to allow or refuse treatment offered by a health professional in a manner that the patient understands and authorises. Consent is an expression of a person's right to determine their own life.

Supported decision-making

People rarely make all their decisions completely independently; they often consult the important people in their lives, and sometimes professionals, to assist. According to New South Wales Communities & Justice (2020), 'assisting, or supporting, someone to make a decision means giving them the tools they need to make the decision for themself'. Unlike a paternalistic approach, where someone else makes all the decisions for a person, supported decision-making is about supporting the person to make their own decision, and in doing so, safeguarding their autonomy. A person's right to make decisions is fundamental to their independence and dignity.

In situations where a person may have some limitation to their ability to make complex decisions because of an intellectual disability, cognitive impairment or injury, the appropriate approach to use is supported decision-making. This helps ensure that decisions about treatment reflect the person's interests and values. Even if you, as a nurse, do not share the person's values, it is important not to try to persuade a person to agree with you simply from a wish to protect them from what you consider to be unwise judgement or wrong values. Everyone – even someone who has an intellectual disability – has a right to make decisions based on what matters to them, regardless of what a clinical judgement might suggest. Protecting a person from making what you think is an unwise decision may seem helpful, but it is very important that any steps you take to intervene are appropriate. If a person isn't allowed to confront a difficult decision or its consequences, their right to be in control of their own life is denied. Furthermore, nurses should accord people with disability 'dignity of risk' (Marsh & Kelly 2018). In other words, nurses acknowledge that someone with a disability has just as much right as anyone else to make their own mistakes and to learn and grow as a result.

Acting without consent

EMERGENCIES

There are occasions when consent is not legally required before treatment can be given. These are rare occasions, when a person is too incapacitated to either consent to or refuse treatment but needs an immediate life-saving intervention. The common law 'doctrine of emergency' (Skene 1997) provides legal protection for clinicians against charges of assault when they provide treatment that they genuinely believe is required in the circumstances, and that is within the clinician's scope of practice. For example, if a person collapsed and became unconscious in the street and was given cardiopulmonary resuscitation by a bystander and then defibrillation by an ambulance officer, then scheduled drugs by hospital staff – remaining unconscious all the while – the bystander, ambulance staff and hospital staff would not have committed assault.

However, a competent person can refuse life-saving emergency treatment, and if the clinician ignores this, then the clinician's actions may constitute assault. If the person in the example above was to become conscious in the ambulance, they could refuse medication at the hospital, despite the medication being life-saving, as long as they were mentally competent. Even if medical staff thought that the patient's reasons for refusing were bizarre, treatment could not legally be given unless the patient could be shown to be incompetent to consent. This principle was made clear in the case of *Malette v Shulman* (1990). Ms Malette was brought to a hospital unconscious and seriously injured. She carried with her a card stating that she was a Jehovah's Witness and refused to be administered blood. The treating doctor administered a blood transfusion and Ms Malette subsequently sued successfully. The court determined that her card constituted valid refusal of the treatment, and further that it was not up to doctors to decide whether or not the patient's wishes were reasonable.

USE OF RESTRAINTS

Sometimes a patient will need to be restrained without their consent in order to prevent harm to that person or to others. However, the wrongful use of a restraint can amount to false imprisonment, and make the nurse applying the restraint liable to disciplinary measures and/or legal action. In addition, a person who is restrained becomes much more vulnerable to other forms of abuse because the power imbalance in the patient–nurse relationship is vastly increased and the person is rendered relatively defenceless. If the patient has a history of trauma, applying a restraint is likely to be retraumatizing (Hammer et al. 2011) and may escalate the problem.

False imprisonment is any action performed against a person's will that wrongfully and intentionally restricts the person's freedom of movement. A person need not be physically restrained to be falsely imprisoned. A person can be restrained chemically through the administration of drugs, or psychologically through the belief that they will suffer an adverse consequence if they try to leave their situation.

Sometimes a person can be restrained by psychological as well as physical means. Consider the following example. Can you see how Ben is being restrained?

LAW AND ETHICS IN PRACTICE

Ben goes to see a local doctor after falling over while intoxicated. After the consultation, the receptionist asks Ben to pay the bill. Ben, still intoxicated, becomes irate and says he is not going to pay. The receptionist picks up the phone and tells Ben that she is going to call the police unless he pays. Ben believes that if he leaves the room the police will be called, so he starts asking people in the waiting room for money to pay his bill so he can leave.

>> **Is the receptionist acting within her legal rights? Is it ever appropriate for a nurse to threaten a patient with arrest by the police?**

Restraints can be used lawfully without consent under the following circumstances:

→ if it will prevent the person from incurring harm to themself – especially if the person is a child (and the harm is serious and imminent)
→ if it will prevent harm to other persons.

While we usually think of restraints being physical (like handcuffs or being locked in a room), a person can be restrained chemically, through the use of sedatives, or psychologically, as we noted above. Wherever possible, a medical officer should be called to assess the patient and to order a suitable restraint in writing before any restraint is applied. Occasionally, a patient may have to be restrained by the nurse or other staff until a medical officer is called. However, the use of restraints of any kind must be legally justifiable and requires extreme vigilance on the part of the nurse. *Restraints have been fatal* (see the example below).

LAW AND ETHICS IN PRACTICE

An agitated elderly woman was tied to an armchair with a bed sheet and a bedside table was placed in front of the chair to further restrict her movement. The woman was left unobserved for a period of time. During that time, the woman continued to struggle against the restraint. She worked her way down in the chair and twisted around, with the result that the bed sheet became wound around her neck. She continued to struggle against the restraint and eventually asphyxiated.

>> **In a situation where you think you need to restrain a patient, how will you know what you can and can't do?**

This case raises legal issues relating to false imprisonment, negligence and possibly assault and battery (see the discussions in Chapter 5). False imprisonment occurs when a person is detained against their will. In the above case, the woman has been tied up so that her freedom of movement is severely curtailed. This may also be a case of assault if, when she was being restrained, there was a direct and intentional threat of physical contact made by the nurse to the woman and the woman had a reasonable belief that the threatened behaviour would occur. Furthermore, because actual bodily contact was made, this may also constitute battery, regardless of whether the woman was aware of the bodily contact. Finally, the nurse's behaviour constitutes negligence because the nurse has not provided care of a standard that could be reasonably expected of her, with the consequence that the patient was harmed, and that the harm could have been anticipated (that is, was foreseeable).

When applying restraints, whether physical, chemical or psychological, the following care should be taken:

→ The type of restraint must be of an approved type and appropriate for the person (for example, an adult restraint would not normally be appropriate for a child).
→ The period of restraint must be specified by the doctor and reviewed frequently.
→ The place of restraint must be appropriate and safe for the patient and other people.
→ The patient should be observed and reassessed regularly, and the medical officer informed of the patient's condition.
→ The workplace's policy should always be consulted.

The use of restraints is permitted legally in some situations – for example, under some sections of the *Mental Health Act* in a state or territory. Nurses working in mental health services, or with patients experiencing certain serious, acute mental health problems, must be familiar with their legal obligations toward their patients. Preventative action is always a better option than a restraint. If an agitated person anticipates being restrained against their will, the agitation will increase and the conflict will escalate. It is always preferable to utilise good interpersonal and communication skills to provide emotional reassurance than to engage in a verbal or physical battle with another person, or to subject a vulnerable person to the risks associated with the various kinds of restraints. Careful observation, timely intervention and a calm approach can sometimes prevent the need for a restraint.

PEOPLE WITH SERIOUS MENTAL HEALTH CONDITIONS

Mental health problems are common afflictions that in many cases require very little, if any, clinical intervention. Many people diagnosed with a mental health condition live productive, successful lives, independently of clinical intervention. However, sometimes a problem can be serious enough to warrant medical intervention without consent. Each state and territory has its own *Mental Health Act* that deals with consent pertaining to persons experiencing profound mental health problems, which the Acts define as 'mental illness' (see the Appendix for a table of relevant legislation).

The various Acts generally define mental illness as a significant disturbance of thought, mood and perception. Consequently, the definition may include dementia or developmental disability in some states or territories. Importantly, the legislation also specifies a range of behaviours that alone *do not* constitute an illness – for example, sexual promiscuity, immoral or indecent conduct, or antisocial or illegal behaviour.

Persons with an acute serious mental health problem and who pose a serious risk to the safety of themselves or others may be detained against their will. This is sometimes referred to as being 'scheduled' (so named after the certificate issued by a medical officer under Schedule 2 of the New South Wales *Mental Health Act 2007*). Involuntary detention should occur only after every effort has been made to avoid the person being admitted as an involuntary patient. It is lawful to use reasonable force to detain a person under the *Mental Health Act*. A fairly common cause of involuntary detention is a psychotic episode: an acute clinical state where the person may hear voices and experience fantastical and disturbing delusions or hallucinations, and overwhelming feelings of paranoia and impending catastrophe. Sometimes a psychotic person is taken to hospital by police or ambulance – usually by force. On arrival at the hospital, the person is restrained physically and by the administration of antipsychotic medication or sedation.

Involuntary detention can occur only after an assessment of the person is made by a medical officer, who determines that no care other than hospital treatment is appropriate and available. The medical judgement must be made on the basis of clear evidence. As soon as possible after admission to hospital, and usually within 24 hours, the person will be examined by another suitably qualified doctor (or, in Tasmania, two doctors), who confirms the assessment. The Mental Health Tribunal in the relevant state and territory is then informed of the admission. An order for involuntary detention has a time limit – typically five days – after which the patient must be reassessed by a qualified doctor, usually a psychiatrist. Patients subjected to ongoing detention must be reviewed by a psychiatrist regularly, typically every three to five days. Patients subjected to longer periods of detention, called 'continuing care orders', are reviewed by Mental Health Tribunals every 28 days. The Mental Health Tribunals also hear appeals against involuntary detention.

People who are being detained involuntarily still have the right to consent to, or refuse, some treatments as long as the person can adequately comprehend the nature and implications of treatment. As for all persons, proposed treatment must be justifiable on the basis of the patient's need. State and territory legislation specifies requirements for consent for invasive procedures, such as electroconvulsive therapy (ECT).

Persons with mental health conditions that are not so serious as to require detention, but that do require supervision, may be subjected to community treatment orders. Community treatment is treatment prescribed by a qualified medical officer (usually a psychiatrist), and provided by mental health professionals in the community. An example would be a supervised medication regime with social and psychological support provided to build capacity in self-care and promote social participation. An order for a community treatment order is made by a magistrate, and is effective for up to six months. Failure to comply with an order may result in involuntary detention.

The United Nations' Principles for People with Mental Illness and the Improvement of Health Care (United Nations 1991) sets out 25 principles pertaining to the fundamental freedoms and basic rights of people with 'mental illness', including standards of care in mental health facilities. Principle 1 states, for example, that:

1 All persons have the right to the best available mental health care, which shall be part of the health and social care system.
2 All persons with a mental illness, or who are being treated as such persons, shall be treated with humanity and respect for the inherent dignity of the human person.
3 All persons with a mental illness, or who are being treated as such persons, have the right to protection from economic, sexual and other forms of exploitation, physical or other abuse and degrading treatment.
4 There shall be no discrimination on the grounds of mental illness... (United Nations 1991: 92)

These principles inform mental health legislation and professional practice across Australia.

REFLECTIVE QUESTION 4.4

Examine your own beliefs about people receiving care for a mental health problem. What exactly do you believe? How might your beliefs affect how you regard a decision made by a person with a mental health problem? Discuss your thoughts with your fellow nurses.

Guardianship

An alternative to preparing an advance care directive is to appoint a trusted friend, relative or legal representative as an 'enduring guardian'. An enduring guardian is a substitute decision-maker for the person, and can be appointed by a person over the age of 18 who has the mental capacity to do so. The enduring guardian is appointed to make decisions in the event that the person loses the capacity to make those decisions for themself (O'Neill & Peisah 2011). A guardian may be given the authority to make personal or lifestyle decisions such as where the person is to live or about their medical treatment and health care. Enduring guardians are not entitled to make decisions concerning financial matters.

Legal guardians are appointed by Guardianship Boards or Mental Health Tribunals in each state or territory, according to that state or territory's legislation. Each follows similar basic principles in determining when guardianship is required, and who can be appointed a legal guardian. There are strict requirements for the witnessing of enduring guardianship and power of attorney appointments, which vary between the different states and territories. In New South Wales, for example, these appointments must be witnessed by an 'eligible witness', such as a legal practitioner.

Guardianship is required when a person has a disability (as defined by the legislation of each state or territory) that prevents the person from being competent to manage certain important areas of their own life where decisions need to be made. The New South Wales Department of Justice and Communities advises the following:

> It is very rare for a person not to have capacity for any decisions. However, this can happen when a person is unconscious or has a severe cognitive disability, for instance.
>
> More often, people lack capacity only in making one sort of decision. For example, a person might be able to decide where they want to live (personal decision), but not be able to decide whether to sell their house (financial decision). They can do their grocery shopping (make a simple decision about money), but not be able to buy and sell shares (make a more complex decision about money). (New South Wales Communities & Justice 2020)

Any individual person's capacity can vary at different times and in relation to different types of decisions, whether or not they have any ongoing condition affecting their cognition. Capacity depends on a range of factors, including:

→ the type of decision being made
→ the complexity of the decision
→ how much information the person has been given
→ their level of understanding, the communication strategy employed, and
→ the amount of stress the person is under (New South Wales Communities & Justice 2020).

For these reasons, a guardianship order will be limited to certain kinds of decisions only, as determined by the Tribunal. Guardians do not have to be relatives of the person, but they are required to advocate for the person and protect them – much as a parent would for a child. When making its determinations, the Tribunal will consider whether the person has a disability within the meaning of the Act and whether the person is unable to make the relevant decisions. It will also consider whether the proposed guardian is acceptable to the person, and whether there are any conflicts of interest. Where there are competing or multiple candidates to be a guardian, the Tribunal can give preference to a friend or neighbour over a close relative if it believes that the friend or neighbour can better advocate for and protect the person's interests. The Tribunal can also order shared guardianship – for example, by giving two siblings guardianship of a parent with dementia. Where there is no appropriate person among the person's family or friends or where there is significant conflict over which family member or friend should be appointed, a public guardian may be appointed. Each state and territory has its own appointed Public Guardian; for example, in Tasmania and New South Wales it is the Civil and Administrative Tribunal, while in Queensland and Northern Territory it is the Office of the Public Guardian (see Appendix for full list).

The making of a guardianship order necessarily imposes a restriction on the person's freedom to make their own decisions in those areas specified in the guardianship order. All states and territories must be satisfied that making a guardianship order is the least restrictive option and is in the best interests of the person (O'Neill & Peisah 2011). Guardians must always act consistently with the person's known interests. For example, it would be improper for a guardian to buy a person clothing in a style that the guardian liked, but the person did not; or worse, to move a person from their home to accommodation that was more convenient for the guardian. The scope of a guardian's decision-making power is set out in the guardianship order. For example, a guardian may have powers to make decisions in respect of accommodation, service provision and medical consent. Nurses should not only familiarise themselves with the guardianship legislation of their respective state or territory but, when seeking substitute consent from a guardian, should also be aware of the scope or extent of the powers that the individual guardian has been given.

Legal guardians may be able to make decisions in relation to almost every area of the person's life for whom they are the legal guardian, including consent to medical treatment. As noted earlier, however, guardians are not automatically granted the right to manage the person's financial affairs. Legislation usually makes allowance for the appointment of a separate financial manager. Under state and territory legislation, guardians can consent only to treatments that are required for the promotion or maintenance of the health and well-being of the person. Guardians cannot consent to any treatment that is for the guardian's own convenience. Nor can guardians consent to 'special medical procedures', such as sterilisation or hysterectomy merely to control normal reproductive function in a person with an intellectual disability. Australian law has repeatedly found against requests for such procedures on the basis that they attack a person's fundamental right not to be interfered with unnecessarily (McIlwraith & Madden 2014).

Individuals with guardians can have widely varying degrees of competency, and be more or less competent in different spheres of life. This means that guardians play different roles in the lives of different people. For example, it is often the case that guardians do not need to be involved in simple health-care procedures, such as taking advice from the local pharmacist, attending a wound clinic or having a dental check-up, but could be involved in consenting to surgery or participation in research. Nurses and other health-care providers need to be sensitive to the fact that guardianship is typically limited in scope, and covers only certain kinds of decisions. Nurses should not regard a person with a guardian as having global deficits in decision-making. Even where a person with a disability displays challenging behaviour (such as being unusually loud, demanding or seemingly erratic), this does not of itself indicate an inability to consent in the particular context.

'NOT FOR RESUSCITATION' ORDERS

From time to time, nurses find themselves involved in a situation where a decision is made not to resuscitate a patient. Orders that a patient is 'not for resuscitation' occur in situations where either the patient has refused resuscitation (such as in an advance care directive, discussed below) or where the patient has a prognosis from the treating doctor that any further medical treatment is futile, or both. If the patient is unable to discuss the issue of resuscitation (perhaps because they are mentally incompetent), a decision should be made by a group comprising the appropriate patient representative(s) (usually family), the treating doctor(s) and a senior nurse directly involved in the patient's care, and on the basis that further treatment is futile.

There are a number of stringent requirements for a 'not for resuscitation' order. The order must conform to the law of consent. Where the patient refuses resuscitation, the patient must be mentally competent at the time of refusing, be adequately informed of the implications of the refusal of resuscitation, and have made the refusal freely and without coercion. A 'not for resuscitation' order cannot be based on the wishes of a patient representative or doctor alone; it must be supported by clear evidence that resuscitation is futile. Once an order is made, it must be very clearly documented in the patient notes and the reasons for the order clearly stated. An order should be reviewed regularly in case there is an improvement in the patient's condition.

Nurses should consult the policy guidelines provided by the Department of Health in their state or territory to ensure that 'not for resuscitation' orders are appropriate and legal.

Advance care directives

A person can exercise their autonomy into the future by preparing an advance care directive. Advance care directives (ACDs, also called an advance health directive or a living will) are orders that are typically, but not necessarily, in writing. They are written by a mentally competent adult specifying the care they wish to receive in the event of becoming critically ill and unable to either refuse or consent to treatment. Advance care directives may be made by:

→ the very elderly, who wish to avoid futile, painful and undignified care in the event of cardiac arrest or significant stroke
→ those with a terminal illness who do not wish to prolong their lives
→ those undergoing dangerous procedures, such as brain surgery, who fear they may end up in a vegetative state or similar
→ those who want to ensure that they retain as much control as possible over future health decisions affecting them.

An advance care directive may be completed by any person who has specific wishes about their treatment in the event of grave injury following an unexpected event. For example, a person may not wish to receive a donor organ or blood transfusion, or to be resuscitated under certain specified circumstances.

The legitimacy of advance care directives is provided by common law, but some states and territories have also enacted specific legislation that sets guidelines and criteria for advance care directives, in order to ensure legal clarity and protection of a person's right to refuse treatment (see the Appendix for a table of relevant legislation).

Because legislation varies between the states and territories, people preparing advance care directives – and the nurses caring for them – should check the legal requirements of their state or territory. This is because, while an advance care directive may meet the common law requirements of informed consent, it can

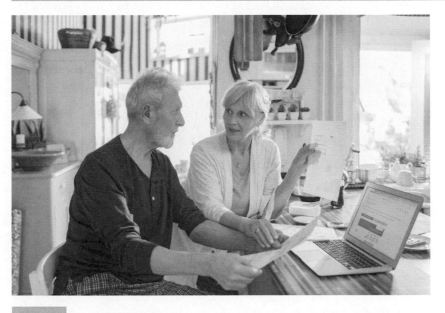

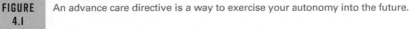

FIGURE 4.1	An advance care directive is a way to exercise your autonomy into the future.

present problems if it does not comply with other legislation. The Queensland University of Technology has a useful website that provides an overview of the relevant legislative frameworks: https://end-of-life.qut.edu.au/advance-directives.

In Victoria, the *Medical Treatment Planning and Decisions Act 2016* gives formal recognition and legal force to advanced care directives, as long as the ACD is prepared in accordance with the requirements of the Act. The Act allows a person to appoint a medical treatment decision-maker and a support person. The aim of the Act is to ensure that people with decision-making capacity can receive medical treatment that is consistent with their preferences and values. The Act allows people to create a legally binding advance care directive so that they can:

→ make an instructional directive, which will provide specific directives about treatment a person consents to or refuses

→ make a values directive, which will describe a person's views and values. A medical treatment decision-maker and health practitioners will be required to give effect to a values directive.

→ appoint a medical treatment decision-maker, who will make decisions on behalf of a person when they no longer have decision-making capacity

→ appoint a support person, who will assist a person to make decisions for themselves, by collecting and interpreting information or assisting the person to communicate their decisions (Department of Health and Human Services, Victoria 2016).

In Tasmania and New South Wales, the legal validity of an ACD is recognised under common law. For an example of its application in New South Wales, see *Hunter and New England Area Health Service v A* (2009).

In general, an advance care directive must meet the following criteria:

→ The person making the directive is competent to consent at the time of making the directive.

→ The directive specifies the treatment that is to be refused and the conditions under which the refusal comes into effect.

→ The person making the directive is informed about the nature of the procedures and treatments being refused, and the consequences of refusal.

→ The directive is witnessed by a suitable, responsible person, such as a justice of the peace, rather than a relative who may stand to benefit from the person's will.

→ The directive is fully voluntary.

→ There exists no other directive that conflicts with the current directive.

→ The directive does not request anything that is illegal.

In general, if a nurse were to follow an advance care directive without taking steps to ensure that it was up to date and expressed the person's current wishes, the nurse may be liable for an action of negligence in the event of the patient incurring a harm as a consequence. Nurses need to know which of the patients in their care have advance care directives in place. They need to be familiar with each individual directive so they can provide the care to which the person has consented, and avoid providing treatment that the person does not want. In addition, nurses need to be confident that advance care directives for patients in their care comply with relevant legislation and policy. An advance care directive cannot request a person to carry out any illegal action. For example, a person cannot request to be given a lethal injection if they sustain profound and irreversible brain damage. A health-care facility should have administrative procedures in place to ensure that it only acts on directives that meet all legislative requirements. It is advisable for anyone preparing an advance care directive to seek professional legal advice.

REFLECTIVE QUESTION 4.5

Sometimes nurses or doctors disagree with an advanced care directive. What would you do if a colleague refused to comply with an advanced care directive?

Conclusion

The fiduciary nature of the nurse–patient relationship requires that the nurse respect patients' authority to make decisions that concern their own lives. In addition to the moral wrong of failing to respect autonomy, treatment given to a person without the person's valid consent can constitute assault. In such a case, the patient may be entitled to take action against the hospital or clinic for any harms incurred as a result of the assault. Nurses who find themselves implicated in an assault may also be subject to disciplinary measures by their employer or their state or territory Department of Health. Chapter 5 will look closely at assault and negligence in the clinical setting.

REFLECTIVE QUESTIONS 4.6

1 Name the three requirements for valid consent.
2 What is implied consent? How do you know if implied consent is present?
3 Under what circumstances can a person be detained in a health-care facility against their will?
4 When can a person with a serious mental health condition give valid consent?
5 Can a legal guardian consent to all medical procedures?
6 What is a restraint, and when would you use one?

Further reading

Australian Commission on Safety and Quality in Health Care (2021). Informed consent. www.safetyandquality.gov.au/our-work/partnering-consumers/informed-consent

——(2021). Person-centred care. www.safetyandquality.gov.au/our-work/partnering-consumers/person-centred-care

Cheng-Pei, L. et al. (2019). What influences patients' decisions regarding palliative care in advance care planning discussions? Perspectives from a qualitative study conducted with advanced cancer patients, families and healthcare professionals. *Palliative Medicine*, 33(10), 1299–1309.

Forrester, K. & Griffiths, D. (2015). *Essentials of law for health professionals*, 4th ed. Mosby Elsevier.

Ho, P. et al. (2018). Addressing challenges in gaining informed consent for a research study investigating falls in people with intellectual disability. *British Journal of Learning Disabilities*, 46(2), 92–100.

Kunneman, M. & Montori, V. (2016). When patient-centred care is worth doing well: Informed consent or shared decision-making. *BMJ Quality and Safety*, 26(7). http://dx.doi.org/10.1136/bmjqs-2016-005969

McIlwraith, J. & Madden, B. (2014). *Health care and the law*, 6th ed. Law Book Co.

Sullivan, M. (2003). The new subjective medicine: Taking the patient's point of view on health care and health. *Social Science and Medicine*, 56(7), 1595–1604.

Cases cited

Brightwater Care Group (Inc) v Rossiter [2009] WASC 229 CIV 2406/09

Dept Health and Community Services v JWB and SMB (Marion's case) [1992] HCA 15; (1992) 175 CLR 218

Gillick v West Norfolk AHA (1986) 1 AC 150

Hunter and New England Area Health Service v A [2009] NSWSC 761

K v Minister for Youth and Community Services [1982] NSWLR 311

Malette v Shulman (1990) 2 Med LR 162

Re Alex [2004] FamCA 297

Rogers v Whitaker [1992] HCA 58; (1992) 175 CLR 479

Watson v Marshall [1971] HCA 33; (1971) 24 CLR 621

X v The Sydney Children's Hospitals Network [2013] NSWCA 320

5 DUTY OF CARE AND PROFESSIONAL NEGLIGENCE[1]

BERNHARD RIPPERGER

LEARNING OBJECTIVES

In this chapter, you will:

→ Gain a basic understanding of the law of negligence

→ Understand the concept of professional negligence

→ Learn how 'duty of care' and 'breach of duty' apply in cases involving health-care professionals

→ Understand how a breach of duty could happen in some common areas of nursing practice

→ Gain an understanding of some legal responses to claims of negligence

→ Understand the concept of vicarious liability and develop an awareness of when someone will be liable for the negligence of another person

A patient attended the emergency department of a major city hospital and was referred to the triage nurse, who performed a brief physical examination. He was placed second on the list of priority patients and was asked to sit in the waiting area. Sometime later, a friend of the patient asked a nurse whether they could go somewhere else for treatment, and was told 'they were free to do so' (*Wang v Central Sydney Area Health Service & 2 Ors* [2000] [21]). The patient left without being seen by a doctor. The following morning, his condition deteriorated and he was taken back to hospital by ambulance. His skull was fractured and he was suffering from extradural haemorrhage, which resulted in irreversible brain damage.

In court, the plaintiff alleged the triage nurse's examination was inadequate and that he was not afforded the priority he deserved, and that the nurse should have attempted to dissuade him from leaving before he had been seen by a doctor. There was extensive expert evidence from a general practitioner, two neurologists, two specialists in emergency medicine and an experienced nurse, who gave evidence about the procedures in an emergency department.

The court held that 'the primary duty which the hospital owed to the plaintiff was to assign him his appropriate priority through the triage system and to observe him in the waiting area in case his condition deteriorated' [76]. That 'assessment had to be made in the light of the other demands upon the department at the time and the available professional resources' [48]. Although it was likely that the plaintiff would have made a good recovery if he had been treated at the hospital when he first attended, the court was 'content to assume that no duty to provide him with medical services arose until he could be accommodated in the treatment area' [76].

However, the court held that there was a duty to provide the plaintiff with appropriate advice when he said that he might leave the hospital and found that if the benefits of remaining at the hospital had been explained to the plaintiff, he would have done so. The hospital failed to discharge this duty, and the plaintiff's present condition was a result of that failure [77]. Accordingly, the plaintiff was entitled to damages.

Chapter 2 explained the main areas of the law, including the differences between civil and criminal law. This chapter will focus on one of the main parts of the civil law that is relevant for nurses: the law of negligence. The law of negligence allows a person to bring legal proceedings against another person to correct a wrong or harm that the other person has done to them. Usually the person who has been harmed (the plaintiff) will seek payment of money (called 'damages') in compensation for their injury from the person whose act or omission caused the harm (the defendant).

This chapter will outline the key parts of the law of negligence, with a particular focus on the special rules that have developed in relation to health-care professionals, including nurses. By understanding how the law applies to things nurses do that can cause people harm, it should be possible for nurses to better avoid acting negligently.

Just because someone is harmed by the actions of another person does not mean the injured person will be able to successfully claim damages. It is only if the person who causes the injury has broken a legal obligation, or duty, that a right to compensation will arise. A breach of a duty imposed by law is known as a 'tort'.

Until recently in Australia, most torts have developed through the operation of the common law rather than through legislation (this process is explained in Chapter 2). This means it is necessary to study some important cases in order to gain a basic understanding of the law of torts.

Some torts have a long history, and they usually involve a breach of a duty not to cause harm to another person by way of intentional conduct (actions done with the intention to cause harm). For example, there are torts of assault (where a person is harmed by someone else making a threat against them), battery (where a person is harmed by someone who intentionally physically interferes with them), trespass to land or goods (entering private land without permission or taking and using someone else's property) and defamation (making statements that damage a person's reputation). The duties that make up these torts can be very similar to criminal laws that protect a person from having their person or property attacked or stolen. This is why the same conduct can lead to a person being prosecuted for a crime by the state and being sued for damages by the victim (again, see Chapter 2 for a discussion of the possibility of multiple legal consequences arising from the same act). Although these 'intentional torts' are important and can be complex (especially the law of defamation), generally speaking it is obvious why physically threatening a person, harming them or interfering with their property is wrong. Some of the more subtle aspects of how these wrongs can occur in a nursing context are discussed in other chapters – for example, why carrying out a procedure without consent can be an assault or battery (see Chapter 4).

The law of negligence

For a long time, the law did not provide much protection against *unintentional* injury, except in some very specific types of relationship. For example, innkeepers were held to be responsible for the loss of any guest's property when the guest was on the premises. However, during the twentieth century the law of negligence emerged, which is based on a more general – but not absolute – duty to take reasonable care to avoid injury to others.

The most famous case in the early history of negligence is *Donoghue v Stevenson* (1932) from the United Kingdom. This case is significant because the court held that a duty of care could exist even where there was no direct, pre-existing legal relationship between two people (such as exists between an employer and employee, or a buyer and a seller).

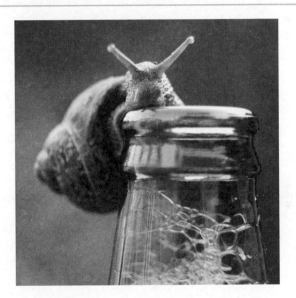

| FIGURE 5.1 | Reform in the law at times goes at a snail's pace – but in this case a snail was responsible for the law of negligence. |

The facts of the case were that a woman (Donoghue) went to a cafe with a friend, who bought her a ginger beer float. Donoghue drank some of the float but then found a decomposed snail in the bottle of ginger beer. She became ill and subsequently wanted to seek compensation. The legal challenge she faced was that, at this time, there was no duty recognised at law which had been broken. Donoghue could not sue the cafe owner, as her friend was the one who had purchased the ginger beer – there was no legal relationship between Donoghue and the cafe owner, and her friend was not injured. For the same reason, Donoghue could not sue the manufacturer of the ginger beer for breach of contract, as she did not buy the ginger beer. The case has a long and complicated history, but ultimately the House of Lords (which at the time also acted as the highest court in England) found that the manufacturer was required to pay damages, as a duty of care existed between a manufacturer and an ultimate consumer. The importance of this case is that the court said there is a general duty of care beyond those limited examples that had already been recognised in the law:

> At present I content myself with pointing out that in English law there must be and is some general conception of relations, giving rise to a duty of care, of which the particular cases found in the books are but instances. The liability for negligence ... is no doubt based upon a general public sentiment of moral wrongdoing for which the offender must pay ... The rule that you are to love your neighbour becomes in law, you must not injure your neighbour; and the lawyer's question, 'Who is my neighbour?' receives a restricted reply. You must take reasonable care to avoid acts or omissions which you can reasonably foresee would be likely to injure your neighbour. Who then in law is my neighbour? The answer seems to be persons who are so closely and directly affected by my act that I ought reasonably to have them in contemplation as being so affected when I am directing my mind to the acts or omissions which are called in question. (*Donoghue v Stevenson* 1932: 44)

The elements of negligence

Ever since the decision in *Donoghue*, the courts have been grappling with the key principles that would justify holding a person responsible for their negligence. Over time, the courts have refined what is involved in determining this question. As the law stands now, a defendant may be liable in negligence if:

→ the defendant owed the plaintiff a duty of care (duty of care)
→ the conduct of the defendant was in breach of that duty (breach)
→ the breach of duty caused the plaintiff loss or damage (damage).

'Duty of care', 'breach' and 'damage' are known as the three elements of the tort of negligence (although sometimes the issue of 'causation' is considered a fourth, separate element).

DUTY OF CARE

It remains true that there is no absolute obligation not to be careless, even if someone may be hurt as a result. Accordingly, the first critical question that has to be answered to determine whether a person is liable in negligence for an injury

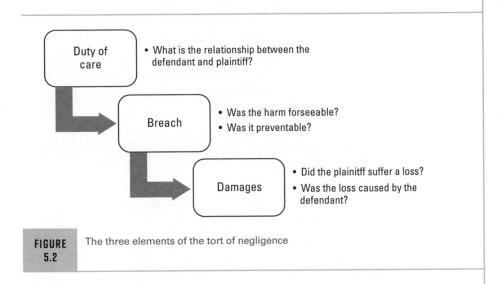

The three elements of the tort of negligence

caused to another person is: does a duty of care exist? The answer to this will depend upon the character, or type, of relationship between the parties.

The courts have identified a range of relationships that are said to give rise to a duty of care. In determining whether a duty of care exists, the court will examine whether the defendant should have foreseen that their conduct could result in injury to the plaintiff. Over the years, certain categories of relationship have been held to give rise to a duty of care: landlord and tenant; solicitor and client; occupier and entrant to private property; and health-care professional and patient. It is easy to see why these relationships give rise to a duty of care, as the person owing the duty is both in a position to be aware of the various risks to the other party in the relationship and can take steps to avoid injury. The situations that may give rise to a duty of care are not closed – the courts can decide that a duty of care exists where previously it was not thought such a duty existed. However, it is important to understand that it is well established that a nurse (including a nursing student undertaking clinical tasks) does owe a duty of care to a patient.

BREACH

A breach of duty exists where the person who has caused harm has failed to take reasonable steps to prevent that harm. The standard of care expected of a defendant is measured by 'reasonableness', which takes into account:

→ the probability and seriousness of the harm
→ the burden of taking precautions against the likelihood of harm, and
→ the social value of the activity that causes the harm.

This is an objective test, so the intention of the defendant is not important. A person who attempts to prevent harm but does so incompetently will still be in breach of their duty. However, because it is an objective test, the fact that a nurse causes harm to a patient does not mean there has been a breach of duty. A failure to eliminate a foreseeable and preventable risk may not be negligent if all reasonable steps were taken to prevent harm from occurring.

CAUSATION

Linked to the question of whether there has been a breach of duty is the idea of causation. Even if a duty of care exists and there has been a breach of duty, the person harmed has to prove the negligent act or omission caused damage. Causation is not used here in a scientific sense, but in a legal sense. The question is not whether the injury was an event that was the direct effect of some act of the person who is said to be negligent, but whether, at law, the person who performed the act or omission should be held responsible for causing the injury.

There are two different aspects of legal causation. The first is a largely factual question, and is often called the 'but for' test – that is, whether 'but for' the negligent act, no harm would have arisen. For example, if a community nurse providing care in a patient's home spills water on the floor and fails to mop it up, and the patient slips and falls causing injury, it can be said that the omission of the nurse caused the patient's injury. The second aspect of legal causation is more complex. It asks whether, even if there is a factual causation, the nurse should be held responsible for the breach. This often involves consideration of the degree of connection between the act or omission and the injury. For example, imagine that the patient in the previous example broke a leg after slipping and falling. This would lead to an ambulance being called to transport the patient to hospital. Imagine, further, that on the way to hospital the ambulance was involved in an accident, causing further injury to the patient. Although this may well satisfy the 'but for' test of causation, it would not be reasonable for the nurse to be held responsible for the further injury that resulted from an unforeseeable event, where the ultimate injury is not part of a causal chain arising from the original negligent act. This means the nurse's negligence in not mopping the floor will not be found to be a cause of the injuries sustained in the accident involving the ambulance.

DAMAGE

Finally, the plaintiff must actually suffer a loss or damage. If the plaintiff can prove damage as a result of negligence, they will generally be entitled to payment of compensation by the defendant. Compensation, called 'damages', is assessed in terms of money. The aim of compensation is to return the person to the position they were in before the injury. The amount of damages they are entitled to recover from the defendant should be no more and no less than the plaintiff's actual loss.

Damages can be for financial losses, such as out-of-pocket expenses incurred because of the injury, such as the costs of replacing damaged property or paying for medical expenses. These are reasonably straightforward to quantify. However, the plaintiff may also (and usually will) recover what are called 'general' damages. General damages are paid to compensate a person for the pain, suffering, disability and loss of enjoyment of life that have resulted from the injury. It can be much more difficult to accurately put a monetary value on this type of loss. It is up to the plaintiff to put forward evidence in support of their claim about the loss they have suffered.

Although in Australia the law of negligence has developed largely through decisions of the courts, in some areas where injuries are common, legislation has become more important. For example, the duty of an employer to take reasonable precautions to prevent an injury to an employee is now largely governed by workers' compensation legislation.

Further, in the early 2000s significant legislative reforms occurred across Australia that both modified and codified much of the law of negligence. The relevant legislation for each state and territory is set out in the Appendix. As a result of these reforms, most cases of negligence now are to be determined in accordance with the legislative provisions (see *Nepean Blue Mountains Local Health District v Starkey* 2016). However, the common law remains very important when it comes to understanding how the courts will apply the legislative provisions in any particular case.

REFLECTIVE QUESTION 5.1

A patient attends a medical clinic and is diagnosed with pneumonia and prescribed an antibiotic. The patient has an unexpected allergic reaction causing short-term kidney failure. Was this negligence?

Professional negligence

DUTY OF CARE

As noted above, the law recognises that a duty of care exists between a health-care professional, such as a nurse, and a patient. This means that the first element of negligence can be met easily by a patient who is trying to sue a health-care professional, such as a nurse, for negligence, provided that, as a matter of fact, they were a patient. Accordingly, most cases of professional negligence relating to health-care professionals involve arguments about breach of duty, causation and damage.

BREACH OF DUTY

As noted above, a breach of duty will be found where a person fails to take reasonable steps to prevent a foreseeable injury. This is sometimes referred to as the 'reasonable standard of care', which exists because of the duty of care owed by the defendant to the plaintiff. This is the standard that applies in most ordinary cases of negligence – for example, a person driving a car must drive in a way that will avoid injury to other road users. However, the law has developed a different approach to determining the standard of care owed by a professional, including a health-care professional such as a nurse, when they are providing a professional service. The nature of this duty of care was examined by the High Court of Australia in the landmark case of *Rogers v Whitaker* (1992). In that case, the High Court confirmed that the duty of care owed by a health-care professional to a patient was a 'single comprehensive duty'. However, because of the nature of this relationship, different factors are to be considered by the court when determining whether there has been a breach of that duty. In particular, the approach taken by the court in determining the reasonable standard of care to be provided in cases involving diagnosis or treatment of a patient will be different from the approach taken in cases involving the provision of advice.

The facts of *Rogers v Whitaker* were that the patient had injured her right eye in a childhood accident and was almost totally blind in that eye. An ophthalmic surgeon advised her that an operation on her right eye would not only improve its appearance but would probably also restore its sight. The patient agreed to the surgery. After the surgery there was no improvement, and in fact the patient developed an inflammation in her left eye that led to loss of sight in that eye as well, leaving her almost totally blind. The patient sued the doctor for negligence. It was not alleged that the surgery itself was performed negligently. The plaintiff's claim was that the doctor had failed to warn her of the risk that she would develop the inflammatory condition in her left eye, and that she would not have consented to the surgery if she had been told of that risk.

Central to the case was the role of the *Bolam* principle in determining the extent of the duty of care owed to a patient. The *Bolam* principle was a rule drawn from an English case from 1957 in which the court said a health-care professional was 'not guilty of negligence if he has acted in accordance with a practice accepted as proper by a responsible body of medical men skilled in that particular art', even though other health-care professionals had adopted a different practice (*Bolam v Friern Hospital Management Committee* 1957). The effect of this rule was that, provided there were a sufficient number of health-care professionals that adopted the practice in question, the defendant would not be in breach of duty. The principle was sometimes said to mean that although 'the law imposes the duty of care ... the standard of care is a matter of medical judgement' (*Sidaway v Governors of Bethlem Royal Hospital* 1985: 881).

In *Rogers v Whitaker* (1992: 12), the High Court agreed that:

> In Australia, it has been accepted that the standard of care to be observed by a person with some special skill or competence is that of the ordinary skilled person exercising and professing to have that special skill.

In this case, the surgeon argued that it had not occurred to him to warn of the risk of inflammation of the other eye, and that there was evidence from other medical practitioners that they would not have given such a warning. Accordingly, applying the *Bolam* principle, this meant he should not be found negligent.

However, the High Court noted that the *Bolam* principle had not always been strictly applied in Australia. In particular, the court went on to distinguish cases involving diagnosis and treatment from those involving the giving of information in order to obtain consent to treatment. It stated:

> Whether a medical practitioner carries out a particular form of treatment in accordance with the appropriate standard of care is a question in the resolution of which responsible professional opinion will have an influential, often a decisive, role to play; whether the patient has been given all the relevant information to choose between undergoing and not undergoing the treatment is ... not a question the answer to which depends upon medical standards or practices. Except in those cases where there is a particular danger that the provision of all relevant information will harm an unusually nervous, disturbed or volatile patient, no special medical skill is involved in disclosing the information, including the risks attending the proposed treatment. (*Rogers v Whitaker* 1992: 14)

In the specific case of *Rogers v Whitaker*, the court held that it would be reasonable for a patient who was blind in one eye to expect to be warned of the risk of becoming blind in the other. Accordingly, the court confirmed that the surgeon was negligent in failing to give that warning.

This decision modified how the *Bolam* principle would be applied in Australia in two important ways. First, although expert evidence of 'accepted practice' would remain important in determining the appropriate standard of care, such evidence would not be decisive of the question of whether a health-care professional was negligent, even in the case of diagnosis and treatment. Second, when it comes to cases involving giving information, the court rejected the applicability of the *Bolam* principle, holding it is a matter for the court to decide what the appropriate standard of care should be. The court held that whether the information given to a patient about risk was reasonable would depend on the circumstances of the patient, not on professional expertise.

As noted in the previous section, the law of negligence has been modified by legislation, including the law relating to professional negligence. This includes setting out how the standard of care owed by a professional in providing a professional service is to be determined by a court. For example, section 59 of the *Wrongs Act 1958* (Vic) states:

Standard of care for professionals

(1) A professional is not negligent in providing a professional service if it is established that the professional acted in a manner that (at the time the service was provided) was widely accepted in Australia by a significant number of respected practitioners in the field (*peer professional opinion*) as competent professional practice in the circumstances.

(2) However, peer professional opinion cannot be relied on for the purposes of this section if the court determines that the opinion is unreasonable.

(3) The fact that there are differing peer professional opinions widely accepted in Australia by a significant number of respected practitioners in the field concerning a matter does not prevent any one or more (or all) of those opinions being relied on for the purposes of this section.

(4) Peer professional opinion does not have to be universally accepted to be considered widely accepted.

(5) If, under this section, a court determines peer professional opinion to be unreasonable, it must specify in writing the reasons for that determination.

(6) Subsection (5) does not apply if a jury determines the matter.

This means that the main idea that formed the *Bolam* principle remains relevant; however, the test now requires that the practice be 'widely' accepted rather than merely 'accepted as proper'. However, section 59 of the Act makes clear that even if the practice is widely accepted, the court may reject that opinion if it considers it to be 'irrational'. This means the court, not professional opinion, maintains ultimate control over whether particular conduct is or is not a breach of duty.

Further, section 60 of the same Act makes it clear that the decision in *Rogers v Whitaker* to reject the *Bolam* principle in cases concerning health-care professionals' giving of information still applies. It states:

Duty to warn of risk

Section 59 does not apply to a liability arising in connection with the giving of (or the failure to give) a warning or other information in respect of a risk or other matter to a person if the giving of the warning or information is associated with the provision by a professional of a professional service.

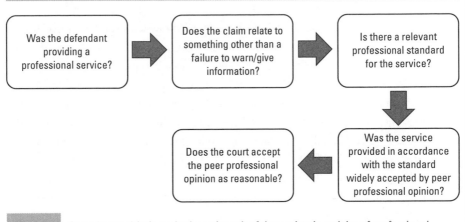

FIGURE 5.3 Steps in considering whether a breach of duty exists in a claim of professional negligence

REFLECTIVE QUESTION 5.2

Why is it important that the court, and not professional opinion, determines the standard of care?

CAUSATION

The case of *Rogers v Whitaker* is also a good example of how the concept of causation can apply to professional negligence. As was discussed above, causation is a legal rather than a scientific question. In that case, the surgery itself was not performed negligently. However, the court was satisfied that 'but for' the failure to warn, the patient would not have suffered the injury. Accordingly, the failure to warn can be said to have caused the injury. Second, the patient was able to satisfy the court that she would not have risked the loss of her sight if she had been given a warning, so there was no reason why the practitioner should not be liable for the failure to warn.

Not all cases are so straightforward. In the context of health care, patients are usually suffering from some condition for which they are seeking treatment or they need some other type of intervention to avoid harm. There are occasions when, despite the best efforts of health-care professionals, treatment is unsuccessful or harm arises that cannot be avoided. This can raise difficult questions about the scope of a health-care professional's liability, which is the second part of the test of causation.

The High Court case of *Wallace v Kam* (2013) shows some of the complexities of causation in professional negligence. In that case, a patient was not warned of two risks involved in treatment. One risk involved a temporary loss of motor function in the legs, due to pressure on the nerves as a result of lying on the operating table for an extended period. The second risk related to permanent paralysis from damage to the spine. The patient suffered the temporary loss of function, but not the paralysis. In court, he said that if he had been warned of the paralysis he would not have had the operation and so he should be compensated for the temporary condition which had in fact resulted. However, the court found that the evidence showed that even if the patient had been warned of the temporary loss of function he would most likely have accepted the risk and had the procedure. Accordingly, the court held the surgeon should not be liable for an injury that was the materialisation of a risk the patient was prepared to take. That is, the failure to warn the patient of the risk of permanent paralysis could not be the legal cause of the temporary condition.

DAMAGE

As noted above, unless a plaintiff can prove damage they are unable to succeed in a claim for negligence. Usually, showing damage involves a comparison between the position of the plaintiff before and after the act or omission said to be negligent. Just as with causation, sometimes damage is relatively simple to prove, even if quantifying the amount of compensation to be paid can be difficult.

For example, in *Rogers v Whitaker* the damage was, in effect, total blindness. This would give rise to compensation for the pain and suffering that resulted from a near total loss of sight, as well as for costs that were and will be incurred in caring for the patient and enabling her to live her life. Damages are assessed on the basis of the actual loss. If this plaintiff had been someone who relied on their sight for their employment, for example, there could be a significant amount of damages awarded for the loss of future income-earning potential. If she lived alone and as a result of her blindness required domestic assistance, this could also be included in the amount of damages.

Although in the case of *Rogers v Whitaker* it might be difficult to put a monetary value on that loss, the fact that the plaintiff suffered damage is obvious. However, as with causation, professional negligence in a health-care context can raise some difficult questions about whether there has been damage. In *Harriton v Stephens* (2006), the High Court faced just such a difficult decision. The case involved a child who had been born with congenital abnormalities as a result of her mother being infected with the rubella virus during pregnancy. The mother's doctor had incorrectly advised her that she was not infected with rubella, and did not arrange further testing. It was accepted that a reasonable medical practitioner would have advised the mother of the risk that a foetus exposed to rubella would be born 'profoundly disabled' (2006: 18). It was also accepted that had the mother been informed of the infection and the risk to her child, she would have terminated the pregnancy.

Accordingly, there was no question that there had been a breach of duty. In order to prove damage, the plaintiff (which in this case was the child, represented by a lawyer) argued that the comparison the court had to consider was between the child's condition as it was now – being profoundly disabled – and what the circumstance would have been if there had been no negligence. However, based on the evidence, if there had been no negligence the child would not exist. The court rejected the claim on the basis that the plaintiff had failed to prove damage. The High Court said this was not a case that involved a difficult comparison – rather, what was involved was actually *impossible*:

> A comparison between a life with disabilities and non-existence, for the purposes of proving actual damage and having a trier of fact apprehend the nature of the damage caused, is impossible. Judges in a number of cases have recognised the impossibility of the comparison and in doing so references have been made to philosophers and theologians as persons better schooled than courts in apprehending the ideas of non-being, nothingness and the afterlife … There is no present field of human learning or discourse, including philosophy and theology, which would allow a person experiential access to non-existence, whether it is called pre-existence or afterlife. There is no practical possibility of a court (or jury) ever apprehending or evaluating, or receiving proof of, the actual loss or damage as claimed by the appellant. (Crennan J, 252–3)

LAW AND ETHICS IN PRACTICE

A patient had been in hospital for 31 days being treated for depression. She was given various medications, including sedatives. During her time in hospital, she was described in notes as lethargic, tired and drowsy. On the morning of her discharge, nursing staff woke her on four occasions, but each time she fell asleep again. When woken at lunchtime, the patient was told the bed was needed for another patient.

While she was in the shower, her bags were packed by staff and the bed stripped. Her car was brought to the door and her belongings were packed into it. While driving home, the patient 'blacked out' and had a car accident. The patient claimed she should not have been allowed to drive home. The defendants (the treating psychiatrist and the hospital administration) said there was no breach of duty because the treatment that was provided was widely accepted by peer professional opinion. This was rejected by the court, which said that the breach of duty was so clear that the issue could have been answered by a layperson. The court also accepted evidence that there was no applicable standard of care for the assessment of the patient's fitness to drive, but rather it was a 'common sense standard' that was to be applied. The court also noted that the health-care professionals involved did not assess whether the patient was fit to drive, but rather left that decision to the patient herself, and all the evidence was that the patient was not in a proper condition to make that assessment. (*Naidoo v Brisbane Waters Administration Pty Ltd* 2017)

》 Why do you think that 'common sense' wasn't used to assess this patient before she was discharged?

Some common types of negligence

The discussion so far has looked at the general principles of negligence in a health-care professional context. The same principles, or elements, of the tort of negligence apply to all health-care professionals – doctors, paramedics and nurses; however, the *standard of care* that is expected of a nurse is that of the ordinary skilled nurse exercising and professing to have the skills of a nurse.

A nurse may be negligent if they do or fail to do something that does not meet the required standard of care and that causes damage to a patient. Nurses have complex and demanding roles. They must have a wide variety of capabilities, ranging from technical skills in using equipment to communication skills in dealing with patients and other health-care professionals. Nurses are not doctors and, although they have significant training and experience, the standard of care they are expected to exhibit is that of a nurse (see the discussion in *State of Queensland v Masson* 2020). Many of the specific challenges that can test the capabilities involved in nursing practice are explored in more detail in other chapters. In this section, however, a few key areas of practice where negligence can occur are highlighted.

USING EQUIPMENT

Nurses frequently use equipment that can be unsafe in untrained hands, such as defibrillators, pacemakers, oxygen cylinders, heat lamps, ventilators, blood warmers and intravenous infusion pumps. Nurses must be familiar with the manufacturer's instructions, and understand the safety procedures associated with equipment they use, such as safe storage, correct positioning and use of alarms. *Nurses should never modify equipment.* They should also be capable of identifying potential problems, such as signs of leakage, damage and contamination (Croke 2003: 58). In addition, nurses should be aware of the effect of working with several pieces of equipment simultaneously.

LAW AND ETHICS IN PRACTICE

Bjorn was working in the intensive care unit, caring for a patient who was receiving several different intravenous infusions, including nitroprusside, a potent vasodilation drug that rapidly lowers blood pressure. All the drugs were being infused by identical-looking pumps. Bjorn wanted to administer a push dose of morphine, but accidentally pushed the nitroprusside pump, causing the patient's blood pressure to plummet so low that the patient had to be resuscitated.

>> **Can you think of another example where a mistake could happen through use of equipment? How might these types of mistakes be avoided?**

COMMUNICATION

Communication failures are likely to be one of the most common sources of potential breaches of duty of care, given the central role of communication in modern nursing care and the number of health professionals involved in treatment – especially hospital-based health care. Nurses can fail to communicate adequately by not seeking medical advice in a timely fashion, not listening to patients' concerns or not passing on information such as details of allergies or pathology results. The Clinical Excellence Commission in New South Wales has introduced the iSoBAR program to improve communication and prevent unexpected patient deterioration (iSoBAR will be discussed in more detail in Chapter 9).

Sometimes being inexperienced or working in an environment with rigid attitudes can cause a nurse to disregard what the patient is communicating (see Table 9.1 for some statistics about clinical errors).

DOCUMENTATION

This is an extension of the failure to communicate adequately. Inadequate documentation can include such things as failure to record administration of medications or fluids, failure to report an adverse drug reaction or failure to report equipment malfunction. In general, any failure of documentation that is needed as part of direct patient care has the potential to result in harm to the patient. Documentation and information management are discussed in Chapter 7.

ASSESSMENT AND MONITORING

All of the above types of failure can lead to failures to adequately assess and monitor patients. In a busy workplace, a nurse's attention can be pulled in many competing directions: towards different patients, relatives, other nurses, doctors, friends, seminars, training events and so on. Consequently, the quality of attention to the patient's condition and needs can suffer. Lack of knowledge and experience can also result in a nurse failing to recognise a serious risk or deterioration in a patient.

The Australian Commission on Safety and Quality in Health Care (ACSQHC) notes that, despite the fact that there are clear, observable physiological signs that precede an adverse event such as cardiac arrest, research consistently shows that warning signs sometimes go unnoticed – or, if they are noticed, such signs are not always acted upon (ACSQHC 2010). Consequently, the National Consensus Statement: Essential Elements for Recognising and Responding to Acute Physiological Deterioration was developed to outline practices that would help prevent the unnoticed deterioration of the patient. The third edition of this document, released in November 2021, has nine 'essential elements' of recognising and responding to clinical deterioration. They are:

1 measurement and documentation of vital signs and other observations
2 diagnosis
3 escalation of care
4 rapid response systems
5 communicating for safety
6 leadership and governance
7 education and training
8 evaluation, audit and feedback
9 systems to support high quality care.

These processes are being implemented across Australia and can be found in programs such as the Clinical Excellence Commission's (2018) Between the Flags (see also Chapter 9).

COVID-19

The global pandemic known as COVID-19 has yet to have any real impact on the fundamentals of the law of negligence; however, the effects of the pandemic on medical professionals and the way services have been delivered over the last few years have the potential to give rise to 'novel' claims in negligence.

The most obvious risk is where there has been a failure to prevent exposure to COVID-19 and a patient is infected. Further, the pandemic has created significant pressures, which have meant that health professionals have had to make difficult decisions, including around the allocation of resources to patients. This may lead to claims about a failure to provide treatment or decisions to refuse treatment to certain patients, perhaps because only limited beds or equipment were available (Gunn & McDonald 2021: 207–8).

It is also possible that there may be vaccine-related injury claims, even though the Commonwealth government has introduced an indemnity scheme in relation to injury asserted to have been caused by the vaccine. Given the possibility of severe adverse outcomes from the vaccine, albeit in a very limited number of patients, health-care professional who administer vaccines will need to take reasonable steps to ensure patients are told of the potential risks of vaccinations.

The expansion of 'remote' care, such as telehealth, may also be an area of risk, with claims arising where it is alleged that there has been inadequate examination or follow-up, or potentially even breaches in relation to privacy and security of health information (Campbell 2021).

In all these areas, courts may be called on to assess the practices and procedures put in place by health-care professionals and hospitals to manage the risk of infection (to patients and staff), and in relation to the allocation of resources and treatment decisions (in the context where there it may be difficult to produce evidence of 'peer professional opinion' in defence of a claim).

REFLECTIVE QUESTION 5.3

Think about the different cases that have been discussed so far, including the case study at the start of the chapter. In many of these cases, simple things could have been done to avoid the injury. Why do you think those things were not done?

Defending negligence

This section will discuss aspects of the law of negligence that can limit the personal liability of a defendant to pay damages. Some of these are technical parts of the law of negligence that a defendant can prove in order to avoid or limit their liability. Others are ways in which a defendant can avoid being personally responsible for paying compensation if found negligent.

EVIDENCE AND THE BURDEN OF PROOF

The previous sections have set out the different elements of negligence. These are things that the plaintiff must prove in order to be successful – referred to as the burden of proof. Most people are familiar with the standard of proof in a criminal case, which is 'beyond reasonable doubt'. For civil proceedings, like a negligence claim, the standard of proof is a lesser one: the plaintiff need only prove the different parts of their claim 'on the balance of probabilities'.

Most of the cases that have been discussed in this chapter feature difficult legal issues that have been examined by the court; however, most cases of negligence are either settled between the parties without going to court, or if they do go to court the major issues in the case are disputes about the facts of the case.

To make a claim in negligence, a plaintiff has to set out what they say are the facts of the case, including what damages they are claiming in compensation. This can be done informally, in what is known as a 'letter of demand'. However, if the matter has to go to court, the plaintiff has to prepare what is called a 'statement of claim'. There are strict rules about how a statement of claim is to be prepared and a court can dismiss or strike out a poorly prepared one, even if there may have been some negligence on the part of the defendant.

After a statement of claim is filed with the court, the defendant will be required to prepare a document in reply, which is called a defence. There is normally a specified period of time in which this must be done; however, the timeframe can be extended, especially if the defendant has to ask the plaintiff for more details about what is alleged to have happened.

The plaintiff is required to prove the facts set out in the statement of claim and demonstrate that the facts prove there has been a breach of duty of care that caused damage. The defence can put forward their own evidence to argue that the facts alleged by the plaintiff are either not true or at least have not been proven on the balance of probabilities. The defence may also put forward evidence and legal arguments to say that, even if the alleged facts are proven, they do not support a finding of negligence.

Because most arguments about negligence are about the facts of the case, it is important that if an incident occurs that may give rise to a claim in the future, steps are taken to preserve any relevant evidence. This can include things such as CCTV footage, but it is also important to think about who may have witnessed an incident and ensure that their details are recorded so that if necessary a statement can be taken from them. Nurses should make a personal record of the details of any incidents of concern that they witness or are involved in as soon as possible after the incident. Most workplaces will have an incident reporting system, and all health services are required to have one as part of their clinical governance arrangements. It would usually be part of an employee's or contractor's responsibilities to ensure any incidents are properly recorded.

In many cases, claims in negligence will not be heard in a court until many years after the event. If steps are not taken at the time to record the facts of the incident, it can create problems in properly defending the claim. For example, in the case study at the start of the chapter, the evidence of the plaintiff's witnesses was preferred to the evidence of the triage nurse. The judge held that he 'found her evidence unreliable in certain respects'. The plaintiff had argued that some of the triage nurse's evidence was fabricated, but also that 'her account was skewed, more or less unconsciously, to place her actions in a favourable light' and, ultimately, the judge agreed that that was the case. The injury occurred in 1988 but the trial did not occur until 1999. In those circumstances, it may be understandable that a triage nurse in a busy hospital would not have a detailed recollection of a brief conversation with a person attending the emergency room. However, the result in this case was that the plaintiff's evidence about what happened was preferred to the evidence of the nurse and the hospital, and as a result the defendant was found to be negligent.

LAW AND ETHICS IN PRACTICE

The law has rules about what evidence can be considered by the court. Not all information or documents are able to be taken to account, particularly if the evidence is irrelevant or unreliable. An example of evidence that is not usually allowed to be taken into account is 'hearsay'. This is when someone wants to use a previous statement by a person to prove what was said by that person was true. For example, if Shirley tells Jane that Roger already had an injured leg before an accident, evidence by Jane that Roger had an injury would be hearsay. This rule exists because evidence given without direct personal knowledge of a fact is usually very unreliable.

One important exception to the rule against hearsay is known as the 'business records' rule. This allows a prior statement by someone that is recorded in a document prepared in the ordinary course of running a business to be considered by the court as evidence that what it says happened. For example, if a nurse has recorded in clinical notes that they had given a patient their medication, this could be relied on in court as evidence that the patient had in fact been given that medication. In this example, if the nurse had merely said in conversation to another nurse that they had given the patient medication, this would be hearsay. This is another reason why good practice around documentation is important – not only does it mean there is less risk of poor treatment outcomes, but the documents themselves can be relied on as evidence to prove that a reasonable standard of care has been provided.

>> **What kind of comments have you heard from a nurse that might be considered hearsay?**

DEFENCES

In addition to putting forward evidence that refutes what the plaintiff says, there are some circumstances where a defendant can try to prove that they have a defence or that there is some other reason why they should not be held responsible. Some defences, if proven, will mean that the defendant will not be liable at all – these are known as 'complete defences'. Others mean that the defendant's liability will be reduced.

Although many of these defences were also part of the common law, legislation has codified and modified them. Accordingly, the discussion below sets out the defences as they now appear in legislation (see the Appendix for the legislation for each state and territory). Where a defence is raised, the burden of proof usually shifts to the defendant to prove the various elements.

Limitations periods

If a person suffers an injury and they want to seek compensation, they must commence legal proceedings within a certain period of time. This is known as the 'limitation period'. Every state and territory has specific legislation setting out the relevant limitation period. The limitation period exists because the law recognises that it may be unfair on a defendant to try to defend a claim that is very old, as there may no longer be reliable evidence about what actually occurred.

Usually the limitation period for negligence is three or six years. However, the period does not necessarily start when the injury occurred. Rather, it starts when the plaintiff knows or ought to have known they may have a claim in negligence. This can, in fact, be many years after the incident and may be only due to receiving legal advice. Further, the court may also allow an extension of time.

Competent professional practice

The role of evidence from professional peers about the standard of care has been discussed above in the section on 'breach of duty'. It is part of the plaintiff's case to prove that the standard of care was not acceptable. However, this principle also acts as a defence – the defendant will need to obtain evidence that their conduct was in accordance with what is widely accepted as competent professional practice (*Boxell & Ors v Peninsula Health* 2019; *State of Queensland v Masson* 2020).

Voluntary assumption of risk

A voluntary assumption of risk refers to a situation where a person pursues a course of action in full comprehension of the nature and the likelihood of its risks, and in full understanding of all advice. This is a complete defence to a claim of negligence.

A person will not be liable where the injury is a result of an 'obvious' risk, which is one that is common knowledge even if there is a low probability of it occurring. Generally, there is no obligation on a defendant to warn a plaintiff of an obvious risk. However, this does not apply in the case of a service provided by a professional. Accordingly, this defence is of limited use in the context of professional negligence.

Good Samaritans

People who, 'in good faith and without expectation of payment or other reward' (*Civil Liability Act 2002* [NSW], s 56), come to the assistance of a person who is injured or at risk of injury ('good Samaritans') will not be liable for negligence. In these circumstances, the usual standard of care is modified from what was reasonable in the circumstances to whether what was done was done in good faith. This protection was introduced because generally at law there is no obligation to give assistance and there was a common perception that a person could be sued if they attempted to provide assistance and injury resulted.

Intoxication

Whether a person is intoxicated will generally not affect whether a duty of care towards them exists, nor the standard of care that is to apply where a duty of care does exist. The mere fact that a person is intoxicated is not enough to give rise to a duty of care towards that person. Further, if a person is intoxicated at the time of injury or death, no damages can be awarded unless the court is satisfied that the injury or death is likely to have occurred even if the person was not intoxicated.

Self-defence and no recovery by criminals

Legislation now makes it clear that a defendant will not be liable for any injury because of something they did in self-defence where they were responding to unlawful conduct. Similarly, a defendant will not have to pay damages if the injury to the person happened 'at the time of, or following, conduct of that person that, on the balance of probabilities, constitutes a serious criminal offence' (*Civil Liability Act 2002* [NSW], s 54).

Contributory negligence

Contributory negligence refers to a situation where a person contributes, through their own negligent act or omission, to the harm that they incur as a result of the negligence of another person. Although originally developed in the common law, contributory negligence is another area where legislation has been used to set out what approach should be taken by the courts (see the Appendix).

For example, section 23 of the *Civil Liability Act 2003* (Qld) states that the 'principles that are applicable in deciding whether a person has breached a duty also apply in deciding whether the person who suffered harm has been guilty of contributory negligence in failing to take precautions against the risk of that harm'. The standard of care that will be applied to the person who suffered harm is that 'of a reasonable person in the same position' (section 23(2)). For example, if a person has been advised to fast before surgery but ignores this and drinks a cup of coffee or eats a snack without telling anyone, they have contributed to a set of circumstances that may result in them incurring harm when they are administered an anaesthetic. Even if the nurse at the operating theatre was negligent by failing to check the time of the person's last oral intake, the person may contribute to the harm arising from that negligence by failing to take reasonable precautions.

Contributory negligence is not a complete defence. If a plaintiff has been found to also have been at fault, this will mean the amount of compensation that the defendant will have to pay will be reduced to that extent. A court will usually make a finding of contributory negligence in percentage terms. However, on rare occasions this amount can be 100 per cent, meaning that although the defendant was negligent, the plaintiff's own negligence was so significant that the amount they should be paid in compensation by the defendant will be reduced to zero.

REFLECTIVE QUESTION 5.4

Why is it important that any incidents involving injury to a patient are carefully recorded?

Vicarious liability, non-delegable duties and professional indemnity insurance

VICARIOUS LIABILITY

Vicarious liability is relevant to nurses because they are usually employees of organisations, and vicarious liability is largely concerned with the protection nurses may have from the payment of financial damages on the basis of their employee–employer relationship.

When negligence is proven, the defendant is required to pay compensation to the plaintiff. Awards of damages in professional negligence cases can be very high, sometimes in the millions of dollars where the injury that results from negligence is catastrophic. This could potentially bankrupt an individual. In practice, most plaintiffs are seeking to actually be paid compensation. This means they will usually seek to sue a defendant who has the capacity to pay.

Generally, a person is not liable for the negligent conduct of another person. Vicarious liability is an exception to this rule. It is a principle of strict liability, where a person is liable for the conduct of another person even if they have done nothing wrong themselves. Vicarious liability only applies in a small number of identified relationships, such as between a principal and an agent (an agent is someone who is given lawful authority to act on behalf of a principal in dealing with third parties – for example, when a real estate agent is authorised to negotiate the sale of a house on behalf of its owner), and between the owner and the driver of a car. The High Court has said that the principles of vicarious liability have not developed logically but rather from judicial perceptions of individual justice and social requirements that have changed over time. Accordingly, the High Court has been very cautious in expanding the scope of vicarious liability.

The best-known example of vicarious liability is where an employer will be held liable for the negligence of an employee incurred in the course of their employment. There are two requirements that have to exist for there to be vicarious liability:

1 The person who was negligent is an 'employee'.
2 The negligence occurred during the course of the employee's employment.

The first requirement usually does not exist where someone is an independent contractor. A person who engages an independent contractor will generally not be liable for their negligence. Whether someone is an employee is a question of law. Sometimes a person who appears to be an independent contractor will be regarded by the court as an employee after careful analysis of all the circumstances of the relationship between the two parties (*Hollis v Vabu Pty Ltd* 2001).

Under the second requirement, an employer is responsible for the negligent acts of an employee only if those acts are connected with what the person is employed to do. If an employee does something that relates to what their employer is set up to do, even if they do it poorly or improperly, this will usually be regarded as something done in the course of their employment. For example, an enrolled nurse who provides care to a patient in a hospital without any supervision may be in breach of the relevant standards and working outside their scope of practice, but this will still usually be regarded as being in the course of their employment. The High Court has said: 'Not everything that an employee does at work, or during working hours, is sufficiently connected with the duties and responsibilities of the employee to be regarded as within the scope of the employment' (*New South*

Wales v Lepore 2003). For example, a nurse who provides a patient with alcohol at their request will probably be regarded as acting outside the scope of their employment. The test concerns whether the act was done as an improper way of doing what the employee was supposed to do, or whether it should be considered an independent act.

Was the person who caused the harm an employee? → Was the harm a result of negligence by the employee? → Was the harm caused during the course of employment?

FIGURE 5.4 What to consider in deciding if vicarious liability arises

Usually it is not a difficult task to determine whether something a nurse has done is connected to the nurse's employment because negligence usually involves someone performing a task or duty without meeting the necessary standard of care. In most cases, an employer will not be held vicariously liable for the intentionally wrongful acts of an employee as these are usually regarded as 'independent' acts. However, in certain circumstances an employer will be held responsible for intentionally wrongful conduct of an employee, such as theft, fraud and even violence, even if those acts are expressly prohibited by the employer. In *Prince Alfred College Incorporated v ADC* (2016), the High Court held that a school was vicariously liable for the sexual assault of a student by a housemaster. Part of the reasoning of the court was that the employer had assigned to the employee a special role in relation to the victim, and the performance of this role provided the opportunity for the unlawful acts. Based on the principle in that case, it may be that a court would hold an employer vicariously responsible for the intentional wrongdoing of a nurse in certain circumstances where the nurse was in a special position by reason of their employment to take advantage of their relationship with the patient – for example, if a nurse were allowed or required to work alone with an elderly patient suffering dementia and they physically assaulted the patient.

It is important to recognise two limits to the 'benefit' of vicarious liability. First, that an employer is found to be vicariously liable merely protects the negligent employee from being financially liable. The fact they were negligent may have other consequences. For example, their employer may undertake a performance review and, in the case of a particularly careless act or if there have been a number of occasions of carelessness, the employee might lose their job. Similarly, negligence could be seen to demonstrate a lack of professional competence and be the basis for disciplinary action under the Health Practitioner Regulation National Law. Second, because the claim still arises from the negligence of the employee, a plaintiff may still choose to name the employee as a defendant personally and pursue them for damages.

NON-DELEGABLE DUTIES

Even where a nurse who is working in a hospital is not an employee or is acting outside their course of employment so that the hospital would not be vicariously liable, it is possible that the hospital could be found responsible for any negligence by that nurse through the legal concept of 'non-delegable duties'.

A non-delegable duty is another exception to the rule that a person is not usually liable for the negligence of another person. It imposes strict liability on a defendant for the negligence of another person. It is called 'non-delegable' because the law has said that the defendant is not allowed to delegate, or pass responsibility on to someone else, to ensure that a reasonable standard of care is provided. The law recognises this duty because of the special relationship of control and vulnerability that the defendant has towards the person under their control.

In the past, a hospital could legally discharge its duty of care to a patient by ensuring that it used competent staff. The idea was that a hospital was merely a custodial institution where health-care professionals could treat patients. This, however, has long been rejected, and no matter what duties are imposed on health-care professionals, there is an overriding and ongoing duty on the hospital as an organisation (*Albrighton v Royal Prince Alfred Hospital* 1980). Accordingly, hospitals must have systems in place to ensure an appropriate standard of care is provided to patients. This can mean that a patient who is injured while in hospital may be able to sue the hospital for negligence, even though no individual health-care professional involved in their treatment was negligent.

The existence of this non-delegable duty is another reason why health-care professionals who work in an institution must take all reasonable steps to comply with the organisation's policies and procedures. It is also a reason why it is important to ensure that all necessary documentation is completed, even if it is routine, because a claim may arise on the basis of a systemic rather than individual failure. (In Chapter 9, we will discuss human factors and system factors in relation to clinical errors.)

PROFESSIONAL INDEMNITY

Recall that earlier we explained that when a claim of negligence is successful, the plaintiff may be awarded 'damages', or compensation, in the form of money. The person found to be negligent must pay the plaintiff that compensation. The most common way by which a person who has been found negligent can avoid having to find the money to pay compensation is through insurance. Everyone would be familiar with motor vehicle insurance that covers a driver for being at fault in injuring a third person (such insurance is compulsory in Australia) or another vehicle (such insurance is voluntary, and is usually up to the owner of the vehicle to purchase). Professional indemnity insurance covers injury that arises during the provision of a professional service.

With the enactment of the *Health Practitioner Regulation National Law Act 2009* (Qld) and the creation of the Australian Health Practitioner Regulation Agency (AHPRA) in 2010, nurses and midwives are now not permitted to practise unless they are covered by professional indemnity insurance. Section 129 of the National Law (Qld) states:

(1) A registered health practitioner must not practise the health profession in which the practitioner is registered unless appropriate professional indemnity insurance arrangements are in force in relation to the practitioner's practice of the profession.

(2) A National Board may, at any time by written notice, require a registered health practitioner registered in a health profession for which the Board is established to give the Board evidence of the appropriate professional indemnity insurance arrangements that are in force in relation to the practitioner's practice of the profession.

(3) A registered health practitioner must not, without reasonable excuse, fail to comply with a written notice given to the practitioner under subsection (2).

(4) A contravention of subsection (1) or (3) by a registered health practitioner does not constitute an offence but may constitute behaviour for which health, conduct or performance action may be taken.

In other words, while it is not a criminal offence to practise without insurance, to do so may expose the nurse or midwife to disciplinary action, such as a charge of unprofessional conduct. If a nurse without insurance (or extensive personal assets) was to be found liable for a substantial sum of damages, the nurse could not compensate the plaintiff, and the plaintiff would simply be left damaged to manage as best they could.

Nurses who are employed by large hospitals and health-care organisations, government agencies or other reputable organisations will normally be covered by their employer's insurance in relation to any vicarious liability for the negligence of an employee. However, other practising nurses may be required to take out professional indemnity insurance. In any case, it is now incumbent upon every nurse to establish that they have the appropriate indemnity insurance protection. Advice on insurance is provided by AHPRA, the Australian Nursing and Midwifery Federation, state and territory industrial unions and the Australian Primary Health Care Nurses Association, among others.

REFLECTIVE QUESTION 5.5

A patient is brought into hospital unconscious. When preparing the patient for transfer to surgery, a nurse steals the patient's wallet and mobile phone. Is the hospital liable for the loss?

Conclusion

The law of negligence is an important part of the civil law in Australia. It allows a person who has been injured as a result of the unintentional but careless conduct of another person who owes them a duty of care to receive compensation. Although health-care professionals owe their patients a duty of care, this does not mean that all mistakes or negative treatment outcomes will result in them being found negligent. Health-care professionals are required to meet a standard of care that is in accordance with widely accepted professional practice. This is just one good reason why nurses must be aware of, and work within, their scope of practice. Careful compliance with policies and procedures will help avoid unnecessary injuries, as well as providing the best possible defence to a claim of negligence.

REFLECTIVE QUESTIONS 5.6

1 In the case study at the beginning of the chapter it was noted that 'extensive expert evidence' was given by a number of different health-care professionals. Why do you think this was needed to help the court decide whether there had been any negligence in this case?

2 Why is it important for a nurse to have 'common sense'?

3 What can you do as an individual to avoid acting negligently?

4 Why is insurance important in the area of professional negligence?

5 What are some of the consequences if you are negligent?

Further reading

Campbell, P. (2021). Recent WA trends in medical negligence and professional regulation. *Health Blog*. www.pmlawyers.com.au/blog/2021/05/health-blog/recent-wa-trends-in-medical-negligence-and-professional-regulation

Cheluvappa, R. & Selvendran, S. (2020). Medical negligence – Key cases and application of legislation. *Annals of Medicine & Surgery, 57*, 205–11.

Croke, E.M. (2003). Nurses, negligence and malpractice: An analysis based on more than 250 cases against nurses. *American Journal of Nursing, 103*(9), 54–63.

Gunn, M.A. & McDonald, F.J. (2021). COVID-19, rationing and the right to health: Can patients bring legal actions if they are denied access to care? *Medical Journal of Australia, 214*(5), 207–8.

Hancy, G. (2017). Strictly liable vicariously. Paper presented at the Australian Insurance Law Association Seminar, Perth, 27 April. https://hancy.net/wp-content/uploads/2017/05/20170427-paper-AILA-Vicarious-Liability-by-Geoffrey-Hancy-barrister-1.pdf

Hobart Community Legal Service (2017). *Tasmanian law handbook*. www.hobartlegal.org.au/handbook.

Kiefel, A.C.S. (2015). Developments in the law relating to medical negligence in the last 30 years. Paper presented at the Greek/Australian International Legal and Medical Conference. www.hcourt.gov.au/assets/publications/speeches/current-justices/kiefelj/kiefelj-2015-0-01.pdf

Nursing and Midwifery Board of Australia (2016). Frameworks. www.nursingmidwiferyboard.gov.au/Codes-Guidelines-Statements/Frameworks/Framework-for-assessing-national-competency-standards.aspx

Trueman, S. (2018). Duty of care: Where does a nurse's responsibility end? *Nursing Review*. www.nursingreview.com.au/2018/02/duty-of-care-where-does-your-responsibility-end

Villa, D. (2013). Breach of duty. *Precedent, 115*, 10–15.

Wheeler, H. (2012). *Law, ethics and professional issues for nursing: A reflective portfolio building approach*. Routledge.

Cases cited

Albrighton v Royal Prince Alfred Hospital [1980] 2 NSWLR 542

Bolam v Friern Hospital Management Committee [1957] 1 WLR 582

Boxell & Ors v Peninsula Health [2019] VSC 830

Donoghue v Stevenson (1932) SC (HL) 31

Harriton v Stephens (2006) 226 CLR 52

Hollis v Vabu Pty Ltd (2001) 207 CLR 21

Naidoo v Brisbane Waters Administration Pty Ltd [2017] NSWDC 372

Nepean Blue Mountains Local Health District v Starkey [2016] NSCA 114

New South Wales v Lepore (2003) 212 CLR 511

Prince Alfred College Incorporated v ADC (2016) 258 CLR 134

Rogers v Whitaker (1992) 175 CLR 479

Sidaway v Governors of Bethlem Royal Hospital [1985] AC 871

State of Queensland v Masson (2020) 94 ALJR 785

Wallace v Kam (2013) 250 CLR 375

Wang v Central Sydney Area Health Services & 2 Ors [2000] NSWSC 515

Note

1 In this chapter, a reference to a 'nurse' as a health care professional assumes a qualified and duly registered nurse (such as an enrolled nurse or registered nurse). There is no doubt that the provisions relating to professional negligence apply to nurses in this sense when performing clinical tasks. However, it is uncertain whether the provisions apply to a nursing student undertaking clinical placements.

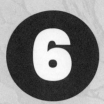

6 CULTURALLY SAFE NURSING PRACTICE¹

KIM ATKINS

LEARNING OBJECTIVES

In this chapter, you will:

→ Describe the role of culture and diversity in nursing practice

→ Explain the concept of cultural safety

→ Describe some ways in which a lack of cultural awareness and safety has impacted on the health of Aboriginal and Torres Strait Islander people

→ Describe nursing practice that is culturally safe

Li Wong, a 67-year-old woman of Chinese origin, presented with abdominal pain and nausea. She had a series of abdominal scans, which showed a growth in her liver; a biopsy confirmed that it was metastatic cancer. When her family was told that she had cancer and would need to have the growth removed and start chemotherapy, they advised the staff that complete truthfulness with Mrs Wong would severely overwhelm her, that their duty as a family was to protect her and that they would make decisions for her. 'She would expect this,' they explained.

The focus of this chapter is culture, and in particular developing nursing care that is culturally sensitive and culturally safe. In the vignette above, Li Wong's family requested that information about her illness and prognosis be withheld from her because she was vulnerable, and they believed she would be severely affected by this information and the implications of it for her future well-being. In their view, emotional stability and well-being were essential to improving health. But to many nurses in Australian culture, the idea of concealing the truth from Li Wong would seem improper. Truthfulness underpins our practices of informed consent. In Australia, a patient is expected to give fully informed consent before treatment is provided, and should be provided with information about the risks and benefits of a procedure; otherwise, the nurse may be liable for assault (see Chapter 5). Truthfulness also forms the basis of clear communication and trust in the nurse–patient relationship. However, in different cultures there is a common expectation that patients will not be told of certain diagnoses, and that the burden of knowledge and decision-making is delegated to family members.

Placing a very high value on truthfulness and the right to know assumes a desire to know the truth on the part of the patient and the community. Not all people or communities hold this desire. In such cases, imposing Western values would be paternalistic, overbearing and disempowering, and would therefore constitute culturally insensitive care.

The presence of different cultures in our community brings about social diversity and requires culturally sensitive and culturally safe care from nurses and midwives.

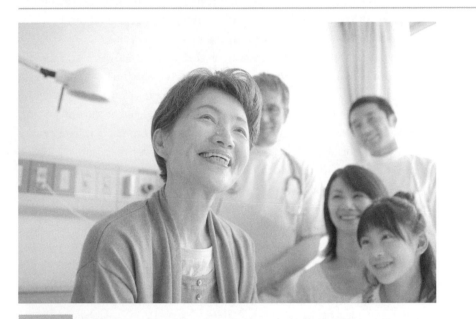

| FIGURE 6.1 | All patients deserve to be treated with respect and dignity while they receive treatment or ongoing care. |

REFLECTIVE QUESTIONS 6.1

1 In the scenario above, what challenges would you expect to face if you were caring for Li Wong, given the vague information she has received?

2 In the scenario, there appears to be a conflict between Western ideas of autonomy and informed consent, and different cultural practices. How do you think this can be resolved in practice?

Considering culture and diversity

The Code of Conduct for Nurses emphasises that nurses should 'engage with people as individuals in a culturally safe and respectful way' (NMBA 2018b: 5). The ICN Code of Ethics for Nurses provides further detail in its expectation that:

> In providing care, the nurse promotes an environment in which the human rights, values, customs and spiritual beliefs of the individual, family and community are respected. (ICN 2021)

Just as the situations of people differ according to age and gender, the beliefs people hold and the way they value certain things also vary in significant ways. Cultural insensitivity can lead to relationship breakdown between nurses and their patients, and between nurses and their colleagues. It can also lead to exclusion, isolation and, in the worst-case scenario, perceptions of prejudice and acts of discrimination. Cultural sensitivity, on the other hand, expresses tolerance and compassion, and is an enrichment of the nurse–patient relationship.

Before we go further, it is important to be clear about what we mean when we refer to culture. The term 'culture' is often taken to mean ethnicity, or to refer to nationality; therefore, when we refer to 'culture', this may evoke images of people from a different country of origin to our own, 'exotic' rituals or different ways of dressing. In this book, we use the word 'culture' in its broadest sense, to refer to characteristic ways by which individuals or groups of people live their lives: their values, lifestyles, how they think about things and interpret them, who they love, the ways in which they approach their health, how they speak and communicate, and to some extent the ways in which they behave. These characteristic ways of going about in the world give a person's experiences meaning and gives their life structure and purpose.

If people were all exactly the same in these things, cultural sensitivity would not be required. However, as we discussed in Chapter 1, being human is characterised by a vulnerability that is experienced by all people in relation to other humans and other things. The ways by which we are affected by our relations with other people and the world around us make us different from each other. Therefore, the concepts of diversity and vulnerability are central to the notion of cultural sensitivity.

The Australian Human Rights Commission (AHRC) refers to human rights as acknowledging 'the inherent value of each person, regardless of background, where we live, what we look like, what we think or what we believe' (Australian Human Rights Commission 2022b). The rights that we take for granted in our everyday lives are based on ethical principles of dignity, equality and respectfulness. They represent objectives of being treated fairly and treating others fairly in exchange. Cultural diversity is not just about ethnicity, then, but includes appearance, language, culture, religion, age, sexuality, nationality, socioeconomic status, physical or mental ability/disability, health status and any other characteristic that might be used to differentiate between groups of people.

Cultural sensitivity requires an awareness that people differ in their beliefs and practices. But knowing that people differ is only part of the equation. What is important to culturally safe care is how nurses think about differences, and how they act in regard to them. Because culture is a fundamental way by which people's lives gain meaning, the requirement for cultural safety is an ethical demand on the nurse. The Aboriginal and Torres Strait Islander Cultural Safety Framework for Victoria, for example, advises that a culturally safe environment is one in which people feel safe from challenges to or denial of their identity and experiences. According to the Framework, cultural safety recognises that meaning is generated culturally, so a meaningful response to a patient's report, questions, requests or complaints will require an awareness of the relevant cultural factors that inform and shape the person's experiences, understanding and behaviour. The more a nurse understands about different cultures, the more appropriate and effective care a nurse will be able to provide. Person-centred care demands awareness and practice of cultural safety in care so patients can exercise their autonomy and put themselves at the centre of their care.

Culturally safe person-centred care should demonstrate the following features:

→ mutual recognition and respect
→ genuine listening
→ shared knowledge and meaning
→ shared decision-making
→ shared resources
→ learning together
→ removing barriers to optimal health and well-being
→ addressing unconscious bias and potential sources of discrimination
→ supporting self-determination
→ shared design, delivery, and evaluation of care.

Cultural safety is also about nurses examining their own attitudes and beliefs, and considering how these attitudes and beliefs might affect their relationships with patients and colleagues. Culturally safe practice requires nurses to not just passively note the diversity of others while going about their own usual practices, but also actively engage in personal and professional reflection about their own culture, attitudes and practices. *This requires nurses to be open to self-reflection and thinking differently.*

Nurses can begin to think in more culturally sensitive ways by reflecting upon the diversity that exists among their own colleagues, families, friends and other social groups.

Cultural safety

Culturally safe practice can be identified by its dedication to inclusion and empowerment and is defined within the NATSIHWA Cultural Safety Framework in Australia in this way:

> Cultural safety is about community and individual empowerment to manage one's own health and wellbeing and social issues. In practice, cultural safety requires health systems to examine their own practices in order to break down the barriers to achieving cultural understanding and responsiveness. (NATSIHWA 2016: 4)

Culturally safe nursing care addresses the quality of health care provided through a lens of communication and access. Nurses are frequently the first health-care professionals a person will encounter, or the health-care professionals with whom a person will have the most contact. The attitude imparted by the nurse, and the way they engage with the person, will directly influence how the person responds to the health service and will leave a lasting impression that may influence whether that person continues contact with the health service, whether they initiate future contact with that service or whether they seek contact with any other service (Crameri et al. 2015; Papps & Ramsden 1996). Therefore, culturally safe nursing practice goes beyond a single encounter with a patient and/or their relative to influence whether or not individuals and communities engage with health services *at all* and the ways in which they do so. Culturally safe practice is underpinned by principles that address:

→ a commitment to fair access to health care
→ an emphasis on the analysis of the use of power and authority in the provision of care
→ a recognition that inequalities and disadvantage exist between individuals and communities
→ an acknowledgement that nurses (and other health professionals) carry their own cultural beliefs and practices, and that these may impact upon patient care (DeSousa 2008: 129–30).

LAW AND ETHICS IN PRACTICE

Peter admits an elderly Indian man, Mr Singh, who is unaccompanied and speaks little English. Peter completes a care plan and, when addressing diet and nutrition, is aware that cultural diversity exists regarding food. Peter's colleagues advise that Indians believe animals are sacred and they therefore don't eat meat. Peter ticks the vegetarian option for Mr Singh and the elderly man receives a series of salads, which are returned to the kitchen largely untouched.

>> **How would you find out what is culturally appropriate care for a patient who does not speak English?**

A problem with the scenario depicted above is that Peter has applied a cultural 'checklist' to Mr Singh. Peter's approach was to judge Mr Singh's needs by reference to a list of supposed cultural attributes – for example:

→ place of birth: India
→ religious beliefs: animals are sacred
→ dietary practice: vegetarian.

Applying 'checklists' of cultural beliefs and customs pertaining to particular cultures reduces the person to a mere stereotype, and seriously obscures their humanity, including what they are owed as a fellow human being. In the case above, the acquisition of information about Mr Singh's beliefs and eating preferences is limited and based on the following assumptions: (1) that all people of Indian origin believe animals to be sacred; and (2) that this means they would all prefer a vegetarian diet.

Bearskin (2011: 552) wisely points out that:

> Cultural competency does not require knowing everything about every culture or needing to abandon one's own cultural identity; rather, it means respecting differences and being willing to accept the idea that there are many ways to view the world.

REFLECTIVE QUESTION 6.2

How differently could Peter have approached the question of Mr Singh's diet? What actions could you take that are different from Peter's?

There is no doubt that awareness of cultural diversity and knowledge about specific cultural practices are valuable to nursing practice. However, myths abound about various cultural mores and who practises them. Confining learning about cultures other than one's own to customs and practices assumes that this knowledge will provide insight into complex human values and social realities. However, this can lead to the checklist approach mentioned above. The danger is that diversity *within* cultures may be neglected. Consequently, the nurse may fail to recognise diversity by reducing all members of a cultural group to a supposed common way of behaving.

As previously noted, diversity is not limited to ethnicity. Among other differences, it also includes gender and sexuality. Experiences with health practitioners that have been reported by people who identify as lesbian, gay, bisexual, transsexual, queer, intersex, queer or divergent in other ways (LGBTIQ+) show widespread intolerance and ignorance, with lasting harmful effects (Smith et al. 2014; Ussher et al. 2020). Smith et al. (2014) found that 81 per cent of young people surveyed (n = 128) who had experienced discrimination due to their gender expression had suicidal thoughts and 37 per cent had attempted suicide, while 70 per cent had self-harmed.

Smith et al. (2014) found that more than half (53 per cent) of surveyed participants had a negative experience with a health professional. Negative results of this experience included avoiding health professionals temporarily or even entirely, while other participants reported fear of complaining in case they were denied treatment (Smith et al. 2014).

Ussher et al. (2020) report that trans women living in Australia experience higher levels of violence than other women, and are subject to pervasive violence both outside and inside the home, including from police. The report also notes that a lack of 'culturally competent information and knowledge about transgender experience' contributes to stigma and discrimination, which in turn plays out in 'serious consequences for trans women's physical and psychological wellbeing' (Ussher et al. 2020: 16).

LAW AND ETHICS IN PRACTICE

The first doctor to whom I made mention of my gender identity locked me in her office alone and left to consult with every other doctor in the surgery about what to do. Without my consent, my GP brought up my gender identity in front of my mother without having ever spoken to me about it (and not knowing whether I had ever spoken to her about it) and a psychologist told me that there was no such thing as a non-binary identity and I was either just a tomboy or possibly a trans man, but only if I had been born in some way intersex. (Smith et al. 2014: 74)

>> What does this experience say about the clinician's attitude to the person's confidentiality, autonomy and family relationships?

In this case, there is more to consider than only a lack of cultural awareness or cultural sensitivity; there are very real moral and possibly legal implications. The clinician involved in this situation utterly failed to respect the person's autonomy and violated their confidentiality, creating an environment that felt unsafe and out of control for the patient. This situation arose as a result of discriminatory and paternalistic attitudes, and this had the effect of excluding and marginalising the patient – and their needs and rights. These kinds of attitudes to sex and gender exist across all social groups and they change slowly. Delivering culturally safe care requires all clinicians to continually reflect on their beliefs and ensure that they set prejudices aside. Nurses should be aware that acts of discrimination may be illegal as well as culturally unsafe. A range of Commonwealth Acts protect Australians against discrimination and promote equal opportunity. Anti-discrimination law in Australia includes the *Sex Discrimination Act 1984*, the *Racial Discrimination Act 1975*, the *Disability Discrimination Act 1992* and the *Age Discrimination Act 2004* (see the Australian Human Rights Commission website, www.humanrights.gov.au). In addition, each state and territory has a range of Acts that protect human rights (see the Appendix for a table of relevant legislation). Nurses have a responsibility to be aware of the most up-to-date legislation in the state or territory in which they are practising.

Practising culturally safe communication

Effective communication in the face of diversity can be challenging if we are not used to challenging our habitual ways of thinking and behaving. Perseverance and careful conversations may be necessary to achieve shared understanding. Being unable to access the dominant language of a society leaves patients feeling powerless and excluded, and being unable to access the language of the patient leaves nurses feeling frustrated. Worse, being unable to access the specific language of health care (which in Australia is English) may render patients more vulnerable to misunderstanding and errors in the provision of health care. Furthermore, the patient may then be blamed for any adverse health outcomes if they are considered to have a responsibility to understand English. Interpreters are available for many patients who speak languages other than English; however, it is extremely difficult to access Indigenous language interpreters, a wide variety of Indigenous languages exist. This makes the training and employment of Indigenous clinicians essential to achieving health outcomes (Wakerman et al. 2019). In 2002, a study of communication in Aboriginal health care found that in encounters between health-care workers and Indigenous patients, what the health workers said and what Indigenous patients heard and understood were often very different. Effective communication was seriously limited, and a shared understanding of key concepts concerning an individual's health was rarely achieved. Non-Indigenous health professionals and their Indigenous patients were not 'on the same page' – or even close (Cass et al. 2002).

Practices of communication need to be flexible, and encompass a range of strategies in order to promote culturally safe practice. For instance, providing information in a nurse's habitual way may not be suitable for all patients, and is not consistent with principles of person-centred care. When developing health information material and ways of communicating this (for example, diagrams or images), it is important that those materials are co-designed with members of the target audience – for example, Aboriginal and Torres Strait Islander (or other specific) communities. Using interpreters is important. Slowing down the process of information-giving is also important. Another strategy might be to break down the information into smaller parts and, after each part is delivered, take the time to discuss the understanding the patient has gained and their perspective on it. In remote area practice, for example, nurses are provided with resources to help improve communication, such as the Central Australian Rural Practitioners Association's (CARPA) *Standard Treatment Manual* (Centre for Remote Health 2017).

Taylor and Guerin (2019) point out how crucial the use of language and particular words or phrases can be in establishing power and, more importantly, diminishing power differences. Language is one way by which meaning is constructed, but meaning is also made in the context of the listener's social reality, so that what is said and what is heard can be different or even offensive. The use of labelling is not uncommon in health-care settings, and the choice of words or terms can be demeaning and alienating to a patient. Even diagrams can be understood differently, and images may have different significance. There may also be hesitation around the use of preferred pronouns of gender-diverse individuals, such as addressing a gender-non-binary person as 'they', or a trans woman as 'she'. The *Australian Government Style Manual* provides the following advice in relation to gender and sexual diversity:

> Inclusive language conveys gender equality and is gender neutral. Respect peoples' preferences around gender and sexual identity with pronoun choice, job titles and personal titles.
>
> ...
>
> Learn the user's preferred pronoun. If it's not clear and you can't ask them, choose gender-neutral pronouns. The singular 'they' is gender-neutral. It avoids specifying a person's gender. (Australian Government 2022a)

Language differences – both verbal and non-verbal – can lead to misunderstandings and misinterpretations of both nurses' and patient's behaviour, and lead to people being unfairly labelled in negative ways as non-compliant, disinterested or even overly intrusive. For example, there are wide differences in cultural practices around 'interpersonal space'. Anglo-Australian culture tends to discourage close physical contact between people who are not close friends or relatives, while among older people in some Chinese communities, touching and even holding strangers in public areas is not uncommon (Sebag-Montefiore 2019). COVID-19 has enforced greater distance between individuals, and this has no doubt contributed to misunderstandings in some settings. In addition, if the nurse is feeling frustrated or is experiencing negative feelings, these may be reflected in their body language, which may be noticed and interpreted. Where there are misunderstandings, the person and the nurse are less likely to trust and cooperate with each other, which can affect the quality of health outcomes.

Clear communication despite language differences is a key to culturally safe practice. When language or cultural differences make communication difficult, operating on assumptions rather than engaging vigilant communication can lead to negligence (see Chapter 5 for a comprehensive discussion of negligence). If you are unsure of what to do, just ask the person what they need, and what you (and others) can do to make them feel safe and in control of their circumstances.

LAW AND ETHICS IN PRACTICE

In the Northern Territory on 14 November 2007, it was reported that a 'tragic sequence of miscommunication' led to the death of a near-blind elderly Aboriginal man who had recently been discharged from hospital following treatment for pneumonia (Ravens 2007). The 78-year-old man was flown to an airport near his community without an escort, and there was no one there to meet him. He was left in 35-degree heat with only a little water and, unable to reach his home, died from a combination of heat exposure, lack of water and pneumonia. His body was found in bushland near the airstrip a week later. His niece accused the Health Department of 'hard-core, systemic racism', and the Australian Medical Association (AMA) subsequently called for an investigation into the state of Aboriginal health care in the Northern Territory (Ravens 2007).

>> **How will you be able to judge whether a hospital policy is racist?**

It was reported that a message regarding the man's discharge had been sent by fax from Katherine Hospital to the local community clinic; however, it was never received. Without confirmation and disregarding a request from the elderly patient's family that an escort be sent with him, the man was flown into a remote area and left alone with insufficient water. The above case is not only an example of unsafe discharge practice, but also of negligent practice, regardless of the patient's cultural identity. However, it is hard to believe that the lack of attention to the impact of the discharge had nothing to do with the patient's Aboriginality (hence the legitimate outcry by family and the AMA).

REFLECTIVE QUESTION 6.3

What assumptions and attitudes characterised the decision by the hospital staff about this Aboriginal patient and the patient's discharge needs? What is the connection between those attitudes and the fatal outcome for this patient?

This is a shocking example of how of some of the social determinants of health affect Aboriginal and Torres Strait Islander people.

Aboriginal and Torres Strait Islander people experience a burden of disease that is 2.3 times the rate for non-Indigenous Australians (AIHW 2020b). While the life expectancy of Indigenous people has increased slightly over the past several years, it is significantly shorter than for non-Indigenous Australians. Aboriginal and Torres Strait Islander men have a life expectancy that is 10.6 years shorter than that of non-Indigenous men, while Aboriginal and Torres Strait Islander women have a life expectancy that is 9.5 years shorter than that of non-Indigenous women (AIHW 2020b). Aboriginal and Torres Strait Islander people also face substantial disadvantage with regard to other key social outcomes, such as employment, income, education and housing (Australian Bureau of Statistics 2018a).

Despite having significantly poorer health, Aboriginal and Torres Strait Islander people do not necessarily have greater access to health care. This is partly related to remote living conditions; however, even where health-care services are provided, they are not always delivered in a manner that makes them readily accessible or effective for the populations they are supposed to serve. For example, there can be specific contextual barriers such as provision of consultations by internet (telemedicine) or visiting services that are infrequent or arrive at times that clash with cultural obligations. Clinics may not have staff that speak the local Indigenous language, or they may inadvertently be intimidating places. Service provision may assume that a mode of treatment delivery suitable to urban-based Australians is also acceptable to Aboriginal and Torres Strait Islander peoples. The relatively low per centage of health-care workers who are Indigenous also affects the ways in which Aboriginal and Torres Strait Islander Australians access health care (Wakerman et al. 2019). Where institutions or services are perceived to be culturally unsafe by individuals or communities, they will be avoided. These barriers were compounded by misinformation on social media during the COVID-19 pandemic, resulting in vaccine hesitancy. This posed a significant risk to people living in some communities.

At the heart of difficulties in successful health service provision to Aboriginal and Torres Strait Islander peoples is Australia's colonial history. With the process of colonisation by Europeans, the lifestyle, traditional food sources and cultural norms of Indigenous Australians were disrupted. Aboriginal and Torres Strait Islander peoples were subjected to oppression and discrimination. Historical attitudes (such as those that underpinned the 1901 White Australia Policy) undoubtedly affected attitudes towards Indigenous Australians and ultimately impacted their social status. Government agencies and church missions practised forcible removal of

Aboriginal and Torres Strait Islander children from their families, believing their interests would be better served if they grew up in European institutions or non-Indigenous families. Such attitudes and acts seriously undermined trust between Indigenous Australians and Europeans. In an attempt to rectify this, then Australian Prime Minister Kevin Rudd formally apologised to Aboriginal and Torres Strait Islander people in 2008 (Australian Government 2008).

When culture is acknowledged and control of service design and delivery is shared, Aboriginal and Torres Strait Islander communities can draw upon their broader conceptions of wellbeing and health, and so can be best placed to intervene, protect, build and evaluate their own wellbeing (CATSINaM 2021).

Practising in a culturally safe way

Indigenous communities have been able to achieve outstanding health outcomes when they design and deliver services that are culturally safe. This is perhaps best demonstrated in their rates of child vaccination, which, at 97 per cent for five-year-olds, is higher than the national average of 95 per cent (Australian Government 2022b). Another example is the Inala clinic in Queensland, which began with 12 Aboriginal patients in 1995 and, at last count, had 6000. In addition to the health of its clients, Inala Clinic has made significant contributions to the research basis of much clinical practice (Queensland Health 2016).

What does it actually mean to practise in a culturally safe way? The provision of culturally safe practice requires a commitment that is both professional and personal. Culturally safe practice consists of cultural awareness and sensitivity, but it also consists of a more political way of thinking about culture that 'pushes health-care professionals to the periphery of understanding the influence of culture on relationships in health care' (Bearskin 2011: 557). In other words, culturally safe practice means taking account of historical and institutional discrimination, and actively advocating for more culturally safe health policies, practices and institutions. Culturally safe practice goes beyond understanding different cultural mores and practices, and requires that nurses reflect on themselves, their language, their prejudices and the impact of their beliefs and attitudes on the patients in their care. Moreover, culturally safe practice requires nurses to actively account for power imbalance in patient–nurse interactions. The skill for nurses in practising in a, but in self-awareness and respect for cultural difference. When nurses practise unsafely, they diminish, demean and disempower people of another culture. However, when nurses practise safely, they recognise, respect and acknowledge diversity.

An important point to note about culturally safe care is that it requires us to move from a 'one-size-fits-all' approach, where everyone is treated the same regardless of their cultural differences, to an approach in which diversity is recognised and our approach to care is mindful and respectful of those differences.

While nurses and midwives in Australia have not yet formally adopted a fully articulated philosophy of cultural safety, as has occurred in New Zealand in relation to that country's Māori people, the Congress of Aboriginal and Torres Strait Islander Nurses and Midwives (CATSINaM) has lobbied for changes to national legislation to require cultural safety to be built into clinical education, training and practice (Keast 2017). In March 2018, a statement was issued by the NMBA that indicated joint purpose in implementing culturally safe practice (NMBA 2018c: 1–2).

REFLECTIVE QUESTION 6.4

Casey has recently been appointed to work in a rural community in Australia. There is a high population of Aboriginal and Torres Strait Islander people living there and she has been asked to prepare a talk to other health professionals about cultural safety. What key points should she include to make an impact on the professional development of others with regard to culturally safe practice?

Understanding one's own culture and social reality requires both personal and professional reflection. This relates to being constantly aware of the dominant values that inform practice. Reflective practice for nurses means developing an understanding of what it means to be a practitioner by being able to link theory and practice (Howatson-Jones 2016: 10). Reflection is the intellectual activity of examining one's experiences and thinking through – judging, analysing and reasoning about – the nature of the experience and one's own actions, thoughts and attitudes in order to understand oneself and one's experiences (Howatson-Jones 2016: 7).

Culturally safe practice requires that nurses be conscious of the cultural values *they* are bringing to the interaction with a patient. This is important because nurses' unconscious attitudes and values can cause them to have negative responses to patients, and these can be observed and sensed by others – even if the nurse thinks they have suppressed them. Negative responses can lead to avoidance of a patient by a nurse, or avoidance of a nurse – or indeed a whole health system – by a patient. When nurses avoid and remain distanced, patients become disempowered and marginal to the health service, and may receive poorer quality care.

Understanding one's own culture and social reality requires both personal and professional reflection. Becoming more conscious of your own culture and values may take time and structured reflection.

Take a notebook and record your answers to the following questions. We encourage you to think analytically about your answers.

→ What do I know about other cultural views of the world?

→ What did I learn as a child about 'us' and 'others', and what kind of words were used to describe others?

→ What do I fear from other people?

→ When caring for a patient of a different culture, what thoughts come into my head? Are these thoughts fair and reasonable? Where did I get those thoughts from?

To assist further reflection in practice, consider the critical questions below. These questions could guide reflection following an interaction with a patient to address the question of whether that interaction was culturally safe.

→ Was the feeling of power equalised in the situation?

→ What pressures were present from a Western culture?

→ Was my use of language acceptable and respectful?

→ Was communication effective? Who else should I have involved in the conversation for the safety of the patient?

→ What cultural values might lie behind the patient's reaction?

→ How could I have managed this interaction in a more culturally safe way?

Practising in a culturally safe way requires nurses in Australia to acknowledge the cultural assumptions that frame all aspects of their work and care. For example, in Australian and other Western cultures, the expression of individual autonomy is strongly favoured, to the extent that we actively protect the human right to determine outcomes for ourselves, including the right to refuse or to withdraw from treatment or research. However, non-Western philosophers such as Glick (1997) perceive the emphasis we place on autonomy as 'culturally biased' since other cultures do not necessarily place the same value on individual rights and self-determination.

Further, the ways in which patients exercise their autonomy may be different in non-Western cultures. Some philosophers claim that privacy and confidentiality are culturally constructed and are greatly emphasised in liberal societies that value individualism and autonomy, such as Australia. By contrast, the role of family in decision-making is often more highly valued in many community-oriented societies (Kuczewski & McCruden 2001). Cultures other than mainstream White culture in Australia may also value individual privacy differently or practise parental responsibility in a different way. That said, patients from different cultures may still be concerned to exercise their autonomy and may be sensitive about the sharing of information beyond the group for which that information is provided. Establishing a respectful, trusting relationship with the patient is the best way to ensure the patient's needs are being met appropriately.

Ensuring culturally safe access to care

There are numerous examples of culture-specific health-care provision in Australia, including separate services for termination of pregnancy, lesbian groups facilitating donor insemination, Italian (and other nationality) aged-care services, migrant and refugee health services, meals on wheels and men's 'sheds' (men's health spaces). In relation to Aboriginal and Torres Strait Islander Australians, governments have funded Aboriginal Community Controlled Health Organisations (ACCHOs) to run their own affairs and have provided specific funding for programs such as the Medical Outreach – Indigenous Chronic Disease Program. Culturally safe practice therefore extends beyond individual nurse–patient interactions to health-care institutions in which care is provided. But further than this, governments have acknowledged that empowerment through funding and independence can ensure that the needs of a particular cultural group are better met. Nurses can influence institutional policies and practices to create more culturally safe environments for patients through challenging culturally unsafe practices and through advocacy, representation and affirmative action. Nurses can also influence government policies and practices through empowering people from other cultures to have a voice and by acknowledging difference and diversity.

Conclusion

In this chapter, we have explored the concept of cultural diversity in the delivery of nursing and midwifery care. Culture pertains to demographic and other characteristics, lifestyles or human ability, as well as ethnicity. Culturally safe nursing care is delivered by nurses who are aware of cultural diversity and are culturally sensitive. Yet culturally safe care goes beyond this remit to incorporating reflective practice, non-discriminatory communication, non-discriminatory access to health care, and advocacy on the part of nurses in challenging culturally unsafe institutional policies and practices.

REFLECTIVE QUESTIONS 6.5

1 What is cultural safety?

2 List three components of culturally safe nursing practice.

3 What immediate implication does the concept of cultural safety have for your expectations of professional nursing practice?

Further reading

Australian Human Rights Commission (2021). Child safe organisations. www.humanrights.gov.au/our-work/childrens-rights/projects/child-safe-organisations

Bearskin, L. (2011). A critical lens on culture in nursing practice. *Nursing Ethics*, *18*(4), 548–59.

Crameri, P., Barrett, C., Latham, J.R. & Whyte, C. (2015). It is more than sex and clothes: Culturally safe services for older lesbian, gay, bisexual, transgender and intersex people. *Australasian Journal on Ageing*, *34*(Supp. 2), 21–5.

DeSousa, R. (2008). Wellness for all: The possibilities of cultural safety and cultural competence in New Zealand. *Journal of Research in Nursing*, *13*(2), 125–35.

Laverty, M., McDermott, D. & Calma, T. (2017). Embedding cultural safety in Australia's main health care standards. *Medical Journal of Australia*, *207*(1), 15–16.

NATSIHWA (2021). The centrality of culture. www.naatsihwp.org.au/policy-position-statement-centrality-culture

Nursing Council of New Zealand (2011). *Guidelines for cultural safety: The Treaty of Waitangi, and Māori health in nursing and midwifery education and practice*. Nursing Council of New Zealand.

Taylor, K. & Guerin, P. (2019). *Health care and Indigenous Australians: Cultural safety in practice*, 3rd ed. Bloomsbury.

Victorian Department of Health (2019). *Aboriginal and Torres Strait Islander Cultural Safety Framework*. www.health.vic.gov.au/publications/aboriginal-and-torres-strait-islander-cultural-safety-framework-part-1.

Note

1 Previous editions of this chapter were authored by Sheryl de Lacey.

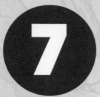

7 PATIENT INFORMATION AND CONFIDENTIALITY[1]

KIM ATKINS

LEARNING OBJECTIVES

In this chapter, you will:

→ Learn about and be able to apply the concepts of privacy and confidentiality

→ Learn about and be able to explain the nurse's legal and moral responsibilities in relation to privacy and confidentiality

→ Learn about and be able to apply nurses' mandatory reporting requirements

→ Learn about and be able to describe the safe use of digital and social media in relation to patient confidentiality

Ross was admitted through emergency services with chest pain, and was found to have suffered a myocardial infarction. He was admitted to the cardiac unit and placed on bed rest with cardiac monitoring. On admission, Kate, his nurse, gathered information from him about his condition and lifestyle to help plan his recovery and rehabilitation. When collecting this information, Ross told her that he was married and had three teenage sons. He added that he also had a long-term and loving relationship with Gill, and together they had a daughter who was seven years old. His wife did not know about his relationship with Gill or about his daughter, and he asked Kate to promise that this would not be disclosed to her. He said, 'I know I can trust you with this information.' He was most concerned that Kate arrange for Gill and his daughter to visit as well as notifying his wife about what had happened to him. Kate briefly described this unusual family situation in Ross's notes, and suggested that discreet management of visitors was required as part of his nursing care. The next day, as she entered the unit, she noticed several nurses – one of them from the neighbouring renal unit – huddled around Ross's case notes. They were whispering and giggling, apparently about her notation regarding his family situation.

This chapter addresses the topic of the information we receive about or from patients and introduces the concepts of privacy and confidentiality in relation to the management of patient information. It also sets out your legal requirements for mandatory reporting, including reporting harmful conduct of health professionals and others.

The above case demonstrates the complexity of caring for people and how easily private and sensitive information recorded about a patient in their interests can result in a breach of confidentiality and unprofessional conduct. Kate appropriately recorded very personal information that Ross had disclosed to her because she judged it relevant to his care. Yet other nurses perceived this to be a source of curiosity and gossip, and in sharing this with a nurse not involved in his care, had acted unprofessionally and breached Ross's confidentiality. Their conduct was therefore unethical, and disciplinary action should have been taken (see the section on mandatory reporting below).

Providing excellent nursing care for a patient requires that each nurse involved in the patient's care acquire relevant information from the patient (or a representative) concerning the patient's symptoms, their lifestyle, their medications, their concerns and their experiences. Therefore, nurses routinely see, hear, read and record things about other people that are not normally discussed outside the health-care setting, and have privileged access to matters of patient privacy. This brings with it certain legal and moral obligations.

As we discussed in Chapter 3, the practice of nursing is subject to the regulatory authority of the Nursing and Midwifery Board of Australia (NMBA), which strongly upholds the professional duty of confidentiality. The Code of Conduct for Nurses in Australia pronounces:

> Nurses have ethical and legal obligations to protect the privacy of people. People have a right to expect that nurses will hold information about them in confidence, unless the release of information is needed by law, legally justifiable under public interest considerations or is required to facilitate emergency care. (NMBA 2018b: 9)

Therefore, managing information about patients is one of the most important ethical and legal roles nurses play in health care and, owing to modern technology (as we discuss below), it is arguably one of the greatest challenges faced by professional practice.

Information, personal care and privacy

When someone consults a health-care practitioner, they are asked to provide information about their current health, their medical history and any symptoms they may be experiencing, as well as other personal information.

LAW AND ETHICS IN PRACTICE

Imagine you are admitted to a hospital for a dental procedure – you are going to have a tooth extracted. The nurse who admits you asks your age, whether you have any allergies, whether you smoke, whether you have had any dental operations previously and whether you have ever had an adverse reaction to an anaesthetic, sedation or antibiotics, or to other medication.

>> **How would you feel about disclosing this information, and then having it recorded in the hospital notes or on a computer?**

There are certain risks involved in having a tooth extracted under sedation, so this information is appropriate and relevant because it relates directly to the procedure and its after-care.

But imagine that, on admission for the dental procedure, you were also asked to provide information about your bowel habits, history of sexually transmitted diseases, whether you rent or own your home, your sexual orientation, whether you are sexually active, what contraceptive you use (if any), how many siblings you have and whether you have had thoughts about self-harm. There is no clinical indication for knowing how many siblings a person has, their sexual orientation or behaviour, or whether they rent their home. Certainly much of this information, while it may be relevant in another clinical setting (such as a family planning clinic consultation), is not relevant to this admission. Because none of this information is directly relevant to a tooth extraction procedure, the questions are unnecessarily intrusive. You would be wise to question why the nurse needs to know this and you may also decline to provide answers. Questions that are intrusive because they are irrelevant to the procedure or care are likely to make patients feel uncomfortable about answering them, let alone having them recorded in notes or on a computer where many others will have access to such private and sensitive information.

Recording information about a patient that is accessible to others and can be taken out of context can put them at risk of prejudice. Further, the way in which information about a patient is recorded and shared with other health professionals can lead to assumptions and judgements, and have a negative impact on their care.

The International Council of Nurses' Code of Ethics for Nurses (ICN 2021: 25) defines 'personal information' in the following way:

> Information obtained during professional contact that is private to an individual or family, and which, when disclosed, may violate the right to privacy, cause inconvenience, embarrassment, or harm to the individual or family.

Nurses and other health professionals are not permitted to collect and/or record any personal information just because they happen to think it might be useful, or because they are curious. There must be a good clinical reason to request private information, and *only* information that is directly relevant to the person's health needs can be collected and recorded – *nothing more.*

The principle of privacy refers to boundaries relating to a patient's body or their knowledge of themselves, their memories and information about their lives or their personhood. When patients exercise their right to privacy, they may select what they reveal about themselves, and they may choose whether and to what extent they will expose their bodies to others for examination or other procedures. They may keep things to themselves – and they have a legal right to do so. Nurses may not threaten to – or actually – withhold treatment or care in order to obtain information from a patient – to do so constitutes coercion. So, in relation to privacy, the choice about what to do, or the extent of private information revealed, is the patient's. However, once disclosed, this also does not mean that the nurse is free to record it for others to read. Discretion must be observed with regard to what, if any, information casually disclosed by a patient ought to be recorded for their benefit, and which information should *not* be recorded in order to avoid unnecessary inconvenience, embarrassment or harm to the patient.

Invasions of privacy are, of course, necessary in the provision of patient care. Washing a patient and taking care of their hygiene sometimes involves quite intimate procedures performed by nurses. However, nurses should acknowledge and take seriously the issue that what may seem like everyday procedures for them may feel more like invasions of privacy for the patient. It is therefore important that a patient's consent is sought prior to performing even simple procedures, and that all steps possible should be taken to ensure their general privacy, comfort and dignity. For example, nurses should ensure that curtains are pulled around beds in acute care settings when the patient is using a bedpan or urinal. These are all measures that indicate professional attention to patients' rights, dignity and privacy, regardless of whether they are young or old, competent or infirm, male or female, rich or poor.

In addition, many people consider information about their health to be particularly sensitive. Information – such as the results of genetic testing that show a person to have inherited Huntington's disease, for example – holds implications for their access to employment and insurance, such as health insurance and life insurance, not to mention implications for the health of their immediate and extended family.

Recent research suggests that although student nurses place a high value on patients' privacy, their own awareness of privacy issues for patients is lower (Kucukkelepce et al. 2021).

REFLECTIVE QUESTION 7.1

While chatting with his nurse, a young male patient, Tua, who is in hospital for a cardiac arrhythmia, confides that he has been feeling sad lately because a good friend has recently died of AIDS. Tua also discloses that he is gay. The nurse makes an entry in Tua's file noting that he is homosexual and that he is depressed because his partner has recently died of AIDS. At shift handover, one of the incoming nurses suggests that Tua be isolated from other patients to prevent them contracting AIDS. The next day, the resident doctor reads the notes and then asks Tua how long he has had AIDS. Tua is furious and signs himself out of the hospital.

What went wrong here and how should Tua's disclosure have been managed by his nurse?

Privacy legislation

In Australia, the *Privacy Act 1988* (Cth) defines personal information as:

> information or an opinion about an identified individual, or an individual who is reasonably identifiable:
>
> **(a)** whether the information or opinion is true or not; and
> **(b)** whether the information or opinion is recorded in a material form or not.
> (Pt II, Div I, s 6(1))

Privacy legislation determines how personal information is collected, how it is used and disclosed, its accuracy, how securely it is kept and the rights of patients to access information about themselves. Nurses are obliged to act consistently with the Privacy Act, just as they are obliged to adhere to any other legislation that applies to nursing. The law on privacy in Australia aims to protect personal information that is held by federal government departments and agencies such as health-care institutions, so that only people who really need to have that information for legitimate legal purposes will have access to it. Personal information is any information that identifies or could identify you. Personal information does not need to include your name and address to achieve this, as a birth date or postcode may be considered sufficient identification.

Information concerning a person's health that is protected by this law includes any notes about symptoms, diagnosis or treatment; specialist reports or test results; appointment and billing details; prescription and pharmaceutical purchases; dental records; genetic information; health-care identifier; and any other information concerning a person's race, sexuality or religion.

Furthermore, the *Privacy Act* protects a person's health information from unexpected uses beyond the sphere of their health care, such as health or medical research (Office of the Australian Information Commissioner 2022a). The Privacy Commissioner has approved legally binding guidelines issued by the National Health and Medical Research Council (NHMRC) concerning the handling of health information for research purposes. These guidelines are laid out in the National Statement on Ethical Conduct in Human Research (NHMRC 2018).

All organisations that provide a health service, other than public health services, are bound by the *Privacy Act*, whether they are private health institutions or small businesses – such as home nursing organisations or agencies, physiotherapists or natural therapists. Public hospitals and health services within individual states and territories of Australia are not covered by the Act, but instead are bound by state or territory legislation, for example, in New South Wales that is the *Health Records and Information Privacy Act 2002* (see the Appendix for a table of state and territory legislation).

Confidentiality

Confidentiality and privacy are related, and are often talked about interchangeably. But while they are associated ethical concepts, they should not be confused, and it is important for nurses to differentiate them. While confidentiality is a practice underpinned by ethical principles, an individual's right to privacy is enshrined in law.

To confide in someone is to trust information to them, or to disclose personal information while relying on their maintaining secrecy about it. Requests to keep information to yourself or to contain it 'between us' are very common. There is a strong cultural or social practice around confidentiality. However, not all information that is confidential (that is, shared only between certain, specified, parties) is required to be kept confidential by law. For example, if a patient asks you not to tell their family that have been outside the ward to smoke a cigarette, you are not under a legal obligation to keep that kind of information confidential. There is nothing private, in the relevant legal sense, of smoking a cigarette in a public place. However, personal information that is specified in the *Privacy Act* of either the Commonwealth or the relevant state or territory must not be shared (except as permitted under the Act), and in that sense it is confidential. Much information about patients to which a nurse will have access will be private and legally required to be kept confidential.

Although nurses are bound by privacy legislation concerning the management of patient information in order to protect patients' rights, a clinical relationship with a patient requires a nurse to have access to certain information about patients. Furthermore, a nurse has a duty to share that information with other health professionals who also have clinical responsibilities to the patient. That said, the right to access this information carries corresponding obligations and duties of confidentiality for the nurse.

The ethical management of patient information is reflected in the ICN Code of Ethics for Nurses, which states the nurse's moral obligation:

> Confidentiality refers to the duty of the nurse to refrain from sharing patient information with third parties unrelated to the patient's care. Confidentiality is a limited duty, sometimes it may be overridden by law or regulation, e.g. mandated reporting of specific diseases. (ICN 2021: 24)

The legal observance of the principle of confidentiality, then, is that information about a patient belongs to the patient. If a nurse considers that this information should be disclosed further, the patient remains in control of whether and to whom it is disclosed. The patient has the right to determine what information is disclosed, to whom and who else besides this person may know it. In this way, the patient's right to privacy is respected. When collecting and documenting information from patients, nurses need to communicate clearly to patients that personal information acquired from them will be documented and available for other health professionals to read. Be aware that, at this point in the procedure, the patient has a right to withhold information, refuse examination or part of an examination, or request that some specific information be withheld from their formal patient record.

Privacy and confidentiality are related to a patient's legal as well as moral right to privacy, and ultimately are framed by the principle of autonomy, which requires that patients be respected as being in charge of themselves, their choices and their actions – provided these do not seriously impinge on the moral interests of others (Beauchamp & Childress 2019; see also Chapter 4). When nurses make promises to maintain confidentiality, they must therefore be aware that maintaining confidentiality is their professional responsibility but may not be justified if the consequences of doing so are harmful to others. For instance, if a patient discloses that they are going to be a suicide bomber and requests this information be kept confidential, a nurse is ethically justified in disclosing this information in the public's best interest. However, if a child discloses to a nurse that they are the subject of sexual abuse, the nurse is required by law to disclose this information in a formal report to child protection authorities and is ethically justified in disclosing the information because it is in the child's best interests (see the section on mandatory reporting below).

THE RIGHT TO CONFIDENTIALITY

The Code of Conduct for Nurses in Australia suggests that maintaining confidentiality is a fluid concept that requires nurses to continually assess the situation and make ethical decisions concerning its maintenance:

> [Nurses] respect the confidentiality and privacy of people by seeking informed consent before disclosing information, including formally documenting such consent where possible. (NMBA 2018b: 11)

Clearly, nurses need to exercise discretion about who needs to know information about the patient for the therapeutic benefit of the patient, as well as the extent of disclosure that will be necessary.

The minimum judgement a nurse must make concerns what information revealed by a patient about their health is relevant to share with other health professionals *for the patient's benefit.* This requires some sorting of information, together with professional judgement about the extent to which it is noted, documented and/or verbalised. Nurses need to differentiate information that should remain confidential from information that may be shared freely with key stakeholders.

REFLECTIVE QUESTIONS 7.2

John is a 63-year-old man who has been admitted to hospital for a hip replacement. While the nurse was helping him to shower, he described pain he had been experiencing in his hip at night when lying on his back. In the conversation about sleeplessness that followed, John also told her how he was plagued with regret about having sold his mother's jewellery when he was strapped for cash. When the physiotherapist arrives, the nurse tells her that John is having pain in his hip and that he can't sleep because he's feeling guilty about his mother's jewellery.

1 Was it appropriate for the nurse to tell the physiotherapist about John's hip pain?
2 Was it appropriate to tell her about the jewellery?
3 What criteria would you use to decide which information was appropriate to tell or not to tell?

Generally, patients perceive that the sharing of information is for their benefit, and they trust nurses and other health professionals to act with discretion concerning confidential information, and to act in their best interests. Trust is therefore an essential component of the flow of information necessary in a patient's care and management. (Trust will also be discussed in Chapter 8.)

THE ROLE AND LIMITS OF TRUST

The rules of confidentiality are rooted in a set of values within nursing and other health-care professions that regard trust as important within the nurse–patient relationship. Confidentiality is vital to the preservation of trust between nurses and patients in that it serves to improve patient welfare. But it does not just preserve trust between individual nurses and their patients, it also serves to promote public trust in nurses and other health professionals in general. Trust, as has been argued extensively, is the moral foundation of the nursing profession (Peter & Morgan 2001: 4; Rutherford 2014). People who seek the help of nurses, or who by circumstance end up in the care of nurses within an institution or in their own homes, are considered vulnerable. Their vulnerability may relate to physical or psychological incapacity, or it may be related to having shared information about themselves that is of a very private or intimate nature.

LAW AND ETHICS IN PRACTICE

Imagine you are someone famous who is well known in public – for example, a rock star, TV personality or politician. You need to attend a special clinic because you have a sexually transmitted disease or a drug addiction, or some other condition that is socially stigmatised. Imagine how vulnerable you would feel about the information that the clinic staff now have about you – even if the information is no more detailed than the fact that you attended the clinic for consultation. You must trust that the staff at the clinic will use their absolute discretion, for this loss of control means you are open to such harms as embarrassment, shame and prejudice. You are reliant on their professional duty of confidentiality for your continued privacy, your personal safety and perhaps your continued career.

》 **What kind of things would you expect the nurses to do and say in order to earn your trust?**

What does it mean for a nurse to be regarded as trustworthy in relation to the possession of confidential information about a patient? Banks and Gallagher (2009: 140) suggest that trustworthiness is a relational virtue. In their view, it is not simply a matter of patients blindly trusting nurses with information; rather, as a relationship forms between nurse and patient, each party establishes the trustworthiness of the other. When a patient reveals confidential information to a nurse in the process of care, this usually indicates that they have judged that nurse to be trustworthy. Likewise, in receiving information from a patient, a nurse usually judges whether this information is trustworthy to act upon in diagnosis and treatment. There are cultural factors at play as well. As Banks and Gallagher (2009: 145) point out:

> Built into the role of 'nurse' is the requirement to be trustworthy, and built into the hospital systems are procedures and programmes for vetting and educating nurses.

Thus, trustworthiness and reliability are elements rooted in the very meaning of what it is to be a nurse, and essential ingredients in the rules of confidentiality. If nurses generally began sharing confidential information indiscriminately and without regard for patients' privacy and human rights, there would soon be a change in the behaviour of patients, and they would be less willing to share their intimate details.

WAYS OF PROTECTING PRIVACY

In order to maintain high standards concerning the management of private and confidential patient information, we must all contribute to being vigilant and sustaining an environment in which patients' privacy is protected.

REFLECTIVE QUESTION 7.3

One evening, for educational purposes, a nurse, Keva, attended an after-hours nurses' meeting in the diabetes outpatient clinic of a hospital in which she is not employed. On the counter-top, a series of patient files were placed ready for the first clinic the next morning. Keva did not open the files, but could hardly miss seeing the patients' names as they were boldly scribed in Texta on the outside. She recognised one file as belonging to her neighbour and, with surprise, realised her neighbour may be diabetic.

Is this acceptable management of patient files?

Within institutions, private patient information is shared in myriad ways, including the use of whiteboards, video-conferencing, fax machines and electronic file transfers. Care must be taken with the handling of paper patient files so that they are not left open where they can accidentally be viewed or left in public places where they are accessible to visitors or others who may be curious. All people accessing a patient's notes should carry some form of identification that authorises them to have access. If they are not displaying this, they should be asked to identify themselves and state their reason for accessing patient files. Information about patients – including discussion of their cases, handovers or ward meetings – should occur in a private and restricted area. This is also the best area for the fax machine.

Inadvertent breaches of confidentiality

Inadvertent breaches of confidentiality are potentially commonplace in health institutions and typically occur through error, complacency, carelessness or thoughtlessness, and they may be intensified by structural or cultural problems in the clinic or hospital environment, including common practices that have gone unchallenged.

Arguably, health institutions exhibit a culture of lax attention to privacy and confidentiality. In a study of medical students more than a decade ago, Jethwa et al. (2009) reported poor observance of confidentiality and practices that breached confidentiality. Patient records were extremely accessible, and it was rare for students and others to be questioned about accessing them (2009: 329). Patient confidentiality was breached through routine practices such as case presentations where identifying information about the patient was copied into notebooks and carried in the doctor's pocket, sometimes discarded into the trash and even taken into the home environment (2009: 330). A more recent study of medical students found an estimated frequency of one breach of patient confidentiality per 62.5 hours. Severe breaches were the most frequent, making up almost 50 per cent of all breaches. Largely, the incidences of breaching confidentiality took place in public areas such as corridors, stairwells, lifts and the cafeteria (Beltran-Aroca et al. 2016).

Common nursing practices give rise to similar issues. Nurses routinely note details about a patient's diagnosis, their immediate care and social observations at staff handover, and carry this in their pockets for rapid reference when at a distance from the office where patient records are stored. This practice also raises the possibility that nurses may lose the paper or inadvertently take it home or discard it into publicly accessible trash. Handover may be communicated by voice recordings, and the recordings mishandled or overheard by other patients or visitors. The nursing practice of handover, while an essential communication among nurses and often involving the patient to their benefit, especially if conducted at the bedside or in the corridor, also runs the risk of confidential information being overheard by other patients, their visitors or other employees, such as cleaners and domestics.

Nurses (and others) who inadvertently breach confidentiality may be subject to disciplinary action by their employer. This may range from a stern 'talking to' but without any documentation to an incident report being lodged and a note being entered in their workplace file. It is unlikely that a nurse would lose their employment over a minor breach, but if the impact of a breach was serious, then a more serious response would be likely.

Practices become routine and are sometimes altered for convenience, particularly in large institutions. However, vigilance is required and practices need constant review to maintain standards of confidentiality. In the recent controversy in Australia regarding the introduction of My Health Record (discussed in more detail below), health-care workers were reported as being concerned about inappropriate access to these electronic health records due to a lax culture of security in which computer logins and passwords were shared and computers left open for long periods, making them accessible to passers-by (Bogle & Willis 2018). Clearly, a concerted effort needs to be made at the individual professional level, as well as at the institutional or management level, to overcome institutional traditions and professional complacency concerning confidentiality.

REFLECTIVE QUESTION 7.4

Jody and Mia are having a conversation about work on the train going home. Mia is debriefing about a patient admitted that day with huge pressure sores and bruises that suggested she had been neglected by her husband and carers. Mia is careful not to mention the patient's name and refers to her by her initials, JK. Mia has taken a photograph of the patient's extensively bruised legs and pulls out her mobile phone to show Jody. She has been careful not to include the patient's face in the photograph. Jody is shocked by the patient's condition and the pair continue to discuss the patient's husband, describing his behaviour and his conversation with the patient.

Has the patient JK's confidentiality and privacy been preserved here? Apply what you have learned about professional duties of confidentiality and privacy and note the reasons for your answer.

There are several myths surrounding the practice of confidentiality. Many health professionals believe that so long as a patient's name isn't mentioned, their confidentiality is protected. However, a person's identity and private information do not rely on name alone, and many other features of a story can identify someone if they are spoken about in a public place. Have you ever noticed in old medical or nursing textbooks photographs of patients as examples of various medical conditions, usually with a black rectangle covering their eyes? A similar practice exists in the television media today, with footage of people with their faces pixelated. This is an attempt at maintaining their privacy; however, it is a poor practice that leaves people vulnerable to being recognised by their other features (such as tattoos, scars, gait, hairstyle or body shape).

Maintaining confidentiality is more complex than it is typically perceived to be and requires nurses to act thoughtfully about sharing any aspect of patient information. For example, in assisted reproductive technology (ART) clinics, patients are sensitive about others in their social network or family knowing about their infertility and their participation in the in vitro fertilisation (IVF) program. A social stigma still exists in relation to not being able to become pregnant, making infertile women vulnerable to social pressure.

LAW AND ETHICS IN PRACTICE

Anne-Marie (a nurse in the ART clinic), Magda (a patient in the ART clinic) and Amy are all members of the same social group. Magda's two friends knew she was having IVF treatment to become pregnant, and they had talked about it together over coffee. So, without checking first, Anne-Marie thought it was okay to tell Amy that she had seen Magda that morning when she came to the clinic for her treatment. However, Magda had experienced pressure from Amy during previous treatments, and had not wanted her to know she was having treatment *at this specific time*. When Amy rang Magda to ask whether she was pregnant from the treatment, Magda learned of the breach of her confidentiality and reported Anne-Marie to the nursing and midwifery board in her state.

>> How can you ensure a clear and safe distinction between what you can say outside of work and on social media, and what you can say in your capacity as a nursing professional?

As a result of her inadvertent disclosure and a formal complaint about her conduct, Anne-Marie was subject to an investigation of her professional practice. This case is an example of the ways in which confidentiality can have subtle undertones, and of how practising confidentiality as a professional nurse requires clear communication, thoughtfulness and sensitivity.

Deliberate breaches of confidentiality

Unlike inadvertent disclosure, a breach of patient confidentiality may be deliberate but ethically unjustified. For example, an anonymous author reported that a hospital in the United Kingdom had initiated an internal review that involved a deliberate breach of confidentiality by a nurse (EMAP Publishing Limited 2010). It was alleged that, after the admission of a 16-year-old girl who requested that the reason for her admission not be revealed (complications following an abortion procedure), a nurse caring for her telephoned the girl's mother to disclose the circumstances of her admission. As a consequence, the patient was thrown out of home because her mother held strong anti-abortion views. It was revealed that the nurse was a friend of the patient's aunt, and possibly perceived some obligation to the family. Yet, perhaps in being concerned to protect her, she effectively breached the patient's trust and in so doing unwittingly brought about an adverse outcome for the patient.

This is an example of a serious and unjustified breach of confidentiality and trust by a nurse. The matter of maintaining confidentiality in the case of a person aged under 18 is a complex one. Whether confidentiality can be maintained as requested, or whether it should be breached for the best interests of the child, depends largely on whether the person is legally considered to be a minor in relation to consent processes. (See Chapter 4 for a discussion of children and consent.) There are circumstances when it is not only ethically acceptable to breach confidentiality, but also a legal requirement to do so.

When can or must confidentiality be breached?

Historically, the rule of confidentiality tended to be viewed as an absolute promise by professionals to protect information about a patient. The medical profession, for instance, promoted practices of patient record destruction to avoid breaches of confidentiality. Lawyers and priests were protected from being forced to disclose potentially incriminating information about a client or member of their congregation. Rather than reveal a source when required by a court of law, journalists were prepared to spend time in jail for contempt of court. This view of confidentiality as absolute has been widely portrayed in movies and television programs. However, it should be noted that there is no legal privilege for information disclosed in confidence to a nurse or other health professional. If necessary, a court of law may order release of that information through a subpoena, through a police officer demand with a warrant, or through a demand issued by a statutory investigative authority by virtue of its statutory powers.

Therefore, as Beauchamp and Childress (2019: 16) point out, in health care the principle of confidentiality is at best *prima facie* – that is, it is not an absolute moral obligation, but may be overridden by more serious moral considerations. This means that if the consequences of maintaining confidentiality benefit the patient at no cost to others, then it is justified. But if maintaining a patient's confidentiality will put others at significant risk, it is not justified. In other words, where innocent people may be harmed by a failure to disclose information that may protect them, the call to breach confidentiality is morally compelling. For example, where health-care professionals are aware that a person who has a positive HIV status is continuing to have unprotected sex, they have a duty to intervene in the interests of the vulnerable person. Importantly, Beauchamp and Childress (2019: 16) also note that 'a prima facie obligation does not simply disappear when overridden'. Rather, an inability to meet an obligation can give rise to 'moral residue'. This concerns things that still require our moral attention, such as feelings of regret or conscience, or the need to apologise or inform a person that we cannot keep a promise we made to them.

'Duty to warn' or 'duty to protect'

LAW AND ETHICS IN PRACTICE

A young student, Poddar, was seen by a psychiatrist for depression after a relationship break-up. During a consultation with his psychiatrist, Poddar expressed his intention to kill his ex-girlfriend, Tarasoff. The psychiatrist was later informed by the patient's friend that the patient had bought a gun. The psychiatrist informed the university police that the patient might be a danger, but did not take it any further, believing it was his duty to maintain the patient's confidentiality. Two months later, Tarasoff was killed by Poddar.

》》 Find out about your workplace policy concerning this kind of situation, where a patient discloses that they intend to harm someone.

This case, *Tarasoff v Regents of the University of California* (1974), is now famous because of its impact on the way health professionals view confidentiality. In the judgment of this case, the California Supreme Court acknowledged the general rule that there is no duty for health professionals to control the conduct of another or to alert those endangered by such conduct. Nonetheless, it also recognised certain exceptions. In this case, neither Tarasoff nor her parents were warned of Poddar's threat, and were therefore unable to take protective action. In its final decision, the court judged that the psychiatrist Dr Moore had a 'duty to warn' Tarasoff of the danger that Poddar posed to her life (Cohen 1978: 153).

The duty to warn raises the possibility that nurses may not keep information confidential if they judge that harm may come to another from doing so. A difficulty arises from this because when a patient trusts the nurse to maintain their confidentiality, they will be more likely to reveal information that is vital to an accurate nursing assessment or medical diagnosis. Clearly, if nurses listened to patients and then spread this information indiscriminately, the public would cease to rate nurses as trustworthy professionals. They would likely tend to be wary about telling nurses anything at all that mattered to their treatment and care. Worse, they may avoid seeking the help of nurses at all. Likewise, other health professionals would grow wary of sharing private information about patients with nurses in the multidisciplinary team. As you can see, there is a risk that the whole fabric of health-care communication may collapse and become ineffective.

On the other hand, proponents of the duty to warn maintain that there is an obligation on the part of health professionals to warn identifiable individuals – and not just the police – of the risk of possible harm. The principles of non-maleficence and justice require that where significant harm to others may result from maintaining patient confidentiality, a nurse should seriously consider a duty to warn, and use their professional judgement to determine whether the benefits outweigh the harms of breaking a confidence.

REFLECTIVE QUESTION 7.5

Adam, a nurse, hasn't seen his friend Raphael in some weeks and calls around to his flat on the way to his afternoon shift. Raphael answers the door looking dishevelled and dressed in his pyjamas despite it being afternoon. Adam is surprised and asks Raphael whether he is unwell. Raphael breaks down and confides to Adam that his long-term partner broke up with him, that he feels 'very blue' and is thinking that life isn't worth it. He has a plan, he says, to 'end it all' and swears Adam to secrecy. He doesn't want to be labelled as having a mental illness. Adam tries to persuade Raphael to see his GP and offers to take him there, but Raphael declines.

What should Adam do?

Mandatory reporting

In some circumstances, nurses are compelled by law to disclose confidential information in order that appropriate decisions can be made for the protection of people in their care. Such disclosures are referred to as mandatory reporting. Although there are some variations between states and territories in Australia, reporting that requires a breach of confidentiality is required by law in the case of:

→ certain deaths, such as injuries involving firearms
→ diseases that seriously threaten public health
→ medical conditions that may result in harm to the public
→ professional misconduct by a practitioner registered with AHPRA
→ all crimes, including abuse and sexual abuse of children, the elderly in an aged care facility, or people receiving services under the National Disability Insurance Scheme (NDIS)
→ a reasonable suspicion of abuse of a child
→ a reasonable suspicion of abuse of an elderly person in an aged care facility, if you are employed at that facility
→ a reasonable suspicion of abuse by an NDIS service provider of a person receiving services under the NDIS
→ unauthorised use of restrictive practices on a person with a disability (under the NDIS)
→ in the Northern Territory, domestic violence.

REPORTABLE DEATHS

The Coroner is an official appointed by the government who determines the cause of death of persons within their jurisdiction. The Coroner is responsible for overseeing an investigation into the manner or cause of death, and confirming the dead person's identity. The Coroner's office maintains death records for its jurisdiction. All Australian states and territories have a Coroner and their own *Coroners Act*, which mandates the reporting of deaths that are unusual, unexpected, suspicious or violent, or where the death involves unnatural circumstances. While they are separate Acts, all require the same criteria as those listed below (see the Appendix for the legislation for each state and territory).

Reportable deaths are those where:

→ the death occurs during a medical procedure or following a medical procedure or anaesthetic, where the death may be causally related to the medical procedure and where the death would not reasonably be expected

→   a medical certificate stating the cause of death has not been signed

→   the person was a patient within the meaning of the *Mental Health Act*

→   the death occurred in custody

→   the identity of the deceased person is unknown

→   the death was unexpected

→   the death was violent or unnatural – for example, suicide, poisoning or homicide

→   the death resulted from an accident or injury – for example, a motor vehicle accident, a sporting injury or drowning

→   the death is otherwise specified in the *Coroners Act.*

The role of the Coroner is to investigate reportable deaths in order to identify the deceased (if unknown), determine the cause of death and make recommendations that lead to a reduction in preventable deaths. Police may assist the Coroner by obtaining information about the deceased person from any witnesses, including health-care staff, family and friends. It is the responsibility of a doctor to report a death arising from medical treatment; however, anyone who becomes aware of a reportable death must report it to a Coroner if they have reasonable grounds to believe it has not already been reported.

When a reportable death occurs in a health-care facility, it is advisable to retain *in situ* all medical and nursing apparatus, such as drains, intravenous cannulae, catheters, nasogastric tubes and endotracheal tubes, as well as any bags or syringes attached to these. However, in special circumstances, if a device presents a danger to staff handling the body, it may be removed. The person's body should not be washed, but left as it was at the time of death in order to allow examination and analysis by a forensic pathologist. The Coroner will also require the patient's medical records, any discharge summary and a death certificate, if it has been issued.

The Coroner's Court

When a death is reported to the Coroner, the Coroner's Court may conduct a coronial inquiry. The purpose of the inquiry is to provide a thorough and impartial investigation of the circumstances in which the reported death has occurred. If the inquiry determines that the death is a criminal matter, the case will be referred to another court for a criminal trial. However, the Coroner does not make findings of guilt against any individual or group.

It is not unusual for deaths that relate to health care to be reported by a doctor or by the police. The Coroner may call health-care practitioners (including nurses) to give evidence at an inquiry. The health-care practitioner may be asked to explain any notes that they recorded about the patient, as well as their recollection of the circumstances. For this reason, it is very important to always make accurate documentation of the care you deliver, and to pay particular attention to accurately recording events surrounding the death of patients in your care. While the Coroner may not find evidence of criminal behaviour, a health-care practitioner can be referred to a disciplinary body and may be liable for a civil action. The Coroner may also make comment and recommendations in relation to the conduct of health-care practitioners and/or institutional practices. The findings of the Coroner are made publicly available on the websites of the Coroner's Courts.

CHILD ABUSE AND NEGLECT

In Australia, there is a legal requirement placed upon nurses as a professional group (as well as other specified people) to report suspected cases of child abuse or neglect. Mandated reporting is a symbolic acknowledgement of the seriousness of child abuse, but it also reinforces the moral responsibility of nurses, along with others who work with families, children and youth, to take action to protect children from harm. Mandatory reporting laws clearly define the types of situations that must be reported to child protection services. Child abuse includes physical injury, emotional abuse, physical or emotional neglect and sexual abuse. As a nurse, you have grounds for reporting suspected abuse if:

→ a person tells you that a child has been abused or neglected
→ a child tells you that they have been abused or neglected
→ your own observations of a child give you reason to believe that the child has been abused or neglected.

Although the people compelled to report, and the types of abuse to be reported, vary between states and territories in Australia, all jurisdictions have mandatory reporting requirements. The threshold for reporting child abuse differs between states and territories (see the Appendix for a table of legislation).

The mandatory requirement to report suspicions of child abuse concerns all children up to the age of 18 years; however, New South Wales is an exception. In New South Wales, it is not mandatory to report suspected abuse in young people aged 16 or 17, and in Victoria it is not mandatory to report suspected abuse in young people aged 17 (AIFS 2020). The Northern Territory's *Care and Protection of Children Act 2007* has specific mandatory requirements relating to sexual activity involving people aged below than 14 years, those aged 14–15 years and those aged 16–17 years.

COMPULSORY REPORTING OF ELDER ABUSE

Elderly people are particularly vulnerable to abuse. An elderly patient's vulnerability may relate to a reduced ability to safeguard their own interests, such as when suffering physical disability or dementia, or it may relate to their feeling of powerlessness about their condition or their stay in an institution, such as an aged-care facility or hospital, or their need to have family or strangers care for them in their own home (Kaspiew et al. 2016). Elder abuse is 'a single or repeated act, or lack of appropriate action, occurring within any relationship where there is an expectation of trust that causes harm or distress to an older person' (WHO 2021). Elder abuse may include financial exploitation, neglect, sexual abuse and/or behaviours intended to harm the individual.

In 2006, it was revealed on the Australian Broadcasting Corporation's *Lateline* TV program that several residents of an aged-care facility in Victoria had been sexually assaulted (O'Neill 2006). As a result, changes were made to the *Aged Care Act 1997* by the *Aged Care Amendment (Security and Protection) Act 2007*. This Act now incorporates compulsory reporting of physical or sexual assaults by staff, residents or others to the Aged Care Quality and Safety Commission (ACQSC). The office must investigate any complaints in a breach of care, including incidents concerning sexual and physical assault.

Allegations or suspicions of unlawful sexual contact with a resident of an aged-care facility or unreasonable use of force with a resident must be reported to the police and the Department of Social Services within 24 hours (ACQSC 2022). Providers of aged care are required to report allegations or suspicions of elder abuse, and must in many instances rely on the moral integrity of their nursing staff to alert them to these circumstances. They are also required to take reasonable measures to protect the identity of any staff member who makes a report, as well as to protect them from victimisation. It has been argued (Kaspiew et al. 2016) that, rather than being confined to those people in residential care, elder abuse should be subject to equal or similar mandatory reporting requirements to those established for child protection in Australia – in other words, there should be a model of protection established for the elderly. This was a subject of debate during the 2019 Royal Commission into Aged Care Quality and Safety (Royal Commission into Aged Care Quality and Safety 2021).

COMPULSORY REPORTING UNDER THE NDIS

People living with disability are subject to high rates of violence, and many are counted among the groups of people who are most vulnerable to interpersonal, organisational and institutional violence (Royal Commission into Violence, Abuse and Exploitation of People With Disability 2022). In 2016, the Australian Bureau of Statistics (ABS) estimated conservatively that people with a disability were sexually assaulted at a rate of at least twice that of the overall national rate, and women were affected at seven times the rate of men (Australian Bureau of Statistics 2016). However, there has never been a formal attempt to estimate the actual rates of violence experienced by people living with disability.

In accordance with the *NDIS Act 2013*, the NDIS Quality and Safeguards Commission requires that all registered NDIS providers notify the Commission of all reportable incidents (including alleged reportable incidents). If you are working in a role where you have registered to provide services to a person through the NDIS, you will be subject to these reporting requirements.

The NDIS Quality and Safeguards Commission advises that for an incident to be reportable, a certain act or event needs to have happened (or be alleged to have happened) in connection with the provision of supports or services. This includes:

→ unlawful sexual or physical contact with, or assault of, an NDIS participant
→ sexual misconduct committed against, or in the presence of, an NDIS participant, including grooming of the NDIS participant for sexual activity
→ unauthorised use of restrictive practices.

If you have a reasonable suspicion that abuse has occurred, you are required to report it to your supervisor immediately. Your service management must report the incident to the NDIS Commission within 24 hours, using the NDIS Commission Portal. If you do not have a supervisor – for example, if you are providing services as an independent practitioner – you are required to report through the NDIS Commission Portal within 24 hours. The exception is misuse of restrictive practices. You have five days to report this.

You can obtain more information about lodging an incident report by contacting the NDIS at reportableincidents@ndiscommission.gov.au or by phoning 1800 035 544 during business hours.

Mandatory or compulsory reporting requirements can create ethical issues for nurses and other health professionals. The trust established in a nurse–patient/family relationship may be damaged by a report to authorities of suspected child or elder abuse. Indeed, the integrity and therapeutic potential of the relationship may be undermined, leaving nurses unable to provide interventions for the 'at-risk' child or older person. There is also a risk that nurses will become less sensitive to patient confidentiality and over-zealous about reporting any signs that might be interpreted as abuse in order to avoid legal liability. On the other hand, if suspicions are not reported, intervention for the person's benefit may not be possible. Reporting is further complicated by power relations in the workplace and diversity in the interpretation of what constitutes abuse.

COMMUNICABLE DISEASES

The Commonwealth government and all states and territories have mandatory reporting of diseases that present a risk to public health, called 'communicable diseases' (see the Appendix for a list of legislation). The Office of Health Protection and Response within the Australian Government Department of Health conducts national and international surveillance of communicable diseases, and provides advice on policies and actions to minimise the impact of these diseases on the community. It is a requirement that the medical officer report any case of communicable disease.

FIREARMS

Each state and territory has legislation that regulates the ownership, licensing and use of firearms. This legislation may include mandatory reporting of firearms injuries (for example, South Australia), but requirements differ between jurisdictions. All states and territories protect health professionals from civil action if they report that a person to whom they have been providing a professional service possesses or has access to a firearm, and the health professional believes that this person may pose a threat to public safety or to the person's own safety. However, some jurisdictions mandate this reporting. In the Northern Territory, section 101 of the *Firearms Act 1996* requires a health practitioner or social worker to report to the police if and why they believe that a person is not fit and proper to have a firearm in their possession or control. In South Australia, regulation 96 of the Firearms Regulations (2017) under the *Firearms Act 2015* requires:

> medical practitioners, nurses, psychologists, professional counsellors, or social workers, to make a report when they suspect that a patient is suffering from a physical or mental illness, and there is a threat to the patient's own safety or the safety of another person from the patient's possession of, or intention to acquire, a firearm. (SA Health 2012)

MEDICAL CONDITIONS CAUSING PUBLIC RISK

Rules pertaining to who can drive a motor vehicle have been developed by a range of medical experts, and agreed to by the driver licensing authorities in each state and territory. These standards are set out by Austroads (2022) in the document *Assessing Fitness to Drive*. A range of medical conditions, as well as treatments, may impair driving ability. These include:

→ disorders involving blackouts or fainting
→ sleep disorders
→ vision problems
→ diabetes
→ epilepsy
→ some psychiatric disorders
→ some heart conditions
→ certain medications.

Individuals suffering from these conditions or taking the medications of concern are legally required to inform the driver licensing authority in their state or territory. Nurses and other health practitioners are advised, but not mandated, to report drivers to the driver licensing authority in their state when they know the drivers have these conditions or are taking such medications. The driver licensing authority deals with all such reports confidentially, and makes the final decision about whether a person should retain a driving licence after they have considered the advice of the person's doctor as well as other factors, such as the driver's accident history and the type of vehicle being driven – for example, a truck, car or public passenger vehicle (Austroads 2022).

MANDATORY REPORTING OF HEALTH-CARE PRACTITIONERS BY HEALTH-CARE PRACTITIONERS

The Australian Health Practitioner Regulation Agency (AHPRA) requires mandatory reporting by all registered health practitioners and their employers when they have a reasonable belief that a practitioner has engaged in 'notifiable conduct' – that is, if the practitioner has:

→ practised the profession while intoxicated by alcohol or drugs
→ engaged in sexual misconduct in connection with the practice of their profession
→ placed the public at risk of substantial harm in the practice of the profession because they have an impairment

➜ placed the public at risk of harm because they have practised in a way that constitutes a significant departure from accepted professional standards (AHPRA 2020a).

The obligation to report requires a nurse to report the notifiable conduct not only of other nurses, but also of other health professionals. However, any report made must take into account 'accepted professional standards', and the reporting party must understand and articulate how the notifiable conduct 'significantly' departs from these professional standards.

In relation to nursing and midwifery, AHPRA has developed guidelines for mandatory notifications of registered health professionals under the National Law. These guidelines advise that:

> Section 237 of the National Law provides protection from civil, criminal and administrative liability, including defamation, for people making notifications in good faith. However, if you make a notification that is vexatious or not in good faith, you may be subject to regulatory action (such as, for example, a caution). The National Law clarifies that making a notification is not a breach of professional etiquette or ethics, or a departure from accepted standards of professional conduct. It is consistent with professional conduct and a practitioner's ethical responsibilities. Privacy obligations do not prevent you from making a mandatory or voluntary notification. (AHPRA 2020a)

In Australian culture, this mandated form of reporting may seem like nurses are invited to 'dob in a mate'. But such a policy is primarily designed to protect the public from harm. This is why the threshold for notifiable conduct and mandatory reporting is high – requiring a 'reasonable belief' founded in knowledge rather than mere suspicion, rumour, gossip or innuendo. Nurses have an obligation to take their role in protecting the public very seriously.

Challenges to maintaining confidentiality

Nurses are required to be vigilant about confidentiality; however, it is sometimes difficult to maintain confidentiality in institutions where the system or culture can interfere. Historically, in commenting on codes of medical ethics, Siegler (1994, cited in Beauchamp & Childress 1994: 330) argued that patient confidentiality is a 'decrepit concept', noting that in practice it is often violated and widely ignored. He cited a case where, despite having had a simple surgical procedure, a patient's notes were accessed by over a hundred people in the process of his care. Thirty years later, Anesi (2012) concluded that if anything has changed, it is that even more people are likely to access a patient's notes and confidentiality faces many more threats.

However, Anesi argues that new ways of addressing confidentiality now exist. This raises questions for nurses in practice: with whom should nurses share a patient's private information? How should they share it – should it be shared verbally, or by email, by SMS text or in nurses' notes?

Siegler (1994, cited in Anesi 2012) argued that information should only be shared on a 'need to know' basis. But how should nurses decide this? The judgements nurses make about who should share patient information, and how widely it should be distributed or how well it should be contained, are complicated by modern technology, such as computers, telephones, video-conferencing and other electronic communication. Anesi (2012) argues, however, that this is a challenge of patient beneficence and not a reason to ignore confidentiality.

COMPUTERISED PATIENT INFORMATION-MANAGEMENT SYSTEMS

Most institutions employ computerised patient information-management systems in combination with paper patient records that can be accessed by various practitioners in the process of caring for a patient. However, in Australia, as in other countries, there is a move towards patient records that are only electronic.

Electronic patient-record software stores a patient's medical history in a way that can be accessed by doctors, nurses and paramedics. This form of storage and access is argued to have several advantages, such as the speed and ease with which nurses and other practitioners can access a person's records. It is also expected to improve safety outcomes when patients are transferred from one institution to another, and will reduce issues arising from poor handwriting.

Electronic patient data are more easily managed than paper files. For example, information can be cross-referenced for internal consistency and accuracy, and all professionals involved in the patient's care can access the same information. Electronic health records can also link clinicians and patients who are geographically distant from each other. One important advantage of a single electronic health record is that the patient record remains intact wherever the patient travels and whichever health-care professional is consulted. On the other hand, it is evident that computerised systems have systematically failed to adequately protect confidential information. In 2018, the personal and medical information of 1.5 million people in Singapore was stolen by cyberhackers (Kim 2018). Medical records are a rich source of personal information and a valuable source of identity theft, likely to fetch a high price on the dark web.

MY HEALTH RECORD

In 2016, the Australian Government introduced My Health Record, a computerised database of individuals' health records that can be accessed and updated by the patient themself but is also accessible to health-care practitioners, who can add information. The Australian Digital Health Agency believes that the My Health Record 'can transform quality, experience and value in Australia's health-care system through a range of important benefits' (Australian Digital Health Agency 2019a). The key benefits claimed for My Health Record are that:

→ adverse drug events can be avoided
→ patient management and outcomes can be improved through clinician efficiency and accuracy
→ the time spent gathering information can be reduced and duplication avoided (Australian Digital Health Agency 2019a).

However, the introduction of My Health Record has been controversial. Following an announcement that everyone would have a My Health Record, members of the Australian public raised many concerns about their privacy and right to determine who had access to their record. Public trust was low, with fewer than two in 1000 people registering for a record when asked to do so (Kemp et al. 2018). Initially, privacy and security measures were minimal and there were risks related to the transmission and storage of digital information. The Australian Government has addressed public trust and concerns about privacy by ensuring security via strong encryption, firewalls, secure login processes and audit logging, and there is currently a process in place for people to opt out of the My Health Record system (Australian Digital Health Agency 2019b).

It has been argued that electronic patient-record keeping is inevitable and offers many benefits to the larger health-care system because these systems are an important source of information for clinical, research and policy questions (Perera et al. 2011). For example, electronic systems may allow 'meaningful use' by providers (such as the Department of Health) in order to monitor and achieve significant improvements in care within and across institutions (Blumenthal & Tavenner 2010). They may also provide increased data protection since they are backed up regularly and password protected. However, electronic records make peering into a patient's records easier because intruders don't have to physically access the patient's paper notes (Anesi 2012). As is evident, for example, from the experience of the government introducing digital records in Australia, privacy of health information is a prominent concern of the public, patients and health-care providers (Pang et al. 2020).

Paradoxically, the very characteristics seen to be sources of concern for health information privacy are also strengths in regulating patient privacy. Electronic records make the tracking of who accesses them inappropriately far easier. In South Australia a hospital audit revealed that nine patients had their records 'spied on' (that is, unauthorised access) by 21 clinicians in a 12-month period. What is unclear in reports of this unprofessional conduct is whether patients were advised that their privacy and confidentiality had been breached (Crouch & Wills 2016). Of these 21 clinicians, 13 had accessed the patient records of Cy Walsh, who had been accused of the stabbing death of his father, a prominent AFL football coach, and admitted for psychiatric care. All 13 clinicians were suspended and disciplined.

Electronic patient information may therefore be more vulnerable to misuse, misinterpretation and, worse, inappropriate distribution via social media. Take, for example, another case of reported professional misconduct. In this case, 49 staff were investigated after accessing information about a patient who had an eel removed from inside him at a major city hospital in New Zealand. Only 13 of those staff were accessing information as part of direct care, and 33 people were found to be merely snooping. Some staff had distributed images outside the hospital, including to the media. All those staff were reported to their respective professional bodies (Johnson 2013). There is significant further research needed to assess the impact of the use of electronic record systems on patient safety, whether that be positive or negative (Li et al 2021).

Electronic patient records exhibit other problems for nurses in the clinical or primary health-care setting. For example, if the electronic system fails for any period of time, it means that staff will not be able to access patient records at all, and this can result in chaos and potential for harm to patients. This occurred in South Australia in 2016 (*ABC News* 2016). Health system administrators have multifaceted protective mechanisms in place to try to avoid this problem.

DIGITAL CAMERAS AND OTHER ELECTRONIC COMMUNICATION

Today, many health-care professionals – including nurses – carry mobile phones, and some institutions provide a digital camera for the taking of images (of a wound, for example) for comparison of healing progress or teaching, or for recording bruises or other forensic evidence. This means that any health professional can become a 'medical photographer' (Burns & Belton 2012). However, it also means that patients are vulnerable to breaches of privacy and confidentiality, since maintaining confidentiality regarding images is more complex and requires nurses to act more thoughtfully as images may be more identifying than text. A further complexity arises if patients and/or their relatives are taking photos or recordings of each other because they may inadvertently photograph other patients. For this reason, personal photography is normally not permitted in clinical settings.

Nurses must also be aware of, and sensitive to, the potential for breaches of confidentiality and privacy inherent in the use of social media. Students of nursing worldwide are being disciplined for inappropriate behaviour on Facebook, and for breaches of patient confidentiality and lapses of professionalism in relation to their 'online presence, footprints or image' (Jones & Hayter 2013).

Telephones are widely used in the provision of health care, especially in rural and remote areas of Australia. It is a very common experience for nurses to answer the telephone and attend to a caller who is inquiring about the welfare and condition of a patient. However, disclosing information via the telephone carries considerable risk. Take, for example, the events following a prank call by two Sydney radio broadcasters to King Edward VII hospital in the United Kingdom. In this now-infamous scandal, the radio broadcasters impersonated the Queen and received intimate details regarding the condition of Catherine, Duchess of Cambridge. They then aired those details on radio. Following this prank, the nurse involved in the disclosure of information took her own life. There followed a revision of telephone protocols, a court inquiry in the United Kingdom, personal harm to the radio personalities and damaged inter-country relations (Evans 2012).

Over the telephone, nurses cannot be certain to whom they are speaking, whether others are listening or whether the conversation is being overheard or even recorded. Similarly, email communication is vulnerable to exposure to others and further distribution – either intentionally or inadvertently. Assessing the identity of phone callers is highly complex, and the call should end in one of two ways: either staff disclose details without any solid proof of the caller's identity, or they refuse steadfastly to disclose any details at all to telephone callers. This latter course of action can make life difficult for relatives living overseas or at a distance when their family member is seriously ill. McKinstry et al. (2009) reported that patients expressed concerns that included anxiety about telephone conversations being overheard due to the use of mobile phones in public places, telephones in open work environments or a lack of privacy in the home. When phoning a patient to relay results or to inquire about their well-being or condition, it is therefore wise, before commencing a consultation, to seek information about whether they are comfortable with their environment. A further concern for confidentiality was the use of telephone answering services and caller identification. Leaving a message, even simply to return your call and a telephone number, may be enough to breach a person's confidentiality (2009: 346–7). The Office of the Australian Information Commissioner (2022b) has advice for clinicians about communications with patients.

SOCIAL MEDIA AND PROFESSIONALISM

In recent years, there has been an increase in the use of social media such as Facebook, Instagram and Twitter. Social media is now widely used, including by many health professionals, with Facebook alone being reported as having almost three billion active users each month (Statista 2022). The rapid growth of social media has given rise to the concept of 'e-professionalism' – that is, professional attitudes and behaviour on social media (Barnable et al. 2018: 28). While Facebook has many benefits for nurses, such as for learning and sharing information, there have also been incidents of inappropriate use of social media by nurses and other health professionals. Such unprofessional activity includes posting private patient information; material such as sexually explicit photos, drinking or drug use about themselves; profanity; and negative comments about patients, colleagues and peers, work environments and the profession in general (Barnable et al. 2018). Boundary concerns have also emerged, with nurses being asked to 'friend' patients or vice versa, raising issues regarding the blurring of personal and professional positions. Nurses need to take great care in accepting a friend request from someone who has been or is a patient, and should not send a friend request to a patient or former patient. It is very important for all nurses to be aware that employers, potential employers and professional regulators may have access to personal Facebook and Instagram postings.

Conclusion

Collecting personal information from and about patients carries important legal and moral obligations. Confidentiality is an ethical concept that is difficult to fully maintain in health-care settings because of the complexities of communication within the modern health-care environment. Confidentiality is at best a *prima facie* right, which means that nurses must exercise informed professional judgement about what information to record, how to protect it and under what circumstances or legal requirements of professional practice confidentiality must be breached. In addition, as Beauchamp and Childress (2019: 16) note, although a prima facie right may be overridden, the nurse nevertheless has some moral obligation toward the patient in relation to the confidential matter, such as providing an explanation or apology.

REFLECTIVE QUESTIONS 7.6

1 Mr Payne, a patient who has recently undergone surgery, is a prominent politician. Gail is allocated to care for him on her shift. She answers the ward phone and a male who says he is Mr Payne's son asks about his condition. Mr Payne is sedated and asleep. The caller explains that he is calling from the United States and is very worried about his father. He wants to know what was involved in the operation his father had that afternoon and what outcomes are expected from the surgery. How do you think Gail should respond?

2 What is the role of the Coroner's Court?

3 Jim, a nurse, observed Sue feeding her elderly and frail mother. When her mother raised her hand and caused Sue to spill the food from the spoon on to her dress, Sue pinched her mother's arm hard enough for her to cry out, and said to her menacingly, 'You do that again you stupid bitch and you won't get any dinner.' What are Jim's mandatory obligations here? What do you think he should do?

4 What are the circumstances in which a report made by a nurse or other health professional is mandatory by law?

5 What is the Australian My Health Record? List the benefits and risks that you are aware of.

Further reading

Banks, S. & Gallagher, A. (2009). *Ethics in professional life: Virtues for health and social care.* Palgrave Macmillan.

Barnable, A., Cunning, G. & Parcon, M. (2018). Nursing students' perceptions of confidentiality, accountability, and e-professionalism in relation to Facebook. *Nurse Educator, 43*(1), 28–31.

Beltran-Aroca, C.M., Girela-Lopez, E., Collazo-Chao, E., Montero-Pérez-Barquero, M. & Muñoz-Villanueva, M.C. (2016). Confidentiality breaches in clinical practice: What happens in hospitals? *BMC Medical Ethics, 17*(1), 52.

Burns, K. & Belton, S. (2012). Click first, care second photography. *Medical Journal of Australia, 197,* 265–6.

Jones, C. & Hayter, M. (2013). Editorial: Social media use by nurses and midwives – a recipe for disaster or a 'force for good'? *Journal of Clinical Nursing, 22,* 1495–6.

Kaspiew, R., Carson, R. & Rhoades, H. (2016). Elder abuse in Australia. *Family Matters, 98,* 64–73.

Case cited

Tarasoff v Regents of the University of California (1976) 551 P.2d 334

Note

1 Previous editions of this chapter were authored by Sheryl de Lacey.

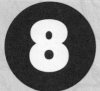

8 'TRUST ME, I'M A NURSE'

KIM ATKINS

LEARNING OBJECTIVES

In this chapter, you will:

→ Learn about trust and how it relates to power and in the nurse–patient relationship

→ Be able to identify the four features of trust

→ Develop your understanding of when it is a mistake to trust, and understand how people may be resistant to evidence of untrustworthiness

→ Develop your understanding of how, through trustworthiness, the nurse can deliver person-centred care

→ Develop your understanding of the patient's right to negotiate treatment, and its limits

Lena is a patient in the medical ward of a hospital. One day she tells her nurse that she is feeling 'a bit out of sorts' because her best friend has left on her honeymoon and won't be visiting her. At handover, the nurse reports that Lena is feeling depressed. The nurse on the incoming shift then writes in the notes that Lena is depressed. The resident doctor reads in the notes that Lena is depressed and informs the specialist doctor the next day, suggesting that he prescribe a medication. In the meantime, he arranges for a social worker to talk with Lena about possible problems at home.

Lena is outraged. She marches to the nurse's station and demands to see her file. She demands to know who has decided she is depressed and who has sent a social worker after her, then insists on seeing the resident doctor. The nurse on duty is not experienced in dealing with an angry patient, and when she calls the doctor she tells him that Lena is 'out of control'.

This chapter will further explore the moral and legal aspects of the nurse–patient relationship, with special attention paid to the role of trust. Lena's situation demonstrates how a patient can be disempowered and rendered increasingly vulnerable through careless use of professional power. Lena's sadness at being parted from her friend (a normal reaction) has been turned into a medical condition (or 'medicalised'), which is then recorded in her file as if it is a fact about her. Then this purported medical condition is used as a reason to pry into Lena's private life – and all without any consultation with Lena herself. When Lena expresses quite justifiable outrage, she is further cast as a problem patient, and her anger is regarded as part of her emotional instability.

Nursing staff have failed in their duty of care to Lena by failing to understand (and record) Lena's actual situation, failing to consult with Lena about her needs and failing to respect her legal rights to be informed about, and to consent to or refuse, treatment. By excluding her from a role in the decision-making process (and by misrepresenting her in official documents), they have failed to observe the moral principles of non-maleficence, beneficence, autonomy and justice. They have also failed to earn her trust. The result for Lena is unhappiness heaped upon unhappiness. The result for nursing staff may be an official complaint by Lena or her family to the Australian Health Practitioner Regulation Agency (AHPRA), followed by disciplinary proceedings. Furthermore, if staff were to administer treatment to Lena on the basis of the misinformation in the patient file and without Lena having met the full requirements for informed consent, they may have committed a trespass or assault. This is definitely not how the nurse–patient relationship should work.

Nurses need to be careful about creating misunderstanding by using common cultural expressions in the clinical context. For example, it is common to remark about some annoying experience that it 'sent my blood pressure through the roof'. Of course, this simply means that the speaker was highly agitated, not that the speaker's actual blood pressure was above the normal range. High blood pressure – hypertension – is a clinical condition that may require medical intervention. Similarly, the term 'depression' is commonly used in non-clinical conversation to describe feeling glum or sad or disappointed. In the everyday situation of conversation, 'depression' does not refer to the *clinical* condition of depression, which involves significant physiological and psychological problems that may require clinical intervention. One of the clinical terms that creates the most significant misunderstanding among patients is the use of the word 'complaining'. In the clinical context, nurses and other health professionals often describe patients as, for example, 'complaining of back pain'. In this usage of the word, they do *not* mean that the patient is whingeing or being a nuisance. They mean that the back pain is a symptom. They are saying that there is something (in this case, back pain) that is causing the patient a problem. They are not saying that the *patient* is a problem! However, when patients hear a clinician say that they are 'complaining', quite understandably they fear that the clinician is saying that they are whingeing or being unreasonable.

REFLECTIVE QUESTION 8.1

Think hard about some of the expressions you commonly use. The context in which you use an expression can change its meaning.

Could any of your expressions be misunderstood by your patients in the context of clinical care? What might be the effect?

In Chapter 3 it was noted that the nurse–patient relationship is one of power. The nurse is in a position of power over the patient because the patient has a need that cannot be met without the assistance of the nurse. The nurse has power to influence treatment and the patient's recovery in ways that the patient cannot. This power brings with it certain responsibilities and obligations that constitute the nurse's 'duty of care'. Because nurses have a legal duty of care, patients are justified in having reasonable expectations about how they will be treated. They have a reasonable expectation that they will be treated fairly, honestly, with respect, kindness, compassion and confidentiality, and that the care they receive will meet a recognised professional standard.

However, patients do not always know what they want or need from nursing care, and sometimes patients or their families can have unreasonable expectations of care. For example, the family of an elderly man with end-stage heart failure may request a heart transplant because family members have little knowledge of the complexity and danger of such surgery, the scarcity of donor organs or the national system of donor organ allocation. More commonly, patient expectations concern access to private rooms in a public hospital and nurses' and doctors' prompt attention. However, one very important and reasonable expectation that patients have of their nurses is *trust*.

Trust and trustworthiness

The Nursing and Midwifery Board of Australia's Code of Conduct for Nurses (NMBA 2018b) recognises the importance of trust in the nurse–patient relationship: Principle 4.4: 'People rely on the independence and trustworthiness of nurses who provide them with advice or treatment' (2018b: 13). The code defines person-centred care as 'collaborative and respectful partnership built on mutual trust and understanding through good communication' (2018b: 17).

The willingness of patients to share information with nurses and other health-care practitioners is directly related to their trust in the practitioner. The ICN Code of Ethics for Nurses (ICN 2021) makes several references to privacy – for example, that the nurse will 'Advocate for the ethical use of technology and scientific advances compatible with safety, dignity, privacy, confidentiality and human rights' (2021: 19) and 'Support the ethical and proficient use of social media and technologies' (2021: 20). Principle 1.4 states that 'Nurses hold in confidence personal information and respect the privacy, confidentiality and interests of patients in the lawful collection, use, access, transmission, storage and disclosure of personal information' (2021: 7). Principle 2.9 states that 'Nurses maintain a person's right to give and withdraw consent to access their personal, health and genetic information. They protect the use, privacy and confidentiality of genetic information and human genome technologies' (2021: 12).

The nurse–patient relationship is not a relationship of choice, so it is quite unlike many other social relationships. In the nursing setting, two people who may have very little in common find themselves sharing a close relationship – for example, through physical care of the body or through disclosure of private information. Different nursing roles involve different degrees and types of closeness, and so present different types of responsibilities. For example, community nurses go into patients' homes and work with them in a fairly informal and highly personalised environment; midwives work in the context of emotionally powerful and very intimate physical contact; and mental health nurses deal with people who may expose their most deeply felt and desperate inner thoughts and feelings.

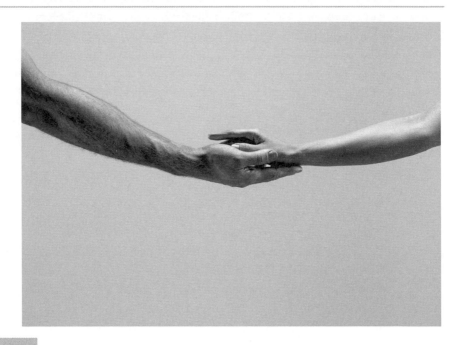

FIGURE 8.1 Trust is a kind of bond with another person.

The diversity and complexity of the clinical relationship provides multiple points of potential misunderstanding or harm. Because the nurse–patient relationship is not chosen, trust and trustworthiness are vitally important in this context where there is an imbalance of power. The patient has to trust that the nurse will protect their interests, and nurses have to be trustworthy to protect the interests with which they have been entrusted, even though the nurse's and the patient's personalities, values and beliefs may differ greatly. A trusting relationship is necessary for a nurse to meet the standards of a duty of care towards the patient. Without a trusting and understanding relationship, the nurse's care may lead to outcomes that the patient considers harmful to their interests (Rutherford 2014). If serious, this can lead to a claim against the nurse of professional negligence (duty of care is discussed in detail in Chapter 5).

Philosopher Annette Baier (1986: 259) describes trust as 'reliance on others, competence and willingness to look after, rather than harm, things one cares about and which are entrusted to their care'. Trusting is a form of collaborative (or social) activity because it allows a person's interests to be cared for by others in ways that the person cannot achieve by acting alone. A trustworthy person has both the competence to look after the things with which they are entrusted and the willingness to do so. We do not entrust the things we care about to people we know to be incompetent to care for them, and a competent person who is not willing to look after the things we care about cannot be trusted either. When acting professionally, a registered nurse meets both requirements of trust. The nurse has the competence to be trusted with a person's health, and the nursing role is an expression of willingness to care for a person's health.

Trust may be described as 'not-so-calculated' risk-taking (Kelly 2003). Trusting nurses can be dangerous because nurses make mistakes, and accidents sometimes happen. However, distrusting is dangerous too. For example, without disclosure of relevant personal information, the safety of treatment cannot be fully assured. It is better, says Kelly, to know 'how to trust wisely, to know who to trust, with what and to what extent' (Kelly 2003: 88). According to this formulation, trusting recognises both the need for some calculation of risk and the limitations of trying to calculate every risk. The risks of trusting arise from the involuntary nature of the clinical relationship, and the fact that the nurse has power over the patient's personal interests.

Trust is not an all-or-nothing affair. We would not trust wisely if we trusted a person beyond their sphere of competence. For example, it would be reasonable to trust a nurse's advice on a wound dressing, but not so reasonable to take the same nurse's advice on building repairs. To ensure that nurses are entrusted only with those things that are appropriate to the nurse's specific role, various checks, regulations and legislation exist, such as the *Health Practitioner Regulation Acts* in the various states and territories (see the Appendix for a table of legislation). Nurses are limited with regard to the kinds of things with which they can legitimately be trusted (for example, clinical practice rather than financial advice); they must undertake ongoing training to guarantee competence (for example, by annual basic life-support testing or credentialling for expanded scope of practice); and nursing practice must be transparent and accountable. These checks and regulations mean a patient does not have to trust each individual nurse, but can have a general confidence that any nurse's practice is safe insofar as it is regulated by institutional and legal protections.

REFLECTIVE QUESTIONS 8.2

1 What do you expect your patients to trust about you?
2 How would you feel if your patients questioned your skill level or knowledge?
3 How easily could you trust someone who had power over your well-being?

Four features of trust

Trust can be characterised by four essential features (Baier 1994):

1 an element of uncertainty
2 an element of risk and vulnerability for the person with less power
3 an element of discretionary judgement on the part of the trusted person
4 asymmetry of power in the trusting relationship.

UNCERTAINTY

Trusting always has an element of uncertainty because we cannot determine in advance what the trusted person will do. In the clinical setting, patients can expect that a nurse will exercise good judgement in relation to their interests, but are likely to lack at least some of the knowledge and skill to specify in advance what their particular health needs will be, and therefore how the nurse will respond. Uncertainty also arises from the unpredictable nature of life itself: all sorts of circumstances can arise that may influence how either the patient or the nurse behaves.

LAW AND ETHICS IN PRACTICE

Gary is a drug and alcohol nurse who has been working with a patient, Jose, for a few months. Jose has been recovering from a drug addiction and is getting married in several weeks. Gary has promised Jose that he will support him up to the wedding and be available during the honeymoon. At short notice, Gary's manager asks him to replace a sick colleague in another part of the state during Jose's honeymoon. Gary tells Jose that he can't be available in person as he promised.

>> Was Jose right to place this kind of trust in Gary? What could Gary have done to maintain trust in this scenario?

RISK AND VULNERABILITY

Trust entails risk because it makes us vulnerable to another person's competence and goodwill. As noted, the trusted person may be mistaken about their competence to take care of your interests. An over-confident new nursing graduate with limited experience may fail to appreciate the complexities of a patient's situation, and also fail to anticipate the ways in which treatment can go wrong. This has numerous legal implications – for example, if the requirements for consent are not met, or if the patient is harmed. As mentioned earlier (and discussed in Chapter 5), any harms to a patient arising from a nurse's lack of knowledge can result in disciplinary action from the employer or AHPRA (or both), or in a claim of negligence against the nurse and the employer.

LAW AND ETHICS IN PRACTICE

Brian was a newly registered nurse doing locum nursing for an agency. He spent two days working in the neonatal step-down unit of a large teaching hospital, which he enjoyed. The following week, he was offered two more shifts at the unit, which he accepted. The unit cares for up to eight newborns, many of whom are premature babies and fed with feeding tubes. Brian easily learned to place a feeding tube correctly. During a staff meal break, Brian was alone in the unit. When it came time to feed one of the larger babies, he thought he would try the baby on a bottle rather than the feeding tube. When the regular staff nurse returned, Brian told her that the baby had fed from a bottle. The nurse was very concerned and explained that the premature babies are fed by a tube because they have not yet developed sufficient gag reflexes, even though they may have strong sucking reflexes. A baby without a gag reflex is at risk of inhaling the feed and ending up with life-threatening pneumonia.

Brian did not anticipate this problem because he lacked sufficient knowledge or experience. In departing from unit procedure, he was acting outside his scope of practice and competency; consequently, he endangered the baby's life.

>> How will you ensure you are working within your scope of practice?

DISCRETIONARY JUDGEMENT

When we trust someone, we give that person power over something we care about in the expectation that the person will take good care of it. At the same time, we have limited ability to control what the trusted person does in relation to our interests. This means that the person has a certain amount of discretionary power: the trusted person has scope to interpret what counts as taking good care of our interests. This can go well, as shown below.

Nick has had abdominal surgery after a car accident. In trusting the nurse to help him mobilise, Nick gives the nurse scope to decide what kind of mobilisation will best help him. Nick would prefer to sit on the edge of his bed and wriggle his toes, but the nurse insists that Nick should walk around the ward. Nick complies with his nurse's advice, even though he thinks she is expecting too much of him. After a couple of days, Nick feels much better and realises that the nurse's judgement was in his best interests.

>> How are you going to earn the trust of your patients?

Or it can go badly, as in the following example.

LAW AND ETHICS IN PRACTICE

Julie is a young, pregnant, married woman on bed rest with unstable hypertension. She complains to her nurse, Eamon, that she is bored and doesn't have anything to read. Eamon offers to go to the hospital newsagent and buy a magazine for her to read. Julie agrees, and asks him to get her something interesting. Eamon returns with a magazine about dirt bike riding (which is a passion of his, but not of Julie's).

>> What does it take to avoid this kind of error of judgement?

Discretionary power brings with it moral obligations of non-maleficence, beneficence and respect for autonomy and justice because it gives the nurse the power to harm as well as heal (recall Chapter 3). As Kelly (2003: 113) notes:

> The paradox of trust is that it is necessary to allow the one we trust this discretion in order to optimise their capacity to take care of the good we entrust to them although this increases their capacity to harm our interests.

In order to avoid the uncertainty, risk and vulnerability associated with giving someone discretionary power, a contract may appear to be a solution. Drawing up a contract with someone (whether in writing or verbally) can reduce the breadth of discretionary power they can exercise. Advance care directives are an example of this approach. An advance care directive is an agreement between the person and the health practitioner that specifies what is to be done to the patient under circumstances in which the patient cannot consent (see Chapter 4). Individuals employing a nurse to provide care in a private home may also draw up a contract specifying what the nurse can and cannot decide for the patient. The more detailed the contract, the less discretionary power the nurse has. However, it is not possible to eliminate discretionary power completely because a contract cannot control for every eventuality. Life itself has an element of uncertainty about it: accidents, electricity failures, roadblocks or natural disasters can all impact what the nurse is required to do in order to deliver care.

ASYMMETRY OF POWER

Giving and withholding information is a way of exercising power in a relationship. In Chapter 3, it was noted that specialist knowledge gives the nurse power, and the patient's lack of knowledge creates dependency on the nurse. The way a nurse shares information is a good indicator of whether the relationship is promoting autonomy or further dependency. Nurses and patients each manage the flow of information between them in order to achieve the outcomes they want. When this is done well, it encourages mutual understanding and cooperation. When it is done badly, it can result in anxiety, conflict or emotional manipulation. As discussed in Chapters 5 and 7, the nurse also has specific legal obligations concerning the management of patient information. Patients must be provided with relevant information about their treatment, including information about alternative treatments; and patients' private information must be treated with confidentiality. The asymmetry of power places the patient in a situation of vulnerability, which is why the clinical relationship requires trust, and also why abuses of discretionary power are possible. The purpose of the power imbalance (in the short term) is to allow patients to have more control over their lives in the long term. The trustworthiness of the nurse corrects the power imbalance over time.

LAW AND ETHICS IN PRACTICE

Pip had surgery on her spine after a period of debilitating illness. In the immediate post-operative period, she relied on nursing staff for the most basic care: feeding, washing, elimination, mobility and pain relief. Her nurses had enormous discretionary power. They decided when and what she ate and drank, which side she lay on, what she wore, and so forth. Pip found her dependency a source of much anxiety and frustration, which sometimes she directed at her carers. Nevertheless, the nurses used their power appropriately by carrying out all that was required to ensure Pip's recovery, and by explaining to Pip the reasons for why they were doing the things they did.

Several months later, Pip is fully recovered, independent and autonomous. In retrospect, Pip can see that the nurses' professional conduct and care in the exercise of their power were necessary to move her from dependency to independence, and through that journey the power imbalance eventually was corrected.

>> **What can you do to optimise a patient's own power to make decisions about the care they will receive?**

The trust and trustworthiness that Pip and the nurses shared was clearly of enormous practical and moral value. The appreciation of that value is an important source of the respect accorded to the nursing profession, as well as being a source of professional and personal self-respect for nurses. Recall from Chapter 1 the idea that the nurse is a mirror to the patient. When nurses genuinely value their responsibilities and treat them with respect, their actions reflect the value they accord to their patients.

Even though the patient is required to trust the nurse at least to a small degree initially, trust is something the nurse has to live up to by being trustworthy. Trustworthiness in the nurse means staying true to their moral and legal obligations to act for the patient's well-being. Trustworthiness is different from friendliness. It is more than simply being nice or agreeable to the patient, or doing whatever the patient wants. It means maintaining high standards of personal moral scruples by never undermining the patient's interests or the nurse's obligations to the patient. Interestingly, being trustworthy can involve arguing with the patient against the patient's apparent wishes.

LAW AND ETHICS IN PRACTICE

Chris is a young man with insulin-controlled diabetes who has been admitted to hospital for stabilisation of his blood glucose levels. Despite his unstable condition, Chris wants to discharge himself home because he is bored in hospital and wants to resume his normal social activities. Chris's nurse tries to convince him that his long-term health interests outweigh his short-term social interests, and that he has more reasons to stay in hospital than to leave.

》 **Is the nurse right to try to convince Chris in this way? Why should Chris trust what the nurse says?**

Nurses need to be careful to distinguish a debate with a patient designed to encourage or provoke the patient to be more reflective about what the *patient* really wants from an argument that tries to coerce a patient to do what the *nurse* really wants. The goals of nursing and medicine do not always coincide with the patient's immediate emotional or cultural needs. This is why nurses must understand the legal requirements of consent, respect individual differences and practise cultural safety. Culturally safe care in relation to Aboriginal and Torres Strait Islander patients should be informed by an understanding of the intergenerational effects of colonisation and ensure shared decision-making (see Chapter 6; also Coombes et al. 2022).

Trustworthiness is different from another common psychological feature of relationships of power, called 'positive transference'. Transference is an *unconscious* process whereby the patient experiences feelings towards the nurse that arise from a powerful past experience, such as the feelings the patient had for their parents (Joyce 2010; Jung 1946). Recall that in the nurse–patient relationship, the nurse always has more power than the patient – similar to the way in which a parent always has more power than the child. Sometimes when the nurse is well liked by a patient who is dependent upon her, the experience of being safely cared for while dependent can produce positive feelings similar to those that the patient felt as a child in the care of their parent. In short, the patient can come to regard the nurse as having all the positive qualities that the parent had. For example, the patient may believe that the nurse is kinder, more generous or more caring than other nurses. The problem here is that such feelings can bring with them a deeper level of dependency than is appropriate because the patient becomes over-reliant on the care delivered by one particular nurse (Burnard & Chapman 2004). In addition, this kind of emotional attachment to the nurse makes the patient resistant to evidence of wrongdoing on the part of the nurse. For this reason, it creates a situation where the patient has increased vulnerability to being abused.

LAW AND ETHICS IN PRACTICE

Glynnis is a hospital nurse caring for a male patient who has recently had a below-knee amputation following years of poorly controlled diabetes. The man, Jeremy, is wealthy, lives alone and suffers from some social anxiety. (He experiences anxiety when meeting new people and mixing in social groups.) Jeremy becomes anxious and upset when Glynnis is assigned to another patient group. Glynnis tells her manager that she should be the one to nurse Jeremy, to stop him making a fuss with the other nurses. The manager agrees, but monitors the relationship. One day, Jeremy is seen giving Glynnis an expensive-looking gold bracelet and earrings. The manager hears Glynnis offer to provide Jeremy with home visits when he is discharged.

 >> Is Glynnis taking advantage of Jeremy's vulnerability, or just acting with compassion? Are there any implications for Glynnis' duty of care?

Principle 4.4 of the Code of Conduct for Nurses (NMBA 2018b) states:

> People rely on the independence and trustworthiness of nurses who provide them with advice or treatment. In nursing practice, a conflict of interest arises when a nurse has financial, professional or personal interests or relationships and/or personal beliefs that may affect the care they provide or result in personal gain. Such conflicts may mean the nurse does not prioritise the interests of a person as they should, and may be viewed as unprofessional conduct.

Glynnis's actions contravened this principle, and she was subsequently disciplined for unprofessional conduct.

To be worthy of trust, nurses need to remain clear-sighted in their own sense of who they are and what they are permitted do professionally, morally and legally. In maintaining trustworthiness, the nurse needs to be steady in their attitude, emotional responses and commitment to legal and professional responsibilities. Trustworthiness rests upon the nurse's fidelity to their scope of practice (recall Chapter 5). Any nurse who works outside their scope of practice is unlikely to act in the patient's best interests because they are failing to work within the following key factors that determine safe practice:

→ the nurse's level of training and demonstrated competence
→ the nurse's scope of practice (which includes the level of appointment at which the nurse is employed)
→ state and Commonwealth legislation
→ the employer's policy framework.

When is it a mistake to trust?

Sometimes we can be mistaken in trusting a person, and fail to realise this because trust can resist evidence of untrustworthiness. This is not just a moral danger for the nurse–patient relationship; it is also relevant to nurse's relationships with their colleagues. Resistance to evidence of untrustworthiness can arise for several reasons (Kelly 2003: 116–26):

→ Old friends have deep bonds of trust that are often forged over long periods of time, and that may have been tested under trying circumstances. Therefore, if someone is accused of wrongdoing in unusual circumstances, an old friend is unlikely to believe the accusation. Individuals often feel that they know enough about their friends to tell whether or not a friend could be guilty of certain kinds of wrongdoing.
→ A lack of self-trust can lead a person to resist evidence of untrustworthiness. For example, a person who doesn't trust her own responses might think that it is unreasonable to doubt their friend ('I'm overreacting') or that they are ignorant ('What do I know?').
→ People can fail to take evidence of untrustworthiness seriously because they hold unreasonable beliefs about the trusted person: 'my doctor would never do the wrong thing', 'my wife is incapable of lying', 'my son does what he's told'.
→ A person may be resistant to evidence due to positive transference (as discussed earlier).

REFLECTIVE QUESTION 8.3

The Tasmanian government has established a Commission of Inquiry into allegations of sexual assault by a paedophile nurse at one of its major hospitals. The assaults are said to have occurred over several years, despite some nursing staff expressing distrust of this nurse.

How would you know whether, in your nursing practice, you were resisting evidence and being too trusting?

Lack of trust

Given the risks of trusting, would it make more sense to distrust rather than trust others? It may be wise to distrust in certain circumstances – for example, where there can be unambiguous evidence of untrustworthiness – but as a general approach to life, and in particular as an approach to the nurse–patient relationship, it is unworkable. Trust is essential to life because we lack the ability to do everything by ourselves that needs to be done to secure our interests and to flourish as persons. Certain fundamental goods of life, such as meaningful communication, security, friendship and love, depend on trust. In addition, many social activities imply trust, such as falling asleep on a train, sending mail, having our cars repaired and using a public library.

Perhaps we should withhold trust until proof of trustworthiness is shown? This isn't much of an option either because it invokes high levels of anxiety and requires equally high levels of alertness and watchfulness. In the absence of trust, all relationships would constantly have to be policed, which is stifling, costly and inefficient (as well as running counter to the nature of a *relationship*). In the end, we would still need to trust the people who would police the relationships, so a world without trust would be a world of rampant fear and paranoia. Rather, we are better off taking the advice to learn 'how to trust wisely, to know who to trust, with what and to what extent' (Kelly 2003: 88).

Truthfulness

Trust and truthfulness go hand in hand. Unless a person's conduct and character are perceived to be truthful, others are unlikely to trust that person. Without a trusting relationship in place, a nurse will be unable to provide the support a patient needs. Nevertheless, the demand for honesty can sometimes present the nurse with a conflict between a patient's right to know and the nurse's duty to minimise the patient's distress. It is important for nurses to communicate effectively and compassionately without resorting to lying or deception, which may be failures of duty of care that result in professional negligence. If a patient is experiencing difficulty comprehending important information, a supported decision-making model might be necessary. This can occur unofficially in the first instance, through the help of the patient's immediate and trusted family, or if necessary through an official process involving guardianship (as discussed in Chapter 4).

For example, someone presented with a diagnosis of cancer almost inevitably feels distressed and fearful. Such a person may even think they are going to die. In these circumstances, a nurse may be reluctant to talk through some aspects of treatment, such as pain and possible disfigurement after surgery, or the side-effects of chemotherapy, in order to protect the patient from the anxiety and distress that may result. However, being truthful in the clinical relationship means accepting responsibility for sharing the pain, shock, anger, grief and despair that can accompany illness and injury by responding with empathy and compassion. A nurse's own emotional maturity plays a part in their readiness to be honest. It is easy to leave bad news to the incoming shift or the doctor, but it isn't always the best or the right thing to do. Recall that in Chapter 1 we pointed out that we are frequently quite unaware of the ways in which our emotional dispositions can function as a kind of background against which our conscious ideas, attitudes and beliefs stand out. For this reason, nurses need to build their own 'emotional intelligence'. Emotional intelligence refers to the awareness and understanding of one's emotional dispositions and tendencies, and the ability to reason about one's emotions in order to have constructive interpersonal and professional relationships (Mestre & Barchard 2017).

Doctors, physiotherapists, and other clinicians can lack emotional maturity and empathy too, and sometimes nurses will find themselves left to deal with the fallout.

LAW AND ETHICS IN PRACTICE

Frank, who suffered from chronic pulmonary disease, was a patient in the high-dependency unit. The medical specialist, a person of few words, visited Frank one morning and, after examining him, said, 'Look, there isn't anything more that we can do for you here, so we'll send you over to the palliative care unit later today.' The doctor then promptly left.

Frank was devastated and sat speechless, believing he had just been delivered a death sentence. Fortunately, his nurse anticipated his misunderstanding and was able to explain that palliative care is also for people with chronic illnesses who need to receive maximal treatment, not just people who are about to die. Nevertheless, Frank was severely shaken by the experience.

 >> **Think about a time when you have witnessed bad news being delivered to a patient. What might a more person-centred conversation be like?**

A patient may have a transient inability to adequately comprehend information – for example, as a result of medication, injury, surgery or emotional turmoil. Under these circumstances, nurses may choose to temporarily withhold information until they feel the patient can take it all in and/or cope with receiving it. However, the nurse is morally and legally justified in withholding the truth *temporarily only*, and then only in circumstances where disclosing it would do unnecessary harm (recall the discussion of guardianship and the conditions for supported decision-making in Chapter 4).

Patients may have a different kind of enduring difficulty comprehending clinical information if they lack health literacy. This will require a different approach, and may entail the nurse taking educative steps to help ensure that the patient develops knowledge of relevant clinical or health concepts and the ability to apply those concepts to their own situation.

LAW AND ETHICS IN PRACTICE

The family of Mrs Popovic have come to realise that she needs to move out of her family home and into aged care. She is physically frail, is forgetful and can no longer prepare food for herself or keep the house clean. The family does not want to discuss this with Mrs Popovic because she will become very distressed. They plan to tell her that she is having a period of respite care at a facility, when in fact she will be there permanently. The family has asked the nurses not to discuss the move with Mrs Popovic.

>> **What are your key responsibilities in responding to this scenario?**

The relevant legal issues here pertain to consent and guardianship. If Mrs Popovic is capable of understanding in broad terms what is being proposed for her, she has a legal right to be fully informed of that, and to refuse to consent if she so wishes, even if her refusal brings her harm. If Mrs Popovic lacks the ability to comprehend the proposed treatment, a robust process of supported decision-making should be introduced. If that fails, it may be appropriate to have a guardian appointed. In any case, any decision about Mrs Popovic's circumstances is legally required to be in her best interests, and not simply in the interests of certain family members. The nurse caring for Mrs Popovic has a legal and moral obligation to act in her best interests and not those of her family. To disregard Mrs Popovic's legal rights by lying to her is not only to fail to respect her, but also leaves the nurse liable to legal action for assault and/or negligence.

Negotiating treatment

We learned two things in Chapter 4: first, that consent must be obtained from a competent patient before that patient can be given treatment; and second, that a competent patient has a legal right to refuse treatment, even if that treatment is life-saving. The nurse is obliged to respect the right of a competent person to refuse treatment or aspects of treatment. The trustworthiness of the nurse depends on respect for this basic principle.

However, a patient's idea of the aim of treatment can differ widely from a health professional's idea of the aim of treatment. For example, a patient with a musculo-skeletal problem might believe that the purpose of her hospital admission is to have a rest, while the nurse believes it is for the patient to have intensive physiotherapy and rehabilitation. The potential difference in understanding between nurse and patient can require that the patient and the nurse negotiate treatment. Therefore, trustworthiness also requires the nurse to be flexible and negotiate to achieve outcomes that are in the patient's interests. Consider the following case.

LAW AND ETHICS IN PRACTICE

Robert is an academic who is used to working late into the night, then sleeping until mid-morning. He is admitted to hospital after a motor vehicle accident in which he sustained abdominal injuries. He is receiving parenteral nutrition because he cannot yet eat or drink. He has become increasingly irritated as a result of being woken early every morning by the day shift nurse, who takes his observations and changes his fluids while other patients are having breakfast. 'Why can't you do this later?' he asks. 'It's torture!'

Consequently, Robert is feeling tired, irritable and gloomy. He is unable to read – one of the few pleasures available to him in hospital – or to converse properly with his visitors. He is lonely and worries about his ability to recover in a timely fashion. He has started to think that the nurses do not really care about him, and he is starting to lose trust in their judgement when they say he is getting better every day. 'Well, I don't feel better. I feel worse every day,' is his reply. A nurse laughs and says, 'Don't be a grouch. Think yourself lucky that you still have all your bits!'

Robert desperately needs sleep and has been unable to adjust his life to the hospital routine. He needs the hospital routine to adjust to him. He cannot understand why the nurse cannot see this.

>> **How might Robert's experiences undermine his ability to trust the nursing staff? How might this affect his cooperation with clinical care?**

There might be a few different responses to the question of why Robert's nurse isn't adapting her routine to his needs. Maybe she is particularly busy; maybe she has other patients with more pressing needs; maybe she is acting under the direction of a more senior nurse; maybe she has personal concerns that are distracting her; maybe she is avoiding Robert. Whatever her reasons, she has a responsibility to deliver person-centred care: care which is geared to the patient's personal needs and preferences, and which promotes the patient's active participation in decision-making. Person-centred care can be identified by asking the following questions:

→ Has the nurse asked the patient about their needs and preferences?
→ Is the nurse working to meet those needs and preferences?
→ Has the patient been encouraged and supported to be involved in planning and making decisions about care?
→ Has the patient been given the option to involve a support person or interpreter during consultations?
→ Has the communication from the nurse been clear and in language the patient can understand?
→ Has the nurse demonstrated respect for the patient as an individual?
→ Does the health-care organisation have clear feedback process? Has the patient been told about these? (Victoria State Government 2018a)

Patient care also has the following goals, which correspond to the various features of personhood (recall the discussions in Chapter 1):

→ *objective, scientific outcomes* – for example, lowering blood pressure or wound healing
→ *psychological and emotional outcomes* – for example, self-confidence, trust in the nurse or the ability to cope with grief
→ *practical personal outcomes* – for example, disease self-management or antenatal preparation
→ *social and interpersonal outcomes* – for example, a therapeutic relationship with the nurse, or being rehabilitated to return to work
→ *moral outcomes* – for example, care given with empathy, respect and fairness
→ *existential outcomes* – for example, where patients feel that the care given is meaningful to their self-conceptions and life – in other words, care given in a culturally sensitive way
→ *efficiency* – for example, providing care in a timely and effective way according to priorities of need.

Each patient will have greater or lesser needs in each of these areas, and each nurse may have greater or lesser capacities in each area. The care Robert is receiving from his nurse is meeting only one or two of these goals. The nurse has been approaching Robert's care from the point of view that it is just one of a list of tasks that has to be completed that day. As long as his observations are stable and his dressings are clean, the nurse can get this task out of the way while the other patients are preoccupied with breakfast and not making demands. Then the nurse can move on to her other tasks during the rest of the morning. There are limited hours in the day to provide all the care that is needed, and the nurse has to prioritise work tasks, especially if help is in short supply. However, the nurse needs to remember that efficiency is only one of the goals of nursing care, and act accordingly. It is important to understand and respond to Robert's situation from his point of view.

In order to respond appropriately to Robert's needs, the nurse needs to place Robert at the centre of care. This move is consistent with what has become known as the person-centred approach to care (ACSQHC 2022b). Using this approach, the nurse organises their workload priorities around the patient's express needs. By contrast, Robert's nurse seems to be working in a way that meets the organisational needs of the health-care institution, while Robert's needs are merely a secondary concern.

Recall that in Chapter 4 the nurse–patient relationship was described as a fiduciary relationship. In a fiduciary relationship, the patient has an active role in decision-making. The role of the nurse within the fiduciary relationship is to provide expert advice in such a way that it maximises the patient's capacity to further their own values and interests. In other words, the nurse–patient relationship – the therapeutic relationship – is a two-way street. The patient takes direction from the nurse, but the nurse also needs to take some direction from the patient if nursing care really is going to support and promote the patient's health and well-being.

There is almost always more than one pathway to a healthy outcome for a patient, and always more than one way to meet a person's needs. Sometimes all that is required is a bit of forethought, planning and collaboration with the patient. In Robert's case, the night nurse could ensure that his parenteral nutrition fluids do not need to be replaced until late morning. Perhaps he could be placed in a single or two-bed room to help him catch up on sleep. A 'do not disturb' sign on the door would help too. Robert may benefit from increased physical activity or occupational therapy. Often patients appreciate the opportunity to take control of their own care. Maybe Robert can be taught to do his own observations or dressings, or to undertake and monitor a physical therapy regime. Working with the nurse through these kinds of shared activities of care could meet Robert's objective, practical, personal, interpersonal and existential needs. Sharing care in this way can improve Robert's relationship with the nurse, increasing his psychological well-being by enhancing his self-confidence and willingness to trust, and also improving the moral quality of their relationship through increased respect and empathy.

THE SCOPE OF NEGOTIATION

In Chapter 4 we noted that treatment cannot be given without consent (except in extreme circumstances), and that consent requires the informed and voluntary agreement of a mentally competent person. Consent is not an all-or-nothing matter.

LAW AND ETHICS IN PRACTICE

A nurse, Jim, goes to his patient, Warren, and says he will take him to the shower, after which Jim will do his leg dressing and then bring him the phone to call his family. Warren says that he will have a shower after lunch, since he had a poor night's sleep, but he would like his dressing done – but after he has had some pain relief. Jim agrees.

>> **Why might not every interaction between patient and nurse proceed in this cooperative fashion?**

Frequently, consent is the outcome of a negotiation: the nurse offers certain activities and the patient agrees or refuses all or parts of that offer. Negotiating care is a normal part of nursing activity. However, how much negotiation is reasonable? How far can a patient's wishes be accommodated before professional standards are put at risk? Consider the following example.

LAW AND ETHICS IN PRACTICE

Marjorie is an active elderly woman receiving community nursing care in her home. She has become dehydrated as a result of a bout of diarrhoea (unusual for her). This morning, she asks you for her usual laxative (psyllium). You tell her you are withholding it because of her dehydration. She becomes upset, saying that she has taken it every day for 30 years and it keeps her healthy. You explain that it may worsen her dehydration, but she demands that you give it to her.

>> **What do you do?**

In Marjorie's case, the nurse knows that by administering psyllium the risk of harm from worsening dehydration is high. Consequently, the nurse's legal duty of care dictates that she should not give Marjorie the psyllium, even in her own home. The appropriate treatment for any patient in any setting is treatment that falls within the nurse's scope of practice and duty of care. While people have the right to engage in whatever (legal) activities they wish, even if it harms them, that right does not impose obligations on others to assist them to participate. And so it is with health care. Patients may have a legal right to activities that do them no good, but nurses are not obliged to assist patients to partake of those activities. In negotiating with Marjorie, the nurse should provide a clear and relevant explanation about the harm she faces by taking psyllium at this point in time, and then involve Marjorie in developing a plan for reintroducing psyllium into her diet.

The problem of challenges to professional standards is less straightforward when the risk of harm is very low – for example, when a patient wants to use an 'alternative' therapy for which there is no objective clinical evidence of therapeutic effect.

LAW AND ETHICS IN PRACTICE

Barinder is a cricketer in hospital for shoulder surgery following repeated injury. Each morning, he asks you to clean his 'Power Balance' bracelet and put it on his unaffected arm.[1]

>> **What do you do?**

While nurses may feel that it is dishonest or unprofessional to administer treatment that has not been scientifically shown to be effective, the objective scientific aspect of care is just one aspect among others – albeit an important one. If the therapy has no effect, then the nurse has no legal concern about causing harm. While the nurse is not under any legal obligation to provide alternative treatment where the patient requests it, there are practical and moral considerations involved. In responding to such requests, nurses will need to decide how administering an alternative therapy sits within the broader context of the nurse–patient relationship, the nurse's scope of practice and the nurse's duty of care. For example, how much time and effort is involved in complying with the request? Will non-compliance cause the patient psychological distress? Will non-compliance amount to a lack of respect for the patient's authority over their own life? Rather than tackle the particular 'treatment' head-on, could this be an opportunity for the nurse to improve the patient's health literacy? In considering these issues, nurses should reflect upon the principles of non-maleficence, beneficence, autonomy and justice discussed in Chapter 3. Rather than criticise ineffective therapies outright, it is often more useful to provide patients with constructive advice about how to look for a quality product from among alternatives. For example, the Cancer Council of Victoria (2022) provides a guide for people with cancer who are considering a range of therapies.

Conclusion

Unless nurses show themselves to be trustworthy by acting with knowledge, compassion, integrity and professional standards, patients will not have good reason to trust them. Recall that a trustworthy person has both the competence to look after the things with which they are entrusted and the willingness to do so. Nurses have a moral responsibility to not only act in such a way that will ensure their patients trust them, but to assist their patients to trust *wisely*. Nurses should always refuse to comply with therapies that they have good reason to believe will cause harms to the patient that outweigh any benefits. Nurses should not be expected to compromise their professional standards or engage in conduct that would compromise their professional self-respect. Patient autonomy does not entail getting whatever the patient wants, and it is quite reasonable to expect that nurses' responses to the demands of patients will be guided by respect for legal, moral and practical principles. At the same time, it is important to understand that trust is also grounded in feeling safe. Lack of trust may arise if a patient, for whatever reason, is not feeling safe, so always look to safety first.

Acknowledgement

This chapter title makes deliberate reference to the title of Dr Martin Kelly's (2003) PhD thesis, 'Trust me, I'm a doctor'.

REFLECTIVE QUESTIONS 8.4

1 Why is trust fundamental to the therapeutic relationship?
2 What are the four features of trust?
3 Why might a lack of self-trust be a problem for a nurse?
4 What is an example of something that would make it difficult for a nurse to be truthful with their patient?
5 How would you know if your trust of a colleague is justified?

Further reading

Baier, A. (1994). *Moral prejudices*. Harvard University Press.

Dinc, L. & Gastmans, C. (2012). Trust and trustworthiness in nursing. *Nursing Inquiry, 19*(3), 223–37.

Luzinski, C. (2012). Trust: A core value of healthy organisations. *Journal of Nursing Administration, 42*(11), 497–8.

Russell, D. et al. (2021). Family caregivers' conceptions of trust in home health care providers. *Research in Gerontological Nursing, 14*(4), 200–10.

Rutherford, M. (2014). The value of trust to nursing. *Nursing Economics, 32*(6), 283–8, 327.

Rydenfalt, C. et al. (2012). Social structures in the operating theatre: How contradicting rationalities and trust affect work. *Journal of Advanced Nursing, 68*(4), 783–95.

Yoder-Wise, P. (2016). Trust in our colleagues. *Journal of Continuing Education in Nursing, 47*(8), 343.

Note

1 In 2010, silicone and plastic wristbands and bracelets called 'Power Balance' appeared on the market, notably at sporting venues, claiming to enhance athletic performance. The bands were worn by several high-profile international athletes, which further enhanced the popular perception of their therapeutic effect. However, after investigating complaints, the Australian Consumer and Complaints Commission chairman, Graeme Samuel, stated that: 'Power Balance has admitted that there is no credible scientific basis for the claims and therefore no reasonable grounds for making representations about the benefits of the product' (Robinson 2010).

WITNESSING AND MAKING MISTAKES

KIM ATKINS

LEARNING OBJECTIVES

In this chapter, you will:

→ Identify factors that lead to clinical errors and incidents

→ Explain what a clinical incident is, and how incidents are managed and tracked

→ Describe the required professional and ethical response to clinical errors

→ Gain insight into the nature of professional self-respect and its connection to trustworthiness

→ Explain the importance of reporting mistakes

→ Describe how you can build integrity through 'Giving Voice to Values'

→ Describe open disclosure policy and processes

Apari had been caring for a diabetic man, Jack, whose blood glucose levels had been difficult to stabilise. One day they would be high, the next day they would be low. By chance, one day Apari saw that a new nurse, Louise, was using the glucometer incorrectly to test Jack's blood glucose. Apari checked Jack's notes and realised that Louise had been recording incorrect blood glucose levels for several days.

Just like everyone else, nurses sometimes make mistakes that can result in harm to others. This chapter looks at how errors can occur in nursing practice and some ethical issues involved in responding to them. The Nursing and Midwifery Board of Australia's (NMBA) Code of Conduct for Nurses (NMBA 2018b) makes a number of statements in relation to the safe conduct of nursing practice – for example:

1.1 Obligations

Nurses must:

a abide by any reporting obligations under the National Law and other relevant legislation …

b inform the Australian Health Practitioner Regulation Agency (AHPRA) and their employer(s) if a legal or regulatory entity has imposed restrictions on their practice, including limitations, conditions, undertakings, suspension, cautions or reprimands, and recognise that a breach of any restriction would place the public at risk and may constitute unprofessional conduct or professional misconduct

c complete the required amount of CPD relevant to their context of practice …

d ensure their practice is appropriately covered by professional indemnity insurance

e inform AHPRA of charges, pleas and convictions relating to criminal offences.

1.2 Lawful behaviour

Nurses must:

…

b comply with relevant poisons legislation, authorisation, local policy and own scope of practice, including to safely use, administer, obtain, possess, prescribe, sell, supply and store medications and other therapeutic products.

2.1 Nursing practice

Nurses must:

a practise in accordance with the standards of the profession and broader health system (including the NMBA's standards, codes and guidelines, the National Safety and Quality Health Service Standards and Aged Care Quality Standards for aged care …)

b provide leadership to ensure the delivery of safe and quality care and understand their professional responsibility to protect people, ensuring employees comply with their obligations, and

c document and report concerns …

The ICN Code of Ethics for Nurses (ICN 2012, 2021) also refers to safe conduct:

2. Nurses and practice

The nurse carries personal responsibility and accountability for nursing practice, and for maintaining competence by continual learning.

The nurse maintains a standard of personal health such that the ability to provide care is not compromised.

The nurse uses judgement regarding individual competence when accepting and delegating responsibility.

The nurse at all times maintains standards of personal conduct which reflect well on the profession and enhance its image and public confidence.

The nurse, in providing care, ensures that use of technology and scientific advances are compatible with the safety, dignity and rights of people.

These statements reflect the expectation that nurses will be aware of and committed to industry-wide standards of safety and quality in their practice. Consequently, one could infer that nurses have a moral obligation to deal with clinical errors and incidents in an open, honest and constructive fashion.

A clinical incident is 'an event or circumstance that resulted, or could have resulted, in unintended and/or unnecessary harm to a [person] and/or a complaint, loss or damage' (ACSQHC 2021a). Some clinical incidents will be the result of clinical error, which is a failure by a clinician to observe the appropriate standards of knowledge and practice. Errors range from the minor – such as doing a dressing more often than is necessary – to a patient's death. Incidents also include far misses – such as misspelling a patient's name on a consent form – and near misses, where something harmful is avoided at the last minute. The causes of mistakes can vary greatly too, from the simple and obvious – such as failing to administer a medication – to complex and systematic problems of workplace culture. How you, as a nurse, respond to your own clinical errors and incidents and those of others is a measure of your professional and moral character and competency.

Factors leading to clinical errors and incidents

Clinical errors are rarely the result of nurses motivated by deliberate carelessness or malice. Rather, clinical incidents are typically the result of several factors in combination, such as a staff member with a lack of clinical knowledge working in an unfamiliar environment during a busy period.

Clinical incidents can be the result of 'system factors' or 'human factors', or both. System factors relate to the coordination of care, routine treatment processes and the application of guidelines and policies. For example, an incident involving the administration of blood products may arise from the absence of a process by which to communicate updates of hospital policy to staff. In its 2020 data, the Clinical Excellence Commission (CEC) in New South Wales reported that the top three system factors in clinical incidents relating to clinical management were:

1 care planning
2 communication
3 workforce (CEC 2020c).

Human factors relate to the judgement and decision-making processes of individual health professionals. The NSW CEC has developed a number of very useful short videos and other publications that explain the role of human factors in clinical settings (CEC 2020a). While the CEC refers to clinical errors in terms of 'slips' and 'mistakes' (see video: 'Errors', CEC 2020a) it can be useful to think of human factors that lead to a clinical error as, broadly three types:

1 skill-based errors
2 cognitive errors
3 rule violations.

Skill-based errors occur when a clinician accidentally omits a step in a familiar task – for example, forgetting to swab an ampoule with alcohol before drawing up a medication or forgetting to check a blood glucose level before administering insulin. Skill-based errors do not occur intentionally. They can result from someone being distracted or interrupted when delivering care, or from fatigue and weariness.

Cognitive errors are errors of thinking and judgement, and are not intentional either. They result from inadequate information or a misinterpretation of a situation or information. Examples of cognitive errors include carrying out a procedure without administering pain relief on the assumption that the patient cannot feel pain because they are unconscious, or giving paracetamol for a high temperature without trying a cool bath or some other less invasive treatment first. With an ageing population and increasing use of technology to treat a range of conditions, nurses are caring for patients with increasingly complex conditions in workplaces that are busy. In this context, cognitive factors can be expected to play an increasingly significant role in clinical incidents.

Rule violations occur when a clinician acts in contravention of a known rule – for example, not washing hands before doing a dressing or not checking the administration of a Schedule 8 drug with another registered nurse. Rule violations are done knowingly, often as short-cuts when working under time pressure.

Consider the following example of an incident involving both system factors and human factors.

LAW AND ETHICS IN PRACTICE

Helen, a middle-aged woman, presented at a rural nurse-led clinic one Sunday morning, complaining of chest pain. The nurse on duty, Sonja, took a brief history, baseline observations and an electrocardiograph (ECG), which showed acute changes. She then rang the nearest medical practice, which was located 30 kilometres away.

There was no doctor on duty, so Sonja rang the emergency department (ED) at the nearest hospital. She spoke with a registered nurse, who advised her to call a doctor and then administer morphine and oxygen. Sonja explained that there was no doctor available, nor any oxygen or medications that she might administer herself. The nurse in the ED put a resident doctor on the phone, and Sonja repeated her story.

The resident doctor said that she should speak to a cardiologist, and attempted to put the call through to the cardiology ward. While this was going on, Helen's situation deteriorated. Her pain worsened and she became short of breath and extremely anxious. There was no cardiologist on duty in the cardiology ward, and the nurse put the call back to the ED. In the meantime, Helen became unconscious after suffering a cardiac arrest. The nurse in the ED advised Sonja to ring an ambulance, which she did.

>> What considerations should inform your decision to ring an ambulance?

A system factor here is the absence of a process for getting urgent medical advice to nurses in isolated rural areas in an emergency. A human factor is the failure of the nurse to realise that she needed to call an ambulance immediately on seeing the ECG changes.

A range of factors make human beings vulnerable to error in professional practice, just as they do in other areas of life. They include:

→ a limited knowledge of certain kinds of situations (you can't know everything)
→ a limited knowledge of possible outcomes (you can't tell the future)
→ the perspectival nature of knowledge (everyone's view of the world is influenced by their own personal perspective)
→ the inherent ambiguity of life (events and experiences often have multiple possible meanings)
→ working under time pressure
→ responding to others' expectations of us (we tend to want to do what we think others would want us to do)
→ not knowing what you don't know (not understanding that a situation requires expertise and knowledge of which you are ignorant)
→ common errors of rational cognition (called 'heuristic biases') (Kahneman 2011).

There are also a number of human factors that are unique to each individual, which arise from the individual's personality and experiences. These may include:

→ under-confidence/over-confidence
→ a lack of relevant life experience
→ low literacy and numeracy levels
→ low self-esteem
→ a lack of role models
→ a lack of respect for authority
→ a lack of objectivity
→ cross-cultural differences
→ internal conflict
→ inappropriate loyalties.

REFLECTIVE QUESTIONS 9.1

1 What kinds of processes can you put in place to make sure your own nursing practice is as safe as it should be?

2 Do you often ask your colleagues to check that you have done something properly, or do you avoid scrutiny in case you are judged to be less competent than someone else?

Tracking and managing clinical incidents

Every health service in each state and territory will have its own mechanisms for monitoring and responding to clinical incidents. For example, each year the CEC reports on the incidence of a range of clinical incidents in New South Wales, reported in the Incident Management System (IMS). The ACSQHC also provides a national *Incident Management Guide*.

In all states and territories, the seriousness of clinical incidents is categorised against a standardised Severity Assessment Code (SAC), the purpose of which is to determine the 'level of investigation and action required' (CEC 2020b). These ratings reflect the level of danger the incident poses to the patient:

→ *SAC 1* refers to incidents involving extreme risk and serious harm, and require immediate action by management. A Reportable Incident Brief (RIB) should be forwarded to the Ministry of Health within 24 hours. SAC 1 incidents are those that result in, or have the potential to have resulted in, death or grave injury.

→ *SAC 2* refers to incidents involving high risk and moderate harm, and require immediate notification to senior management. Detailed investigation is required. An example is an incident where a patient has fallen in a bathroom and sustained a broken femur and suspected concussion.

→ *SAC 3* refers to incidents involving medium risk and minor or no harm. Management must be notified as soon as possible and management responsibility for review must be specified – for example, an incident where a patient has been administered a wrong medication but does not experience a serious reaction.

→ *SAC 4* refers to incidents involving low risk and very minor or no harm, which are managed by routine procedures – for example, an incident where a patient has suffered a skin tear while being moved (WA Health 2019).

The severity of clinical incidents in NSW public hospitals is set out in Table 9.1 (CEC 2020b). The overwhelming majority of incidents are of the less serious kind.

As a result of monitoring and investigating clinical incidents, a number of strategies have been introduced nationally to increase patient safety. These address both system factors and human factors. For example, the Between the Flags program was introduced by the New South Wales CEC in 2010 (CEC 2018).

TABLE 9.1 Clinical incidents by SAC rating

SAC RATING	JAN–DEC 2020
SAC 1	509
SAC 2	3 192
SAC 3	71 161
SAC 4	113 378
No SAC allocated	6 333
TOTAL	195 023

Source: Adapted from CEC (2020b).

It is modelled on Surf Life Saving Australia's approach of watching carefully and making sure swimmers remain in the safe zone. It involves a multivalent strategy to ensure processes and structures are in place to identify those at increased risk, carefully monitor patients, identify early and late warning signs of deterioration and appropriately escalate care (CEC 2018; Pain et al. 2017).

Another strategy currently in use in different states and territories is the iSoBar program, which was piloted and evaluated by the Australian Commission on Safety and Quality in Health Care (ACSQHC 2022a). This is a communication strategy that aims to ensure accuracy of patient information and the appropriate response, especially when handing over to incoming staff at shift changeover or after transport. It has six elements (Porteous et al. 2009):

1 *Identification* – introduce yourself and your patient.
2 *Situation* – explain the situation.
3 *Observations* – describe observations accurately; include not only vital signs but intravenous therapy, drains and dressings.
4 *Background* – provide patient information about diagnosis, treatment, test results, allergies and other relevant issues.
5 *Agreement on a plan* – establish what the situation requires. Do you want advice or urgent intervention?
6 *Reading back* – check for shared understanding to make sure you are all clear about who is doing what, and by when.

While such strategies cannot eliminate clinical incidents and errors completely, they can provide a safety net for clinicians and patients to help reduce the impact of system failures and human factors.

When mistakes happen: The professional and ethical response

RESPECT AND SELF-RESPECT

It is important to deal effectively and ethically with clinical errors and incidents, not simply because they can cause harm to patients who are already vulnerable but for the sake of professional self-respect.

The ICN Code of Ethics (ICN 2012, 2021) makes two relevant statements in this regard: 'The nurse demonstrates professional values such as respectfulness, responsiveness, compassion, trustworthiness and integrity' (Element 1) and 'The nurse carries personal responsibility and accountability for nursing practice' (Element 2).

Living up to these values and personal responsibility entails a level of self-respect. Self-respect means considering yourself to be worthy of high regard; it is the belief that you are a person worthy of being treated well by others (recall Chapter 1 on respect for our common humanity). We develop our self-respect by living up to the standards of conduct we set for ourselves. When we live up to our expectations, we feel a sense of self-worth and we gain self-respect. When we fail to live up to our expectations, we can feel embarrassed, humiliated or shamed. Although making mistakes – and particularly making our mistakes known to our peers – can feel embarrassing, humiliating or shameful, it is important to recognise that those negative feelings can have a powerful positive effect on us by motivating us to want to do better in the future, and so can restore self-respect quickly.

We can respect both people and the roles they occupy. When we treat police officers, teachers and health-care professionals with respect, we act in a way that shows we value those roles. The role of a police officer deserves respect because it is demanding and requires discipline to uphold the law and help the victimised in society. We respect teachers because we recognise and value their specialist skills and commitment to helping us learn, and health-care professionals deserve respect because they willingly undertake demanding studies and difficult work in order to support and care for the incapacitated. In each case, these activities contribute to goods that are of value to every member of society, regardless of whether any particular individual directly uses those services. We all benefit from living in a society that has a system of law and order, shares knowledge and understanding, and cares for the incapacitated.

The individuals who fill these roles deserve respect not simply because the role itself is valuable but, importantly, when they as individuals live up to the standards of their profession. Every profession has certain expectations about what counts as doing the job well, and when a person lives up to those standards, they become worthy of professional respect. Likewise, when individuals fail to live up to their profession's standards, they fail to be worthy of the profession's respect. For example, one can undertake the role of nurse in a satisfactory or unsatisfactory manner. When the role is carried out in an unsatisfactory manner – for example, when a nurse fails to exercise due diligence and care – that nurse is no longer worthy of the respect that is accorded to them in virtue of belonging to the nursing profession.

REFLECTIVE QUESTIONS 9.2

1 Do you think you deserve respect because you are a nurse?
2 Can you have self-respect in some parts of your life but less self-respect in other parts?
3 What can you do to maintain your self-respect?

As discussed in Chapter 1, the Western cultural tradition – which includes mainstream Australian culture – advocates respect for all persons. While religious Enlightenment philosophers believed it was the presence of God that made each person intrinsically worthy of respect, non-religious philosophers have argued that we should have respect for our common humanity because we are all equally vulnerable, flawed and capable of succumbing to suffering. On this view, the successes of some individuals and the failures of others depend upon luck as well as hard work (Williams 1981). Because we are each the product of forces beyond our control, which we did not choose (for example, our country of birth, our genes, our parents and their skills, and our social circumstances), no person can be said to be intrinsically or naturally morally superior or inferior to any other. Respect for our common humanity, then, is a recognition that any one of us could have turned out just like any other person if we were subject to similar circumstances. Respect for our common humanity implies self-respect since each person is a member of that common humanity.

Whatever one's particular beliefs regarding this matter, the idea of universal respect for persons has always been fundamental to ethics and law in Australia. Universal respect for persons places legal constraints upon what individuals can do to each other, and gives rise to obligations towards each other. For example, people are not to be sold, or employed for less than a legally defined minimum wage or subjected to unwarranted force or coercion. In addition to legal constraints, respect gives rise to moral obligations concerning how we are to act towards our fellow human beings. For example, we have a moral obligation to give assistance to someone in need, to refrain from interfering with the person's pursuit of their own interests as long as they do not cause harm to others and to refrain from exploiting those in any particular situation of vulnerability. Each of the four principles of bioethics – non-maleficence, beneficence, respect for autonomy and justice – rests on the idea of respect for our common humanity (recall Chapter 3).

WHEN A PERSON LACKS SELF-RESPECT

Chapter 1 explained that a person's sense of self is formed out of relations with other people from birth and continuously throughout life. Self-respect is not a naturally occurring trait, like having teeth or a voice. It is a socially acquired capacity. We each acquire the ability to value ourselves as persons as a result of being valued by other people. If other people do not respect you, then you will find it hard to respect yourself, and if you do not respect yourself, you will find it difficult to know *how* to respect other people.

People who lack self-respect often behave in ways that puzzle people with healthy self-respect (Dillon 1992). For example, they seem to readily accept treatment that others would regard as insulting or humiliating. In her research, philosopher Robin Dillon describes a range of behaviours that stem from a lack of self-respect, such as self-deprecation and self-betrayal. She describes a lack of self-respect as giving rise to a servile personality – one that:

> willingly accepts abuse from others because he believes the right to fair treatment must be earned through merit and accomplishment, and he knows he is thoroughly inadequate in those departments. He does not understand that certain treatment is his due as a person regardless of his failures (or successes). (Dillon 1992: 126)

A person who lacks self-respect might, for example, be disappointed at not receiving praise from the boss while a less effective colleague does, but will not regard it as unjust if they believe their efforts are never as important as someone else's. In other words, a lack of self-respect leads someone to believe they cannot expect to be treated as the equal of others.

If respect for oneself as a person is compromised, it is very difficult to feel worthy of respect in any specific role (Dillon 2001). That means that individuals with low self-respect are at high risk of being exploited or manipulated by others (for example, by bullies or unscrupulously ambitious colleagues). This is because such individuals regard themselves as appropriate objects of inferior treatment. People who lack self-respect often accept that it is reasonable to expect high standards of conduct from other people, but they do not regard *themselves* as being able to meet those same high standards (Benson 2000). Consequently, such individuals are not surprised when their efforts are considered to be of a low standard by others. In fact, they may expect to be criticised for their efforts, regardless of what their work is like on any objective standard. Consider the following example.

LAW AND ETHICS IN PRACTICE

Alicia is a university student who works hard on her assignments and achieves consistently high marks, but she is never satisfied with her work. She believes that her assignments are full of the kinds of mistakes a good student would have been able to avoid. Some of her classmates become annoyed with Alicia because they think she is constantly fishing for compliments and seeking attention.

>> **Do you know someone like Alicia? Are you a bit like Alicia?**

The reality is that many students like Alicia genuinely cannot see what is good about their work, and may even come to regard their good grades as the result of incompetent teachers or a corrupt education system that pushes students through simply for financial benefit.

Low self-respect can present in two extremes of behaviour. Some people will be unable to muster the motivation to try very hard to succeed. These people may find themselves moving from job to job after a succession of professional failures or interpersonal conflict. Others (like Alicia) will strive harder to improve, but without ever feeling satisfied with their efforts.

While it is important to recognise that every nurse makes mistakes, some nurses who lack self-respect are particularly vulnerable to making mistakes. Nurses whose lack of self-respect gives rise to a 'don't care' attitude are at risk of failing in their duty of care because their expectations of their own professional conduct fall below the normal standard. Such nurses are at risk of being drawn into unprofessional conduct in a number of ways – for example, by failing to recognise situations that are morally dubious, or by not intervening when wrongdoing is witnessed or, worse, by actively participating in wrongdoing out of cynicism. When nurses do not respect their own work, they are less likely to respect their colleagues or their employer, and so are less likely to report clinical errors and incidents or expect problems to be redressed.

Jay was scouting for an operation in the operating theatre. Scouts don't wear sterile gowns or gloves; they use a no-touch technique to place sterile equipment on to the scrub nurse's sterile field. When opening a packet of sponges on to the sterile trolley, Jay noticed that one sponge brushed his hand before landing. He shrugged to himself and ignored it, although he knew it had contaminated the sterile field.

》》 What would you do if you saw this happen?

Healthy self-respect requires that you have standards that are neither too high to reach nor too low to matter, and for that you need to have a realistic and well-balanced self-image, a conception of yourself as basically a good and able individual who is willing to take advice from and correction by other good and able people in order to live up to the standards you consider worth having. And for that you need to be able to establish relationships with people who treat you as worthy and support your sense of being valued. Here, workplace culture plays a powerful role in producing quality professionals. (Workplace culture will be discussed shortly.)

Reporting errors and incidents
ADMITTING YOUR OWN MISTAKES

Jang was nursing Cameron, a football player who had undergone surgery for a shoulder injury. Cameron's shoulder and arm were strapped, and he had some pain, which made mobility difficult. Cameron asked Jang for assistance in getting back to bed. Jang was in a hurry to meet a colleague for lunch, and rushed Cameron getting into bed. As a result, Cameron twisted his shoulder and experienced a severe burst of pain. 'Watch what you're doing, you're too rough', said Cameron. Jang stopped and apologised, then continued more carefully.

At lunch, Jang told his colleague, Emily, what he had done and that he 'felt bad about it'. Emily admitted that she had done a similar thing once, and that Jang should go back and talk to Cameron again to show he really did recognise the harm he had done and to show that he could be trusted to take more care in the future. Jang agreed.

Feeling embarrassed and anxious that Cameron would be angry with him, Jang nevertheless went and spoke with Cameron. Cameron was surprised at first, but said, 'Because I'm a footballer, everyone thinks I'm big and tough, but I know how hard it can be to admit when you're wrong – that takes guts. Good on you, mate – and thanks.'

》》 What personal characteristics does Jang show in admitting his mistake to his patient?

An important source of professional self-respect for nurses is the trust that patients have in them, and the good outcomes that nursing practice brings when it is done well. When nurses make a mistake, their trustworthiness can be called into question because they have failed to live up to their responsibilities. Recognising this, the nurse's sense of self-worth takes a blow. This blow to self-respect is why people often prefer not to report their mistakes: it means admitting that they have not been good enough. However, concealing a mistake can be a doubly negative experience because the nurse not only has to live with feelings of not being good enough; they have to live with the knowledge of being deceitful *as well*.

Admitting to a mistake demonstrates important moral qualities that patients and colleagues value, such as courage, humility, honesty, accountability and integrity. It also demonstrates genuine kindness, compassion and remorse towards those who may have been harmed by the error. It is a recommitment to putting the patient at the centre of nursing care, and brings the nurse's conduct and values into line with normal professional standards. In admitting an error, nurses do not hold themselves above their patients or colleagues; they show themselves to be the patients' moral equal. When nurses show these moral qualities, they are giving their patients and colleagues *more* reasons to trust them. For one thing, everyone can see that the nurse is not the kind of person who deceives others. Nevertheless, many errors go unreported.

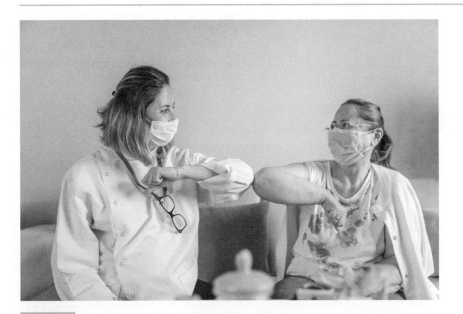

FIGURE 9.1 When nurses show their commitment to doing the right thing, they give their patients good reasons to trust them.

Making a mistake is often regarded as a weakness and gives rise to feelings of shame. This is one reason why we all feel an aversion to reporting our mistakes. It is normal for a nurse to feel an aversion to reporting a mistake for the following kinds of reasons:

→ not wanting to make trouble (for oneself or others)
→ fearing a punitive response/shame/legal action/sacking
→ fearing that the patient will lose trust in the nurse
→ fearing public trust in nurses will be undermined
→ not wanting to be judged by colleagues
→ lacking support from colleagues/management
→ thinking that reporting will just make things worse for everybody.

All these factors have force when admitting your own mistakes, but some relate equally to reporting the mistakes of others. Further factors come into play when considering reporting the mistakes of others – one is loyalty, which will be discussed shortly. However, it is *not* reasonable for a nurse to feel an aversion to reporting a mistake for the following reasons:

→ believing that the harmed person will get over it
→ disliking the harmed person
→ being cynical – for example, seeing what you can get away with ('How hopeless is this place?')
→ thinking 'that is just how things are done here'
→ thinking that patients/management/doctors expect too much anyway
→ showing ignorance ('I don't want to get involved')
→ thinking that reporting will create more work for them.

REPORTING THE MISTAKES OF OTHERS

When a colleague makes a clinical error and then tries to conceal it, such conduct threatens the bonds of professional loyalty, which can give rise to cognitive and emotional distress for the nurse witnessing the error. This is partly why mistakes can go unreported: it is extremely uncomfortable to discuss a colleague's failings openly. At the same time, it must be recognised that, on rare occasions, a staff member may report another's mistake in an effort to obtain or exploit some advantage over that staff member. Because this can happen, reporting another's mistake risks raising the suspicion that the reporting nurse may have a personal grudge against the person being reported. A fear of being suspected in this way can be a disincentive to reporting. It takes a person of strong character and moral integrity, confident in their values and obligations, to respond appropriately to the mistakes of others. Recall the case of Apari at the beginning of this chapter, who discovered that Louise was testing blood glucose levels incorrectly.

LAW AND ETHICS IN PRACTICE

When Apari raised the issue with Louise, she became indignant and said, 'Don't tell me how to do something as simple as a blood sugar level. Do you think I'm an idiot or something?' Apari responded calmly, saying, 'I know that you are new here, and there are a lot of different machines around and it isn't hard to get confused about how long to leave the blood on the test strip. I'll show you how this one works, and we can let the doctor know what has happened so that Jack can get the right medication dosage.'

Apari and Louise went together to explain the mistake to the doctor, and noted this in Jack's file. Apari arranged to meet with Louise later in the day to show her how to use the various testing devices on the ward. Louise asked Apari to follow up with her in a few days' time to make sure that she was confident in using them safely. Although she felt embarrassed about her incompetence and her hostility, Louise was grateful that Apari was supportive and sensitive. Apari felt relieved that Louise could be trusted to ask for help if she needed it. Later that week, Louise met with the clinical manager and explained what had been happening, and how Apari had supported her.

>> **What personal and professional characteristics has Louise shown in working with Apari to address Jack's care?**

Note that Apari was careful not to undermine Louise's self-respect in his response. He did not insult her by calling her 'stupid'. He maintained respect for her humanity by responding with compassion and understanding, and by offering a way forward together. Apari did not treat her as if she were merely 'a cog in the machine' or some kind of servant contracted to the hospital. Nor did he respond competitively by using her mistake to make himself look better than her. Apari's focus was on patient safety and quality nursing care, and he was smart and humane enough to see that Louise (and her patients) needed someone to support her to lift the standard of her care. Apari's support provided Louise with an opportunity to restore and maintain her professional self-respect. She now has the confidence to ask for clarification about how glucometers (and other devices) work wherever she is posted. When individual nurses support each other to provide quality care, the whole health-care system benefits.

Workplace loyalty is a hugely influential factor when it comes to reporting colleagues' mistakes. Workplace culture has a role to play in either facilitating or impeding the exercise of moral capacities needed to deal with clinical errors.

Organisational environments that recognise and reward moral and psychological capacities – such as honesty, courage, accountability and trustworthiness – will retain nurses with those qualities, and nurture those qualities in less morally mature nurses. Accordingly, the quality of nursing care and professional self-respect that is possible within those organisations will be high. Strategies such as the 'Magnet' program aim to do exactly this (Jones 2017; Jones et al. 2019).

On the other hand, organisational environments that fail to support the moral capacities of their nurses can expect to provide poorer quality care because nurses will fail to trust each other, fail to report incidents and fail to provide the requisite support for each other to redress mistakes. Healthy workplaces have *effective* policies and practices in place that support staff to report errors and that protect staff from punitive responses or victimisation as a result of reporting. This is essential because, as Chapter 7 pointed out, reporting of some incidents – for example, suspected or known child abuse – is mandatory. In an effort to promote reporting, most states and territories have specific legislation to protect 'whistleblowers' – that is, to protect employees who report wrongdoing and corruption within an organisation in relation to matters of public interest (see the Appendix for a table of legislation).

REFLECTIVE QUESTIONS 9.3

1 Have you seen a nurse do something that you thought was wrong for a patient? How did you feel? What did you do?
2 Did you feel loyal to the nurse or to the patient?

How you respond to a colleague who admits to an error will have a powerful effect on the willingness of all staff to disclose mistakes. If your reaction expresses anger, contempt or derision, you will become an obstacle to the acquisition of the moral and psychological attributes required for effective ethical practice – both in yourself and in others.

LAW AND ETHICS IN PRACTICE

Brian, a new nurse in the ward, comes to you in an anxious state and tells you that he has just given a patient, Bob, the wrong sleeping tablet. The medication he has administered is very similar to the prescribed medication, and Bob is unlikely to suffer any medical problem as a result.

Unfortunately, there had been a mix-up involving Bob's medication the previous day, when a new doctor wrote the wrong name on Bob's medication chart. Consequently, Bob was very irate and has stated that he will be writing a letter of complaint to the director of nursing concerning the poor care he has received.

>> **What do you do?**

Nurses experience loyalty not only to fellow nurses, but to a range of different people: other colleagues, patients, employers and their own professional ideals. At different times, these loyalties can come into conflict with each other (Lagerwey 2010). Consider the following situations.

LAW AND ETHICS IN PRACTICE

Noula, an enrolled nurse, has started arriving late for work, seems tired and distracted, and is easily irritated. One day you notice that she does a poor job of a patient's dressing. When you speak to her privately about this, Noula tells you that she has been diagnosed with cancer and is going through a rough patch. She asks you not to tell anyone.

》 **What do you do?**

You are nursing Harry, a middle-aged man recovering from surgery for a gunshot injury. One day, Harry complains to your manager about the quality of your nursing care. He shows the manager the dressing you did earlier that morning, which is now falling apart. You can see immediately that the dressing has been interfered with.

》 **What do you do?**

You notice that a clique has formed in the ward where you are doing rotation. There are three nurses – Heather, Jill and Stephan – who roster themselves on the same shifts together so that they can get together at work. They also socialise outside work hours. Whenever you are rostered on with them, you find yourself having to pick up the jobs that they neglect, including caring for their patients at times. When you complain to them about this, they laugh at you. You complain to your clinical manager. When she asks them about their conduct, they deny any problem and demand evidence that they have done anything wrong. They say that you are unfriendly and demanding.

》 **What do you do?**

Sometimes the answer to a question of conflicting loyalties is easy. Patient safety is more important than being one of the gang. But sometimes conflicting loyalties are difficult to resolve. An example of this is the case of Noula. One way to address a case of conflicting loyalties is to ask yourself: 'Who is relying on me most of all to realise an essential human good?' (Ricoeur 1992: 190–4). The answer to this question will tell you where your greatest moral responsibility lies. A nurse's moral responsibilities are greatest to those who are most vulnerable to the nurse's power. That will usually be the patients. Colleagues almost always have more power, and therefore more options, than patients. However, in certain situations colleagues may have less power and fewer options than other colleagues, and employers frequently have more power and more options than individual nurses. Working through these issues of power, responsibility and loyalty can be challenging.

Workplaces have their own local professional cultures, which can vary enormously depending upon the personalities of staff, level of staffing, rate of staff turnover, leadership styles, workloads, conduct and influence of doctors, management competency and general resourcing. Local culture plays a big part in influencing the loyalties that form in the workplace. For example, in workplaces with incompetent management, workers may be more loyal to each other than to the organisation; in workplaces with high staff turnover, loyalties may be stronger towards patients than colleagues; and in workplaces with very high workloads, staff may be more loyal to each other than to patients.

Workplace culture inevitably affects individual nurses' conduct because human identities are dynamic and constantly influenced by relations with other people and the social context. It is a feature of human personhood that we look to others to reinforce and legitimate our identities. That is one reason why we tend to form strong relations with people who like the same sorts of things that we do: they share, and reflect back to us, our views of who we believe we are. In the example of Heather, Jill and Stephan, you are on the outside because you do not reflect back to them their own view of themselves. One of the best ways to maintain strong professional ethics is to build relationships with other nurses who share high ethical and professional standards.

A practical program to build ethical capacity has been developed in business studies in the United States. The program is called 'Giving Voice to Values' (GVV) (Gentile 2010). Rather than trying to teach people about ethical theories, GVV assumes that people have ethical values already, and that what is needed is the ability to *act* on those values when potentially unethical situations arise. To this end, GVV tries to tap into people's positive emotions, since we more readily act from emotion than cool reason. In recognising that people have values upon which they want to act, GVV proposes the following practical steps to build capacity to speak out when you witness wrongdoing.

BE ABLE TO ARTICULATE YOUR BROADER PURPOSE IN THE WORKPLACE

Being able to express your purpose in the workforce means being clear in your own mind about why your job matters to you. When you have a strong sense of why work matters to you (that is, why work is a good in your life), and you are able to express that, you will find that you have a firm position from which to speak, and you will be far less bothered by self-doubt. Work is important to people because it can be:

→ a form of social inclusion
→ a source of peer recognition
→ a source of respect and self-worth
→ a source of a sense of purpose in life
→ an expression of political or spiritual commitment
→ a means of becoming skilled
→ a means of supporting oneself and one's family
→ a means of contributing to the solution of difficult problems
→ a way of being happy.

RECOGNISE THAT SPEAKING OUT IS A CHOICE

Often it is too easy to make excuses for not speaking out, instead of treating it as a real choice. When you do act on your values and speak out, it is empowering because you experience your own strength of character and your ability to have an effect in the world. Even if you cannot change the behaviour of others, you can show yourself that you are not a victim of your circumstances or others' bullying. Recalling situations where you have spoken out previously can give you strength to speak out in the future. In addition, hearing from other people about instances when they spoke out can be powerfully motivating.

NORMALISE CONFLICT

Engaging in conflict is something we are discouraged from doing from a young age. It is often regarded as impolite to openly disagree with another person, even when that person's views are offensive and nasty. Because we tend to avoid conflict, we often find ourselves poorly equipped to deal with conflict when it occurs, and this can be a further reason to avoid confrontation. It is possible to learn how to manage conflict and confrontation calmly and effectively, but this requires practising the necessary skills.

FRAME YOUR RESPONSE – PLAY TO YOUR STRENGTHS

One of the most effective skills we can develop when it comes to building our capacity to speak out is the ability to 'frame' a conflictual situation in such a way that allows us to act on our strengths. Framing means contextualising the situation in your mind in order to highlight those features to which you can best respond. In facing a situation of conflict, you need to be able to tell yourself – with conviction – how speaking out is an expression of who you truly are. Gentile (2010: 108) notes that:

> A knowledge of oneself allows the crafting and embracing of a desired self-image … a significant enabler of values-based action is the clarity, commitment and courage that is born of acting from our true center, finding alignment between who we already are and what we say and do.

This opens up the possibility of speaking out for a whole range of personalities, not just the overtly courageous. For example, if you are fearful and risk averse, these can be precisely the emotions that motivate you to speak out if your patients' welfare is threatened.

BE READY FOR RATIONALISATIONS

Part of the skill set that prepares you for speaking out involves being ready for the ways in which others may try to justify their behaviour in order to discourage you from speaking out. This means being familiar with common 'rationalisations'. To illustrate, consider the example of a colleague asking you to conceal a medication error, particularly if the patient has experienced no apparent harm. Your colleague may say that loyalty to your colleagues is more important than filling out an incident report. In other words, your colleague may try to frame the situation as a conflict between two 'rights': loyalty to your peers and telling the truth. This can disguise the fact that the conflict is actually between a wrong and a right – namely, dishonesty and professional integrity. As Gentile (2010: 177) notes:

> Once we recognise that attempts to persuade us to violate our own values are often framed in this way, we might recognise that our colleague is not showing the same loyalty *to* us (by not respecting our personal integrity) that he or she is asking *from* us.

Gentile (2010: 176) identifies four types of conflicts that are typically evoked as rationalisations:

1 loyalty vs truth – for example, if you report the error you are being disloyal to your colleagues
2 individual vs community – for example, if you report a colleague the whole team will lose its bonus
3 short term vs long term – for example, reporting the error might look good in the short term, but it will harm the hospital's reputation in the long run

4 justice vs mercy – for example, if you report the error, a colleague will lose their job, and they have a lot of problems right now.

BUILD YOUR COMMUNICATION SKILLS

Communication skills are central to speaking out effectively. This includes being able to understand your opponents' perspectives and being willing to understand more about their motivations and what is at stake for them in the situation. This will give you more conceptual resources to imagine a creative solution, as well as helping to foster empathy and other emotional links to your opponents, which can build long-term relationships after the conflict is resolved.

A very important practical communication skill that Gentile (2010: 9–13) argues is fundamental to the GVV approach is 'prescripting' your responses to situations in which you may find yourself, where your values are challenged. This means imagining a situation, writing down how you would like to respond to that situation, then practising that script. While this may seem artificial, it is actually a valuable, effective method that prepares you well for speaking out. Anticipating the rationalisations, and having a ready response, can make a real-life situation more familiar to you, and bring it more under your control. Feeling in control allows you to express yourself more confidently, thoughtfully and effectively. So practising your script and your responses is a very powerful way of supporting your personal integrity and professionalism.

LAW AND ETHICS IN PRACTICE

You are about to undertake a placement at a small hospital. Other students have warned you to look out for a certain staff member who they say is 'slack'.

>> **What might you do?**

Professional conduct and professional collegiality are characterised by respect for nursing work, as well as respect for the nurse who does the work, personal accountability, commitment to high standards of practice, objectivity and fairness. These characteristics should form the basis of professional loyalty. When professionals are loyal to their standards and work ideals, they value those standards both in themselves and others. The presence of those values in colleagues gives them professional value and standing, and makes them worthy of professional respect and loyalty. In our professional identities as nurses, we need to form close relationships with those colleagues who respect what we do – namely, uphold those professional values.

Managing clinical incidents and complaints

A variety of processes exist for dealing constructively with clinical errors in the workplace, such as:

→ ward meetings, where poor patient outcomes are discussed openly and constructively
→ regular confidential, individual meetings with all staff members where sensitive issues can be discussed
→ 'drop boxes' and forms for anonymous reporting
→ open disclosure processes (see below).

COMPLAINTS MANAGEMENT AND OPEN DISCLOSURE

This book has emphasised the role of communication in the clinical relationship. Part of being a good communicator involves being responsive to complaints. The CEC received 16 039 complaint notifications during 2020. Complaints were overwhelmingly of a minor nature – that is, SAC 3 and SAC 4 (CEC 2020b).

The three most common ways that complaints are resolved is typically by:

1 making an apology
2 providing an explanation of the care or concerns
3 providing feedback to the clinician(s) involved.

Being treated with dignity and respect, and being provided with emotional support, are central to patient-centred care (Berghout at al. 2015). The Australian Commission on Safety and Quality in Health Care (ACSQHC) has described that 'being treated with dignity and respect, reducing anxiety and having staff available to provide emotional support, are central to how patients perceive their care'. The commission established a national standard that requires clinicians to actively involve patients ('consumers') in their care, not only to improve their experience, but also to improve safety (ACSQHC 2018).

Open disclosure

Clearly, respect and emotional support are central not only to clinical care, but also to the management of complaints. In this spirit, all states and territories of Australia have implemented an open disclosure process consistent with the Australian Open Disclosure Framework developed by the ACSQHC (2013). Open disclosure is defined as an open discussion with a patient (and/or relative) about an incident that resulted in harm to that patient while they were receiving health care:

> The elements of open disclosure are an apology or expression of regret (including the word sorry), a factual explanation of what happened, an opportunity for the person to relate their experience, and an explanation of the steps being taken to manage the event and prevent recurrence.
>
> ...
>
> Open disclosure is ... an ongoing discussion and exchange of information that may take place over time. (ACSQHC 2013: 4)

The open disclosure process is an attempt to give recognition to the harms and injustices done to vulnerable people in hospitals without becoming involved in a legal process that is expensive, time-consuming and often beyond the resources of the complainant. It is hoped that this non-legal process will provide a satisfactory alternative to legal action and will encourage staff to report clinical errors and incidents. It is important to understand that participation in open disclosure does not preclude a person with a complaint from pursuing legal action for damages.

Historically, hospitals have been reluctant to express regret for clinical errors and incidents in the belief that this is an apology, and therefore an admission of legal liability for any harm that may have occurred (Studdert & Richardson 2010). The Open Disclosure Framework does not refer to an apology; rather, it uses the language of 'regret'. The fine distinction between an expression of regret and an apology is probably unimportant to many victims of clinical errors and incidents, who simply want and need recognition of the harm and injustice they have suffered.

The open disclosure process is inappropriate for some kinds of clinical incidents. If there are reasonable grounds to suspect that the incident is the result of deliberately dangerous activity, senior management must be notified immediately and disciplinary processes activated. Untimely, unexplained or suspicious deaths must be reported to the Coroner (see Chapter 7).

The open disclosure process

Open disclosure requires the skills of specially trained professionals, and is not to be attempted by junior or inexperienced clinical staff, or those who do not have the relevant managerial and legal responsibilities.

The open disclosure process commences with the recognition that the patient has suffered unintended harm during treatment. As soon as a harm has been recognised, the patient should be given prompt clinical care and protected from further harm. The incident should then be reported, either in person or by telephone to the responsible manager, or through some other established reporting procedure at the hospital. Many hospitals now utilise an electronic incident reporting system that automatically notifies management via urgent email.

The level of response required by an incident will be determined by the impact or consequence of the incident. Where the impact is low (where the patient does not require a higher level of care), the process normally ends with a disclosure of the incident and an expression of regret. Where the impact is high (where the patient requires a significantly higher level of care), a more complex and lengthy process follows (see Figures 9.2 and 9.3).

Depending on the severity of the incident, it may be necessary to collect evidence to assist in an investigation. Evidence may include broken equipment, samples of medications or other substances. Nurses involved in incidents are advised to make careful and detailed records of the circumstances of the incident, any people involved and, if witnessed, a description of the incident. There may also be a requirement to notify the relevant statutory authority – for example, if the incident involved child abuse or unprofessional conduct of a health professional.

LAW AND ETHICS IN PRACTICE

Will is admitted to the medical ward for care of a leg wound following a fall at home. After 10 days of dressings, his wound swab shows that he has a hospital-acquired infection.

>> **Does this require an open disclosure?**

A discussion about the incident is conducted with the patient as soon as possible after the identification of the incident. That discussion should be led by the most senior health professional responsible for the care of the patient or a senior manager, who needs to possess excellent interpersonal and communication skills. At that time, the patient may feel frightened or anxious, angry, confused or any combination of these and other powerful emotions, so careful consideration should be given to the patient's clinical, emotional and psychological state. It may also be appropriate to involve a support person of the patient's choosing.

During the discussion, the senior professional will express regret for the harm experienced by the patient. In general, the expression of regret should not involve attributing blame to, or criticising, anyone. Nor should it speculate about the possible causes of the incident or admit liability. However, all known facts relevant

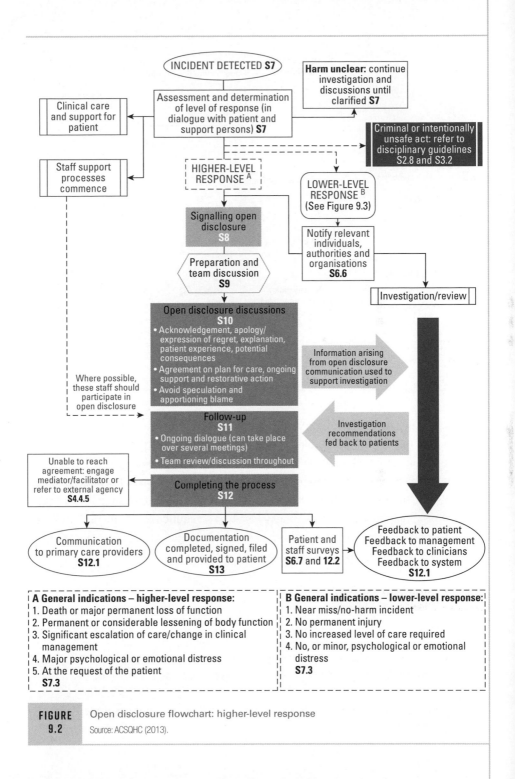

A General indications – higher-level response:
1. Death or major permanent loss of function
2. Permanent or considerable lessening of body function
3. Significant escalation of care/change in clinical management
4. Major psychological or emotional distress
5. At the request of the patient
S7.3

B General indications – lower-level response:
1. Near miss/no-harm incident
2. No permanent injury
3. No increased level of care required
4. No, or minor, psychological or emotional distress
S7.3

FIGURE 9.2 Open disclosure flowchart: higher-level response

Source: ACSQHC (2013).

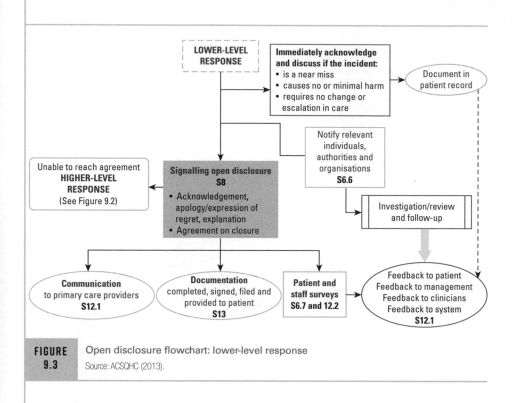

FIGURE 9.3 Open disclosure flowchart: lower-level response

Source: ACSQHC (2013).

to the incident should be made available to the patient and the support person unless there is a legal requirement to do otherwise. The patient should also be informed about what will follow from the incident – for example, whether there is going to be an investigation and how long it is likely to take. The patient should also be informed of all other available courses of action, including legal redress. On completion of an investigation (where that is required), the patient is informed about the findings of the investigation and further advised of any other avenues of action remaining open to the patient.

LAW AND ETHICS IN PRACTICE

Ali calls the 1800 mental health helpline, crying and saying that she is distressed and thinking of taking some pills to stop the pain. The person she speaks to tells her that all the helpers are very busy, but someone will call her back tomorrow. Ali is found by her husband, having taken an unknown quantity of pills. He is very angry about the helpline.

>> Does this warrant open disclosure? If so, to whom is the expression of regret made?

Open disclosure discussions with patients are highly sensitive and need extremely professional handling. Successful resolution of an incident depends upon health professionals possessing personal and moral qualities of trustworthiness, integrity, respect, patience, compassion, commitment and humility. These qualities take time, experience and peer support to acquire, and nursing practice is one of the best places in the world to find them.

As always, nurses must be aware of the policies of their workplace, and the relevant national standards that govern nurses' professional practice.

Conclusion

Everyone makes mistakes. Admitting to a mistake takes moral courage, and the exercise of moral courage can be a potent force for restoring professional self-respect and patient trust. Nurses who admit to mistakes deserve the support of their colleagues and employers. The open disclosure process attempts to do justice to the victims of mistakes – who usually include the person or persons who made the mistakes in the first place.

REFLECTIVE QUESTIONS 9.5

1 Describe the three types of human factors that lead to clinical errors.
2 What are 'system factors' and how can they cause clinical errors?
3 What are some of the benefits to the nurse of admitting mistakes?
4 What practical things can a nurse do to build their capacity to admit and report errors?

Further reading

Cleary, S. (2017). Whistleblowing: What leads a nurse to make the call? *Nursing Review*, 12 December. www.nursingreview.com.au/2017/12/whistleblowing-what-leads-a-nurse-to-make-the-call

Crigger, N.J. (2004). Always having to say you're sorry: An ethical response to making mistakes in professional practice. *Nursing Ethics*, *11*(6), 568–76.

Harrison, R., Walton, M., Smith-Merry, J. et al (2019). Open disclosure of adverse events: Exploring the implications of service and policy structures on practice. *Risk Management and Healthcare Policy*, *12*, 5–12. https://doi.org/10.2147/RMHP.S180359

Rait, J.L. & Van Ekert, E.H. (2011). Legal aspects of open disclosure II: Attitudes of health professionals – findings from a national survey. *Medical Journal of Australia*, *194*(1), 48.

Russell, D. (2018). Disclosure and apology: Nursing and risk management working together. *Nursing Management*, *49*(6), 17–19.

Vines, P. (2011). Apologising for personal injury and other civil harms: Changes in Queensland. *Australian Civil Liability*, *8*(2), 162–4.

10 ISSUES IN ABORTION AND EUTHANASIA

KIM ATKINS

LEARNING OBJECTIVES

In this chapter, you will:

→ Identify the current legislation pertaining to abortion and euthanasia in each state and territory

→ Explain some of the reasons why some people are for, and others against, abortion and euthanasia

→ Describe how the principle of autonomy relates to abortion and euthanasia

→ Distinguish between different types of euthanasia

In Western Australia in October 2012, 81-year-old Herbert Erickson pleaded guilty to murdering his partner in a mercy killing. His partner had suffered a stroke on top of a severe form of paralysis that confined her to a wheelchair. The court heard that the couple loved each other and had made a murder–suicide pact. Mr Erickson had unsuccessfully tried to electrocute himself immediately after killing his partner. He was granted bail on account of his age. One month later, he reported to police as usual, returned his library books, then drove to a nearby beach and killed himself. (Spooner 2012)

Issues relating to life and death go to the heart of human experience and the value we place on our own existence and that of others, especially in those relationships we care about most. This is no doubt because we are mortal and we know we are all going to die at some point in time. Our mortality makes us fundamentally vulnerable. This book has considered ethics in the context of human vulnerability. We are vulnerable because we can be affected by things across the lifespan, and we can be affected by things because we are physical beings – part of the world around us and subject to the passage of time. Consequently, a life can come to an end at any time. For this reason, death is not only completely normal, but inevitable. Nevertheless, death is typically regarded as something regrettable. As philosopher Bernard Williams notes, our experience of being alive is essentially of having an open-ended and indeterminate *future*. From this perspective, death is 'an abrupt cancellation of indefinitely extensive possible goods' (Nagel 1979: 9–10).

Perhaps because of our mortality, it matters to us – as individuals and as a society – how we die. It is not unusual, for example, to hear expressions such as 'a terrible way to die' (meaning that a person has died in a way that no one would want to) or 'it's a blessing that he died' (meaning that death brought a peaceful end to suffering) or 'a good death', which usually means that a person has died in a way that they considered humane and would have wanted. These considerations give rise to some philosophical reflections: Is death always a harm? And if it is not always a harm, can death sometimes be a good thing (Luper 2009)?

The value we attach to ways of dying is directly related to the value we attach to personhood, which is why we typically attach greater value to human deaths than to the deaths of plants or animals. While there are laws that prohibit cruelty to animals and protect some species of animals, there is no equivalent of the concept of murder in relation to animals. Murder is regarded with such seriousness not only because it is the destruction of something living, but because it is the destruction of a self-aware, self-determining (that is, autonomous), free being.

Attitudes toward death, and issues of personhood and autonomy, lie at the centre of bioethical debates about the ending of human life, whether this concerns abortion or euthanasia. Against this backdrop, this chapter provides an overview of the main legal and ethical considerations relating to abortion and euthanasia. While nurses may have a special interest in the morality of abortion and euthanasia, the nurse's role is clearly prescribed by law. Failure of a nurse to act within the law and within a proper scope of practice can result in serious disciplinary action, including criminal charges of assault or even manslaughter.

REFLECTIVE QUESTION 10.1

Recall the discussion on personhood in Chapter 1. Try to articulate your own understanding of personhood. Share these thoughts and values with your colleagues, and try to bring out the reasons behind your views.

Arguments in favour of abortion and euthanasia typically share a common concern with personal autonomy. They maintain that rational, adult individuals should be free to decide for themselves what to do with their bodies and their lives without interference from other people or the state. This view is sometimes called the 'harm principle' (Mill 1975). This is the idea that any particular expression of personal freedom should be restricted only if it actually harms another person. Both opponents and proponents of abortion and euthanasia often maintain that their view encompasses the harm principle. Those opposed to abortion or euthanasia may emphasise the harms that can come to particularly vulnerable people, such as the elderly, the terminally ill, disabled people or single women. Proponents of abortion or euthanasia may argue that laws can be created in such a way as to protect such people – for example, from being manipulated by greedy relatives or being forced to end a pregnancy due to poverty. Much of the debate around abortion and euthanasia concerns how successful the law can be in protecting vulnerable people from harm while respecting the autonomy of individuals.

Australian law and abortion

LAW AND ETHICS IN PRACTICE

In Queensland in 2009, a young woman (assisted by her partner) was charged with procuring her own unlawful abortion when she and her partner arranged for a relative living overseas to send them a supply of the drugs misoprostol and mifepristone, which they used to terminate the pregnancy (*R v Leach and Brennan* 2010). The abortion was considered unlawful because it was not performed to protect the woman's health but rather in order to avoid becoming a parent.

Despite this, the couple were found not guilty as a result of two anomalies in the wording of sections 225 and 228 of Queensland's Criminal Code. Section 228 refers only to surgical procedures of abortion, and not the use of drugs, while section 225 outlaws the use of drugs that are noxious to a woman's health, and does not refer to the effects on the foetus. Consequently, the woman and her partner were found not guilty.

>> **What do you think is the moral difference, in this case, between protecting the woman's health and protecting her from becoming a mother?**

The term 'abortion' refers to the termination of a pregnancy, either spontaneously (as a result of accident or illness) or intentionally (as the result of a procedure). An intentional abortion can be carried out either by means of a surgical procedure or by the administration of a medication, such as mifepristone (also known as RU486). Abortion is legislated by the states and territories of Australia, not the Commonwealth government. Nurses have a responsibility to be aware of the most up-to-date legislation in the state or territory in which they are practising (see Table 10.1 below, and the Appendix for legislation relevant to your jurisdiction).

Abortion was unlawful in all states and territories under the Crimes Acts until amendments were introduced, beginning with *R v Davidson* in 1969 in Victoria (also known as the Menhennitt ruling, after Justice Menhennitt). Justice Menhennitt ruled that an abortion could be lawful if it was performed in order to protect the health of the woman from a serious danger. Abortion law reforms in other states and territories have drawn upon the arguments put forward in the Menhennitt ruling. South Australia amended sections 81 and 82 of the *Criminal Consolidation Act* in 1969, and in the New South Wales District Court Justice Levine ruled similarly in the case of *R v Wald* in 1971. In Queensland in 1986, Justice McGuire made a similar ruling in the case of *R v Bayliss and Cullen* (Petersen 2011).

With the *Termination of Pregnancy Act 2021* introduced to South Australia, abortion law reform has continued across Australia. In 1995 in the Supreme Court of New South Wales, Justice Kirby ruled that, in determining the lawfulness of an abortion, considerations of the impact on a woman's mental health should extend beyond the period of the pregnancy to include her mental health after the child's birth – that is, 'the effects of economic or social stress that may pertain either during pregnancy or after birth' (*Ces v Superclinics Australia Pty Ltd* 1995). This principle has formed the core of all subsequent abortion legislation.

In Victoria, the *Abortion Law Reform Act 2008* made abortion much more accessible by allowing appropriately authorised registered nurses or pharmacists to provide a medical abortion to a woman who is up to 24 weeks pregnant. For an abortion after 24 weeks, a second practitioner must agree that the termination is in the patient's best interest. Abortion by an unqualified person remains a crime.

In Tasmania, the *Criminal Code Act 1924* was clarified in 2001 to give definition to an *unlawful* abortion (and thereby distinguish lawful from unlawful abortions). Legislation was updated in October 2013, and permits a doctor to perform an abortion up to 14 weeks' gestation at the request of the woman. A woman who is more than 14 weeks pregnant must have the approval of two doctors who agree that the abortion is in her best interests. One of the doctors must have specialist training in obstetrics, and the woman must undertake counselling.

Following the case of *R v Leach and Brennan* in 2010, Queensland legislation was amended to include medical abortions and to define a lawful abortion as one performed for the purpose of protecting the woman's health. Penalties for unlawful abortions in all states and territories are severe, and can involve life imprisonment.

History of Australian abortion laws

To understand current Australian abortion laws, it is useful to know something of the cultural context in which they arose. When lawful abortion was first legislated in Australia, the prevailing social attitude towards women was one in which motherhood and domesticity were regarded as their natural and proper destiny. Motherhood was almost compulsory for sexually active women, since positions of power such as law-makers and doctors were overwhelmingly occupied by men, who arguably benefited from women's domesticity. During those times, a woman who rejected the ideal of marriage and motherhood was often considered morally and emotionally suspect.[1]

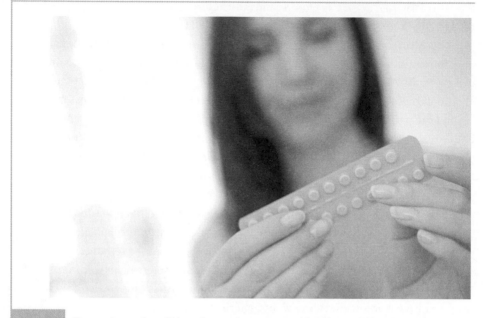

The contraceptive pill has given women greater control over their reproductive capacities, and has prevented the need for many abortions.

Social attitudes slowly changed, and the ready availability of the contraceptive pill gave women increasing control over their reproductive capacities. Being able to defer parenthood allowed women time to participate more fully in public life through study, employment, artistic endeavours, travel and other pursuits. Yet, despite the increasing social recognition of women's autonomy and right to self-determination, discussions about abortion – even from pro-abortion representatives – are often paternalistic and downplay a woman's authority over her own body. This can be seen, for example, in the repeated claim that a decision for abortion is *always* emotionally difficult for *any* woman. This attitude assumes that women are naturally and necessarily predisposed to value conception and pregnancy. The reality is that women experience a range of responses to conception and abortion, depending upon their personal circumstances.

Moral issues

The question of the legal and moral status of a foetus cannot be separated from the question of its relation to the woman's body, and consequently the extent of a woman's personal autonomy (Mackenzie 1992). This underpins the complexity of the ethics of abortion.

Despite the fact that termination of pregnancy has been protected by law under a range of circumstances for some time, the question of women's legal access to abortion is still not settled once and for all. Some sections of society – particularly people with strong religious views – remain opposed to abortion, and continue to lobby politicians to make all abortions unlawful.

At one end of the spectrum of views about abortion, extreme opponents maintain that a foetus is a person with legal and moral rights, making its destruction both immoral and criminal. At the other end of the spectrum, some maintain that a foetus is entirely part of a woman's body, and therefore always subject to her autonomous control. In between are a range of views concerning which kinds of abortions are permissible under what kinds of circumstances, and for what kinds of reasons (Isaacs 2003).

Philosopher Peter Singer (1995) argues that before a woman's right to have an abortion can be defended, it must first be shown that the foetus is not the kind of being that warrants protection from destruction. In short, he proposes that because a foetus lacks rationality and conscious awareness of itself, it is not a person, and therefore does not warrant the same protections as a person.

Against this view, others argue that although a foetus is not actually a person, nevertheless it is a *potential* person, and for that reason it should be protected (Tooley 1972). This view is sometimes based on the concept of the 'sanctity of life', which is the idea that all human life is sacred, and taking a human life can never be justified except to prevent a greater evil (Glover 1977). On this view, there is no higher value than a human life; therefore, any kind of deliberate killing of human life is wrong.

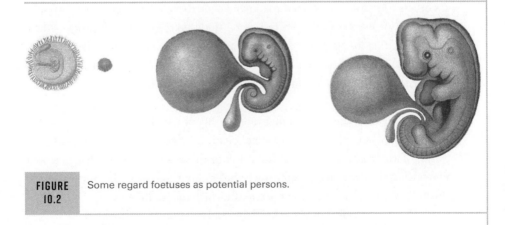

FIGURE 10.2 Some regard foetuses as potential persons.

This raises the question of whether *all* foetuses have the potential to become persons (Hershenov & Hershenov 2015; Lizza 2007). Some foetuses simply never make it through gestation, while others do so only with the help of complex technology. This suggests that potentiality is not a property of the foetus, but rather a property of society. With the development of life-support technologies for premature babies and technologies to treat foetuses *in utero*, the difference between a foetus that has the potential for life and a foetus that doesn't is to be found in technology rather than as a feature solely of the foetus itself (Berkich 2007; Singer & Dawson 1988).

Some ethicists take a different approach, arguing that rather than looking for value *within* the foetus, we should look to the foetus's place in its immediate surrounding world in order to judge its value. On this view, there is a spectrum of value from conception to birth, such that a foetus acquires greater moral value the more it develops (Warren 1989).

To illustrate, consider the situation of a single woman who does not want to become a mother, and consequently has a medical abortion from her doctor very early in the pregnancy. The existence of her foetus is very brief and simple. It exists in a narrow set of relationships consisting only of the woman and her doctor. Such an existence may not be regarded as significant, and therefore its death may not be regarded as significant either.

Compare this to the foetus of a woman who, with her partner, sets out to become a parent. This foetus will be highly valued from conception onwards by the woman, her partner and their circle of family and friends. As the pregnancy becomes more visible, the foetus becomes a greater object of concern for others as well. The needs of the foetus as a future child of the woman become a consideration for others – for example, when the woman negotiates public spaces (such as public transport), or seeks to obtain life insurance, undertakes air travel or seeks medical treatment. This foetus, being an object of regard and value to a wide section of society, has a very significant and complex existence within a broad set of family and social relationships, and for these reasons one might argue that its death could amount to a harm.

To summarise, there are a range of views about whether the death of a foetus is a harm. For some people, every foetal death is a harm; for others, some deaths may be harmful but only under certain circumstances – and there is disagreement about what circumstances matter. Nevertheless, abortion is legal in every state and territory of Australia in the circumstance in which the health and well-being of the woman are significantly threatened by the continuation of the pregnancy.

Nurses' responsibilities

Unless a nurse is qualified, credentialled and employed to provide pregnancy counselling, that nurse should refrain from initiating a discussion of a woman's decision regarding termination of pregnancy. The nurse's responsibilities in providing care for a woman who is having a lawful abortion are no different from the legal and moral responsibilities that relate to any other kind of lawful clinical procedure. The nurse is obliged to maintain a duty of care to the patient. If a nurse has a deep moral conviction that prevents them from providing the necessary care, the nurse should ask to be assigned other duties and should not seek to influence the clinicians who are providing the woman's care. Like all clinicians, nurses with a conscientious objection are bound by the usual legal and moral requirements of confidentiality and professional standards.

Table 10.1 provides an overview of abortion legislation in the states and territories of Australia.

TABLE 10.1 Overview of current abortion legislation

STATE/TERRITORY	ACCESS
ACT *Medical Practitioners (Maternal Health) Amendment Act 2002*	Only a registered medical practitioner may carry out abortion. It must be carried out in a medical facility, or part of a medical facility, that has been given ministerial approval to perform abortions.
NSW *Abortion Law Reform Act 2019*	Abortion was removed from the *Crimes Act* in 2019. Abortion is legal up to 22 weeks' gestation. After 22 weeks of pregnancy, abortions must occur in a hospital or approved health facility, and be carried out by a specialist medical practitioner who has consulted with another practitioner. A woman under 16 years of age may give valid consent to an abortion without her parent's or guardian's knowledge if the doctor judges that she understands the implications of making the decision.

»

STATE/TERRITORY	ACCESS
NT *Termination of Pregnancy Law Reform Act 2017*	Abortion is lawful up to 23 weeks' gestation with the agreement of a second doctor, giving regard to: a) all relevant medical circumstances; and b) the woman's current and future physical, psychological and social circumstances; and c) professional standards and guidelines. Abortion can be performed at any stage of a pregnancy if the treatment is given in good faith for the purpose only of preserving the woman's life.
Qld *Termination of Pregnancy Act 2018*	The Termination of Pregnancy Act came into effect in December 2018. Under the Act, a medical practitioner may perform an abortion on a woman who is not more than 22 weeks pregnant. For a woman who is more than 22 weeks pregnant, an abortion can be performed if the doctor believes it is necessary and has consulted with another doctor who also believes it is necessary. The doctors must give consideration to all relevant medical circumstances, the woman's current and future physical, psychological and social circumstances, and professional standards.
SA *Termination of Pregnancy Act 2021*	This Bill has not yet come into effect in South Australia. When it is enacted, an abortion will be lawful up to 22 weeks and six days' gestation. Under the Bill, an abortion is lawful later than 27 weeks if approved by two doctors and performed in a prescribed hospital by a legally qualified medical practitioner, where both doctors believe that the termination is necessary to avoid serious injury to the pregnant person, or to save the life of another foetus, or because there is a significant risk, of serious foetal anomalies. An abortion after 27 weeks may be performed in an emergency situation. The pregnant woman must have been resident in South Australia for at least two months before the abortion.
Tas *Reproductive Health (Access to Terminations) Act 2013*	Abortion is lawful up to 14 weeks' gestation with the approval of one qualified medical practitioner. After 14 weeks' gestation a second doctor with specialist training in obstetrics must agree the termination is in the patient's best interests. Counselling for the woman is compulsory.
Vic *Abortion Law Reform Act 2008*	Abortion is lawful with the approval of a qualified medical practitioner, nurse or pharmacist if the pregnancy is less than 24 weeks' gestation. After 24 weeks' gestation, a second practitioner must agree that the termination is in the patient's best interest. The abortion must be performed by a qualified person.
WA *Acts Amendment (Abortion) Act 1998 and Health Act 1911*	Abortion is lawful if performed before 20 weeks' gestation. It must be performed by a medical practitioner who believes in good faith that the continuation of the pregnancy would involve greater risk of injury 'to the physical or mental health of the pregnant woman' than if the pregnancy were terminated, or that the woman will suffer 'serious personal, family or social consequences if the abortion is not performed'. Informed consent for abortion occurs when a medical practitioner other than one performing or assisting with the abortion has provided counselling to the woman about the medical risk of continuing the pregnancy, and offered opportunity of referral for counselling prior to and following a pregnancy termination or carrying a pregnancy to term. After 20 weeks of pregnancy, 'two medical practitioners who are members of a panel of six appointed by the Minister' have to agree 'that the mother [or foetus] has a severe medical condition'. These abortions can only be performed 'in a facility approved by the minister'. Women under 16 years of age 'may apply to the Children's Court for an order' to proceed with an abortion if it is not considered suitable to involve their parent(s). The woman must be offered counselling before an abortion can be performed.

The nurse's professional role, as always, is to:

→ obey the law
→ practise only within their scope of practice
→ uphold their duty of care.

You overhear a colleague talking with a young woman who has just returned from the operating theatre after the termination of her pregnancy. Your colleague appears to comfort the patient, saying 'There's no need to feel bad; you did the right thing.'

>> **When would this conversation fall within a nurse's scope of practice?**

Australian law and euthanasia

In May 2018, the *ABC News* network in Australia reported the case of award-winning scientist, Dr David Goodall, aged 104, who travelled to Switzerland after being accepted into a voluntary euthanasia program. In Switzerland Dr Goodall spoke to international news media about his support for voluntary euthanasia, saying that his life had ceased to be enjoyable, and that he wanted to exercise his own choice about how and when he died. Dr Goodall emphasised the value he placed on being remembered as someone with his mental processes intact: 'If they remember me in possession of my senses, but only in part, that would be good' (Hamlyn 2018). With the support of his family, Dr Goodall was assisted in his endeavour by a pro-euthanasia group called Exit International (EI), led by Australian doctor Philip Nitschke.

Other people have not had this option. Consider this submission to the Victorian Parliamentary Inquiry into End of Life Choices:

> Eleven years ago, my mother had a stroke and took seven months to die. As her principle [sic] carer I divided my days into good days and bad days. A good day for me was when she said 'John, I want to die'. A bad day was when she said 'John, please kill me'. That was the only thing in her whole life that she had ever asked of me, and I didn't love her enough to do it because of the legal consequences. Eventually she starved herself to death. Now I live with the guilt: callous, cruel and selfish before God and my mother, but innocent before the law. (Parliament of Victoria, Legal and Social Issues Committee 2016)

The meaning of the word 'euthanasia' has Greek roots, and translates loosely to 'good death'. The word has come to refer to the act of ending a person's life in a situation of intolerable suffering or terminal illness, also called 'mercy killing'. Implicit in the concept of euthanasia is the idea that there are worse things than dying. In other words, from this perspective, death is not always a harm.

As noted in Chapter 4, it is legal in Australia to refuse life-sustaining treatment. However, this is an option only for people who have the capacity to make their wishes known at the time of treatment or beforehand – for example, through a properly prepared advance care directive.

Laws allowing physician-assisted deaths have existed in the Netherlands and some US states since 1984 (Quill & Greenlaw 2008; Singer 2005). However, in a number of states and territories in Australia, with the exception of Victoria, Western Australia and Tasmania, it is a criminal offence to assist someone to die, or to instruct a person on the best means of ending their own life. Despite this, EI claims to have been providing euthanasia workshops in Australia for a number of years (Hamlyn 2018).

In 1995, the Northern Territory government passed the *Rights of the Terminally Ill Act*, which legalised medically assisted voluntary euthanasia at the request of a terminally ill person. That Act was overturned by the federal government in 1997, through an amendment to the *Federal Parliament of the Northern Territory (Self-Government) Act 1978* (Cth). This was possible because, under the Australian Constitution, the territories (the Northern Territory and the Australian Capital Territory) have a different legal status from the states. However, during the short life of the legislation, at least two people (Robert Dent and Janet Mills) exercised their rights and died under the Act (Alcorn 1997). Bills to legalise euthanasia continue to be put before state and territory parliaments, but currently euthanasia attracts criminal charges punishable by imprisonment.

In June 2016, the Victorian Parliament released the final report of its *Inquiry into End of Life Choices* (Parliament of Victoria, Legal and Social Issues Committee 2016). The report was the result of a long engagement with community members and experts to comprehensively consider the range of legal, moral and social issues relating to end of life choices in Victoria. The Parliamentary Committee took submissions from individual members of the public, professional bodies, advocacy groups, clinicians, academics and a range of other groups. It also considered practices and legislation in other states and territories of Australia and internationally. It recommended that:

> The Government should introduce legislation to allow adults with decision-making capacity, suffering from a serious and incurable condition who are at the end of life to be provided assistance to die in certain circumstances.
>
> This should include amending the *Crimes Act 1958* to provide the exemptions necessary to protect health practitioners who act within the provisions of assisted dying legislation. (Parliament of Victoria, Legal and Social Issues Committee 2016)

In 2017 the Victorian Parliament passed the *Voluntary Assisted Dying Act*. Under the Act, from June 2019, people who meet strict criteria were able to access voluntary assisted dying (Victoria Health 2018). Under the Act, a request for assisted dying must come from a competent, consenting adult, who has been assessed by two doctors who deem the person eligible. The two doctors must themselves have been trained and assessed as meeting specific legal requirements before they can provide this assessment. The assistance takes the form of a medication that is prescribed after the assessment. Further authorisation is required before participating doctors can prescribe the medication. The medication is normally self-administered, but a doctor who has been authorised under the Act and has been issued with a permit may administer it.

Doctors or other clinicians who do not wish to participate in voluntary assisted dying are able to register their conscientious objection, which makes it legally permissible for them to refuse to participate in or provide information about assisted dying (*Voluntary Assisted Dying Act 2017*, Part 1, section 7). *Nurses are not permitted to give access to, or administer, the medication.*

The *Voluntary Assisted Dying* guidelines formulated by the Victorian state government (Victorian State Government 2018b) outline that people choosing to access voluntary assisted dying must meet the following requirements:

1   They must have an advanced disease that will cause their death and is:
    –   likely to cause their death within six months (or within 12 months for neurodegenerative diseases like motor neurone disease) and
    –   causing the person suffering that is unacceptable to them.
2   They must have the ability to make and communicate a decision about voluntary assisted dying throughout the process.
3   They must also:
    –   be an adult 18 years or over
    –   have been living in Victoria for at least 12 months
    –   be an Australian citizen or permanent resident.

In addition, the guidelines state that a person cannot request voluntary assisted dying in an advance care directive.

The Victorian legislation has influenced the development of legislation in other states:

→ Western Australia (*Voluntary Assisted Dying Act 2019*)
→ South Australia (*Voluntary Assisted Dying Act 2021*)
→ Tasmania (*(End-of-Life Choices) Voluntary Assisted Dying Act 2021*)
→ Queensland (*Voluntary Assisted Dying Act 2021*).

Each state is in the process of implementing its legislation, and each has a different timeline. You will need to check when your state's legislation comes into effect, and what processes are in place.

In New South Wales, a private member's Bill was introduced to the Legislative Council in 2021, but it lapsed in April 2022 (www.parliament.nsw.gov.au/bills/Pages/bill-details.aspx?pk=3891). The current NSW Premier has announced that he will allow a conscience vote in parliament on the issue (ABC, October 2021).

Because the ACT and the Northern Territory have a different legal status than the Australian states, they have been unable to enact legislation around euthanasia following a ban on such legislation by the federal government in 1997 (see discussion earlier regarding the *Rights of the Terminally Ill Act 1995*).

The Australian government has created the 'End of life law for Clinicians' website (https://palliativecareeducation.com.au/course), which provides training for clinicians.

Types of euthanasia

Two types of euthanasia are commonly discussed. The first concerns situations where a person consciously intends to bring about their own death. This is called 'voluntary euthanasia' because the person seeks euthanasia willingly and voluntarily. An example of voluntary euthanasia could be a situation where a man in the end-stages of a terminal illness asks his friend or doctor to give him an overdose of morphine in order to hasten his death.

The second type concerns situations where the person is unable to express their views about euthanasia because they are unconscious or cannot communicate effectively. Such situations have attracted the most concern precisely because of the difficulty involved in determining consent. Even if an unconscious person had clearly stated on previous occasions that they were in favour of euthanasia, they would be unable to consent in their current circumstances. These cases are called 'non-voluntary' because the person has neither actively consented to nor explicitly refused euthanasia. Given the drastic and irreversible nature of euthanasia, people are wise to be cautious in cases of non-voluntary euthanasia. Note that 'non-voluntary' is different from 'involuntary'. 'Involuntary' refers to a situation where the person has *expressly refused* a proposed course of action. Involuntary euthanasia is murder.

A more problematic distinction is sometimes made between active and passive euthanasia. Active euthanasia is where something is done (an act) to bring about death. Passive euthanasia is where nothing is done (sometimes referred to as an omission), resulting in the person's death. An example of active euthanasia might be a situation where a large dose of morphine is administered and the person dies of an overdose. An example of passive euthanasia might be a situation where antibiotics are withheld and the person dies of an infection. Some have argued that, unlike actively killing, withholding treatment is morally acceptable because it does not involve the carer or clinician doing anything to the person (Rachels 1994).

To illustrate what is at stake in arguing for a difference between 'killing' and 'letting die', philosopher James Rachels (1994) points out that others have argued there is no moral difference between killing and letting die because there is no real difference between an act and an omission. In other words, it is possible to do something through an omission. For example, by *not* shaking someone's hand, we do something: we insult the person. In arguing for this view, Rachels asks us to consider two situations:

1   Smith stands to receive a large inheritance if his young cousin were to die. One evening when the child is in the bath, Smith goes in and drowns the child.
2   Jones stands to receive a large inheritance if his young cousin were to die. One evening when the child is in the bath, Jones sees the child slip and hit his head, then begin to drown. Jones does nothing. The child dies.

While this is a rather dramatic and emotive example, its aim is to illustrate a significant moral point, namely that there is no real difference between actively killing and letting die because the intention in both cases is that the child dies. The fact that Jones let the child die is simply irrelevant. On this argument, once we accept this distinction, we can longer maintain that there is a moral difference between active and passive euthanasia. Rachels argues that there is no moral difference in actively ending a person's life or withholding the means of sustaining a person's life because the intention in *both* cases is to bring about death. After all, if the intention of withholding treatment was not to bring about death, there could be no point in doing it.

THE DOCTRINE OF DOUBLE EFFECT

The 'doctrine of double effect' is a moral argument that aims to absolve a carer from responsibility for a patient's death where that death results from high doses of pain medication (or, conceivably, death arising from other forms of treatment for the relief of pain and suffering).

Sometimes a person who is in the final stage of a terminal illness requires increasing doses of painkillers, typically morphine. A side-effect of a high dose of morphine is respiratory depression, which can lead to death. This means that as pain and medication requirements increase, so does the risk that administering pain relief will kill the person. Consequently, there has been a serious concern, especially among clinicians with religious convictions, that they may find themselves responsible for a person's death.

According to the doctrine of double effect, in a situation where a patient's death follows the administration of morphine to relieve their pain, it is only the carer's *intention* in giving the morphine that is morally important. The morphine has a double effect – that is, relieving pain and killing the patient. However, the two effects can be distinguished morally on the basis of the carer's intentions. If a carer *only* intended to relieve pain, they are not morally responsible for the person's death. The doctrine of double effect relieves the carer of responsibility for the patient's death, so long as the administration of the painkiller was necessary to relieve the person's pain.

This argument has less relevance since palliative care research has cast doubt upon the role of morphine in hastening death. Palliative care specialists have maintained that careful adjustment of morphine doses in response to increasing pain does not hasten death; rather, it is the illness that kills (Ashby 1997; Palliative Care Australia 2022).

Why not suicide?

Some may wonder why people who want to die do not simply choose suicide. In fact, many people do. In 2020, the Australian Institute of Health and Welfare (AIHW) reported that:

> In 2020, the highest suicide rate for males occurred in those aged 85 and over (36.2 deaths per 100,000 population), high rates of suicide were also recorded in males aged 40–44 and 50–54 (both 27.1 per 100,000). Males aged between 40–54 accounted for over one-quarter (27%) of deaths by suicide for males. The highest suicide rate for females was in those aged 45–49 (9.6 deaths per 100,000 population) accounting for the highest proportion of deaths by suicide for females (10.9%). (AIHW 2020a)

Pro-euthanasia advocates say that it is difficult, if not impossible, for an elderly, disabled or incapacitated person to access a humane, effective means of ending their life. In general, non-violent means – such as a drug overdose – are often unreliable, and the person risks ending up in a much worse state of dependency, perhaps with severe permanent injury or brain damage. This leaves only violent means, such as shooting or falling from heights, which are appalling to contemplate and have serious detrimental effects on others. Furthermore, information about suicide is difficult to obtain, partly because Commonwealth legislation prohibits the provision of such information to persons seeking to commit suicide (*Criminal Code Amendment (Suicide Related Material Offences) Act 2005*).

REFLECTIVE QUESTION 10.4

What are your professional responsibilities if a terminally ill patient tells you that they are going to kill themself rather than die of a debilitating illness?

Why choose euthanasia?

People in Australian society have a range of views about death and dying, and those views include support for euthanasia. People who support euthanasia do so for a range of reasons, and under a range of circumstances. These include:

→ a wish to avoid finding oneself in a situation of prolonged hospitalisation and dying

→ a fear of uncontrollable pain at the end of life

→ a wish to avoid being forced to endure extreme old age while being unable to experience interests or pleasures

→ a wish to avoid being forced to live with dementia

→ a wish to avoid being forced to live with profound loss of bodily functions

→ a wish to remain in control of one's life to the very end.

ARGUMENTS FROM AUTONOMOUS ADULTS

Many proponents of euthanasia argue that, as competent, autonomous adults in a democracy, we are each entitled to make our own decisions about our lives (even if others find our decisions repugnant), as long as we do not harm others. According to this line of reasoning, one should be free to determine for oneself the manner and timing of one's death. So, just as we plan for our aged care and funerals, we should also be able to plan for our manner of dying. As a moral principle, we should always act from the right sorts of reasons, and so a decision to end one's life should also be based on good reasons.

At an individual level, one way by which we might distinguish a good reason from a poor one is by distinguishing transient desires from deep convictions. Philosopher Gerald Dworkin (1993) proposes that we can do this by making a distinction between experiential and critical interests. Experiential interests are those things that give us passing pleasure – for example, disco dancing, camping or going to the movies. Typically, these are interests that can be substituted by other interests. For example, if a person who has enjoyed dancing sustains a knee injury, they might take up playing a musical instrument instead. Experiential interests may also be short term. For example, a person may enjoy wilderness hiking in their youth, but give that up without serious regret when they are elderly.

Critical interests, on the other hand, are the things to which a person has a deep and abiding commitment, and that go to the heart of a person's sense of who they are – their identity. Dworkin argues that critical interests give our lives meaning and value, so they are the things that make one's life worth living. If we lose things that are of critical interest to us, we may judge our lives not to be worth living. Critical interests can include things such as a commitment to a relationship with our intimate companion and/or children, political or religious convictions and professional identity. Whereas it is possible to forgo many of our experiential interests without significant impact, it is not possible to forgo one's critical interests without profoundly negative and life-changing consequences. This idea is illustrated dramatically in Arthur Miller's (1974) play *The Crucible*, where John Proctor is falsely accused of witchcraft. When asked why he does not simply say he is a witch and thereby save himself from being hanged, he says 'Because it is my name! Because I cannot have another in my life!' In other words, for Proctor to disown who he really is would be a kind of self-destruction: he is who he is, and no one else. Clearly, he does not consider that living a life in which he is regarded as a witch would constitute a life worth living.

In Dworkin's (1993) view, life-changing decisions should always be motivated by critical interests, not experiential interests (see also Dale 2021). In general, then, a decision for euthanasia could not be justified on the basis of losing an experiential interest, such as the ability to play tennis or drive a car; however, it might be justified on the basis of losing the ability to be the person you understand and value yourself to be, which amounts to losing the kind of life that you believe is worth living. From this perspective, death (due to euthanasia) may not be a harm if it were a response to the loss of a life that one considered worth living, because the harm would already have been done.

REFLECTIVE QUESTION 10.5

Think about your own life. Can you identify your own experiential and critical interests?

When is euthanasia not justified?

People on both sides of the euthanasia debate are concerned that vulnerable people may be pressured into ending their lives prematurely for a range of unacceptable reasons. This is especially concerning in a society in which the mass media are saturated with messages that over-value youth and beauty, and repeatedly raise unsubstantiated concerns about the social burden of an ageing population. Morally troubling reasons for euthanasia include:

➜ feeling that being old or dependent makes a person worthless or undignified

➜ feeling that being old or dependent makes a person a burden on their family, especially if their family members are elderly

➜ feeling temporarily swayed by passing but powerful emotions

➜ mistakenly believing that one's health is worse than it actually is

➜ fear of *future* pain, disability or dependency.

Having relationships in which one feels valued and safe is the best protection against acting on ideas such as these. Nevertheless, even trust can be misplaced. There is a concern that the sick or elderly may be emotionally manipulated to end their lives prematurely by unscrupulous relatives or acquaintances who stand to receive an inheritance or some other benefit. For this reason, some people consider euthanasia too dangerous to allow.

Some people object to euthanasia on the grounds that, even though autonomy may give a person the moral right to end their own life, other persons can be harmed in the process, and this harm cannot be justified by appeals to individual autonomy. Euthanasia is not merely an action of a free individual; it requires assistance from another person, and the effect on that person of bringing about a death – despite their being willing – may not be entirely predictable. The prospect of death can give rise to powerful emotional responses (such as anxiety, anger, grief and guilt), and requires some maturity to manage. It is not difficult to imagine that deliberately killing another person might come to be a harm to some persons who assist another to die.

Others have argued that the legal provision of medical assistance to die introduces an element into the doctor–patient relationship that can undermine trust and the therapeutic nature of that relationship in cases where patients may be having suicidal thoughts and/or impulses (Williams 2018). Williams argues that permissible killing runs counter to the demands of medical ethics and clinical governance to provide patient safety (2018: 286).

LAW AND ETHICS IN PRACTICE

You are caring for Vera, an 83-year-old woman still living at home with assistance from a community nurse and her son, who is 60 years old. She has been admitted with congestive cardiac failure. She is expected to get some improvement from new medications, but will remain short of breath and shaky, and will need further assistance if she is to stay at home. She can reasonably be expected to live only for a few more months. Gasping for breath, Vera asks you: 'Why won't you let me die?'

〉〉 **What do you do?**

It has been argued that the legalisation of euthanasia would make it easier for society to accept other sorts of killing. Philosopher and doctor Grant Gillett (1995) argues that there is a subtle relationship between ethics and law. Writing about the Northern Territory's *Rights of the Terminally Ill Act 1995*, Gillett expressed concern about the legislation changing what society considers normal and reasonable conduct, with the effect that objections to other kinds of killings will gradually be eroded.

It is important to understand that what constitutes a good reason for one person may be a bad reason for another, and what represents a critical interest for one person may be considered superficial by another. Australia is a multicultural society where people hold differing value systems, and this makes it very difficult to reach consensus on some moral issues, such as euthanasia.

Nurses' responsibilities

Nurses risk serious criminal charges if they act outside the professional scope of practice in assisting a person to die. It is essential that where voluntary assisted dying is available, nurses are aware of the authorised processes, and of the nature and limitations their own roles if they become involved. The nurse's professional role, as always, is to:

→ obey the law
→ remain within their scope of practice
→ maintain their duty of care.

LAW AND ETHICS IN PRACTICE

You are caring for Tom, a 52-year-old man with extremely advanced cancer who is receiving palliative care. He has been in and out of consciousness for the past few days, he is not taking food or water, and his breathing is shallow and barely perceptible at times. His family tell you that that they expect him to die at any moment. One day Tom becomes increasingly restless, and his sister, who is visibly upset, asks you to give him another dose of morphine.

》 **What do you do? Would there be professional consequences for you if you gave him another dose of morphine (even if it had been prescribed by a doctor) and he subsequently died?**

Conclusion

Abortion and euthanasia are topics that capture significant public attention and emotion. For this reason, they can seem to be the really 'big' issues in health care.

However, they concern experiences that occupy only a very small part of nurses' professional lives. Philosopher David Seedhouse (2009) likens ethics in health care to an iceberg: issues such as abortion and euthanasia are the tip that attracts our attention, but the significant mass of ethical issues lies beneath the surface, and nurses neglect them at their peril.

REFLECTIVE QUESTIONS 10.6

1 How does the principle of autonomy relate to abortion and euthanasia?
2 What are the three key professional responsibilities of the nurse relevant to abortion and euthanasia?
3 What kind of reasons are given to support the legalisation of euthanasia?
4 What kind of reasons are given against the legalisation of euthanasia?

Further reading

Dworkin, G. & Bok, S. (1998). *Euthanasia and physician-assisted suicide.* Cambridge University Press.

Francis, L. & Smith, P. (2013). Feminist philosophy of law. In E.N. Zalta (ed.), *The Stanford encyclopedia of philosophy*, Spring. http://plato.stanford.edu/archives/spr2013/entries/feminism-law

Goodnight, A. (2019). A life worth living: Value and responsibility. *Journal of Philosophy and Medicine*, *44*(2), 133–49.

Gordon, J.-S. (2008). Abortion. In J. Feisner & B. Dowden (eds), *Internet encyclopedia of philosophy*. https://iep.utm.edu/abortion/

Khatony, A. & Fallahi Rezaei, M. (2022). Comparison of attitude of nurses and nursing students toward euthanasia. *Nursing Ethics*, *29*(1), 208–16.

Wainer, J. (ed.) (2006). *Lost: Illegal abortion stories.* Melbourne University Press.

Cases cited

Ces v Superclinics Australia Pty Ltd [1995] 38 NSWLR 47

R v Bayliss and Cullen (1986) 9 Qld Lawyer Reps 8

R v Davidson [1969] VR 667

R v Leach and Brennan [2010] QDC (Cairns), unreported 14 October Everson DCJ

R v Wald [1971] 3 NSWDCR 25

Note

1 Even as late as the 1980s, British Prime Minister Margaret Thatcher famously proposed establishing institutions to house single mothers and their children, suggesting that women who transgressed the moral norms of womanhood needed to be removed from society.

11 ETHICS OF AGED CARE: AUTONOMY UNDER THREAT AND THE NURSE AS CAPACITY-BUILDER

REBECCA RIPPERGER

LEARNING OBJECTIVES

In this chapter, you will:

→ Understand and be able to respond to the challenges to a person's autonomy that are posed by ageing

→ Understand how issues of autonomy are relevant to elderly people and nurses in their everyday interactions

→ Learn techniques that can be employed by the nurse to provide support to and promote autonomy in aged persons

→ Understand what constitutes elder abuse, and how elderly people are vulnerable to abuses

In November 2012, two artists – a theatre-maker and a puppeteer – resided for seven days in a dementia-specific unit of an aged-care facility in Tasmania. In that time, they engaged closely with the 23 residents, their families and the staff to create an in-house experience that became a site of social interaction, conversation and inclusion. The installation they created involved building a small shack-like structure. A range of materials and fabrics were used to cover the frame. The little shack housed a display of changing treasures that could be viewed through the windows: flowers potted in gilded teacups, decorative quilts, dolls, hanging lanterns, puppets, coloured sea horses, an old suitcase, a treasure chest. The communal room in which the shack stood was decorated with spray-painted life-sized paper figures. The installation developed out of the relationships formed in the aged-care facility, and was built around themes drawn from the residents' lives – past, present and future. The doors of the shack opened out to create a performance space and each resident had the opportunity to experience a performance designed specifically for them. The residents determined for themselves their own levels of participation – whether it was to simply witness the construction, to tell their stories providing inspiration, to make suggestions about what materials could be used or to assist with the construction itself, and ultimately to experience their own unique performance.

An evaluation of the project showed an improvement in residents' levels of participation and social engagement generally as well as improvement in their appetites and behaviour. Families enjoyed watching their loved ones' participation and found a new focal point for conversation and connection to them. Staff found stimulus for interaction with the residents about their lives (Creature Tales Tasmania 2012).

Some of the philosophical and ethical aims of this book are most acutely demonstrated in examining the challenges facing the nurse in the area of aged care. We have proffered a conception of human identity as embodied and socially constructed: our embodiment makes us vulnerable to being affected by, and consequently responding to, other people and our environment in both positive and negative ways. That is, it is by virtue of the fact that we are embodied that we engage with others and the world. It follows from this that our individual autonomy is fundamentally tied up with our relations with others. It is through the opportunities or barriers created by us and others, as we participate in society as a whole, that we each can experience (or be denied the experience of) freedom. This means that my being free is built upon the liberties of others. Therefore, my freedom is contingent on me also recognising and respecting your freedom. We have argued that it is this interrelation of the self with others that allows us to develop personhood, which itself allows us to care.

We have seen that, in navigating the morass of possibilities in human relationships, ethics requires that we strive for the ideal of the good life in which all human beings can flourish, and in which everybody's personal liberty is respected. Indeed, the enshrining of the individual's right to liberty, understood as the freedom to exercise their autonomy, has been shown to underpin our legal systems (Habermas 1996). We identified that it is the role of the law to regulate certain social interactions in order to ensure that people are treated fairly, and we have argued that in order to do this in a morally justifiable way the law must also aim to recognise and protect equality. This means that the law has an inbuilt bias towards promoting the capacities of people (and not merely restricting us in certain ways). Accordingly, we have examined the role of the duty that exists in the nurse–patient relationship, which requires the nurse, whose knowledge and expertise places them in a position of power, to build capability in the patient in order that they may exercise autonomous decision-making.

In general, in advanced capitalist societies such as Australia, there is a tendency to regard ageing in a negative light. The importance society attaches to productivity as a measure of value, and the decline of traditional family and community structures, have seen societal attitudes towards the aged shift, from respect (and even veneration) to a more general disregard or devaluing of the possible contributions of the elderly. As has been discussed previously, autonomy is a function of our relationships. Accordingly, these social attitudes towards ageing, in combination with the specific vulnerabilities experienced by the elderly as physical and mental capacities deteriorate, give rise to a unique set of challenges to their autonomy. In particular, in addition to the problems created by changes in the

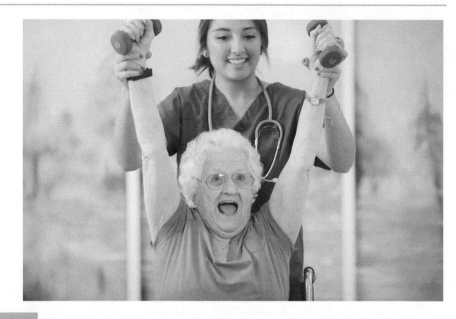

FIGURE 11.1 Nurses can play a substantial role in supporting and promoting the exercise of autonomy.

person's physical and mental capacities, significant issues arise with the challenges posed by the elderly person's *experience* of their own decline and reduction in autonomy. This gives ageing a particular experiential dimension that younger people typically are not aware of until they experience their own loss or disability. It is in this context that the role of the nurse as a builder of capability and a supporter of autonomy becomes most significant.

While there are limits to the therapeutic benefit that a nurse can provide to a person's physical health, nurses can play a substantial role in supporting and promoting the exercise of autonomy in the face of physical changes, especially in the context of ageing. We will see that, just like the artists who created an open and inviting environment that provided opportunities for residents with dementia to exercise choice and engage, so too nurses can play a critical role in creating the interpersonal conditions that allow for a positive and enabling experience of autonomy.

By the end of this chapter, the nurse should come to appreciate that ethical issues, and the need for ethical decision-making, arise in everyday interactions and are not reserved solely for consideration in the context of major life decisions. Indeed, the approach taken here identifies the everyday ethical interaction of the nurse with the patient as being critical to the very foundation of autonomy. That is, without appropriate recognition of a person's capacities, reinforced in daily interactions, autonomy can be undermined, making it impossible for a person to suddenly act 'autonomously' when faced with an ethical dilemma. This approach will also be shown to be consistent with shifts in thinking both internationally and nationally (Joseph 2015).

How ageing challenges autonomy

At the biological level, ageing is characterised by a gradual decline in physical and mental functions as a result of accumulated molecular and cellular damage that takes place over time (World Health Organization 2022). In humans this tends to begin at the end of the peak growth period that occurs in their twenties (Carnes et al. 2008). Although there is no consensus globally on the specific age at which a person becomes 'old', a person is generally considered 'aged' when these processes of decline begin to affect their mobility and mental acuity to a degree that obviously impacts their normal activities of living. A decline in mobility, agility and flexibility results from a loss of bone density, muscle strength and coordination. Diminished memory and duller reflexes are the result of decrease in nervous system function. Old age is also often accompanied by a reduction in hearing and visual acuity, as well as an increase in diseases such as Alzheimer's or other forms of dementia, arthritis, heart disease, stroke and cancer, which can all potentially contribute significantly to debility.

This process of deterioration in a person's physical and possibly also mental integrity poses a significant threat to their ability to function in the world in an autonomous way. Poor vision may result in a person no longer being able to obtain a driver's licence or to cook for themselves. Lack of mobility may mean that a person can no longer do their own shopping or banking. A person who has experienced a stroke may require assistance with even the most basic activities of daily living, such as toileting, dressing, showering and eating. Dementia may result in the restriction of a person's freedom of movement and their decision-making, as concerns for their safety may result in them being institutionalised and in others making both major and minor life decisions for them.

HOW 'CHALLENGED AUTONOMY' IN THE ELDERLY CONFRONTS THE HEALTH-CARE SECTOR

It is not the intention of this chapter to present a picture of 'typical old age' or to deal in stereotypes of elderly people as being necessarily or inherently infirm.

Indeed, according to the World Health Organization's (2015) *World Report on Ageing and Health*, although ageing is characterised by an increased risk of disease and a general decrease in capacity, among the aged population there is a wide variation in levels of capacities and capabilities. Accordingly, government policy on ageing needs to reflect that diversity (World Health Organization 2015).

As the aged population increases – and is predicted to continue to do so significantly (Australian Bureau of Statistics 2018b) – there will be a corresponding increase in the proportion of elderly patients within the broader population of health service recipients. Advances in medicine and medical technology are extending the lifespan, and in doing so are also increasing the number of patients with multiple morbidities who are presenting to hospitals with complex needs (Fallon et al. 2016). Although many elderly people enjoy good health, between 2013–14 and 2017–18, there were large increases in hospital admissions for people aged 65 and over – on average, an increase of 6.3 per cent each year, which was faster than the population growth for this age group (around 4.1 per cent each year) (AIHW 2019). This age group, which makes up around 15 per cent of the population, accounts for around 42 per cent of hospital admissions (AIHW 2019). The increase of elderly patients with complex conditions has been accompanied by a rise in the incidence of dementia. According to the Australian Institute of Health and Welfare (AIHW), there were between 386 200 and 472 000 Australians living with dementia in 2021, with these figures projected to more than double by 2058 (AIHW 2022). As a result of these developments, health-care workers are now seeing much larger numbers of older, frail consumers of health care who have complex health needs *and* may often have diminished capacity to make decisions for themselves.

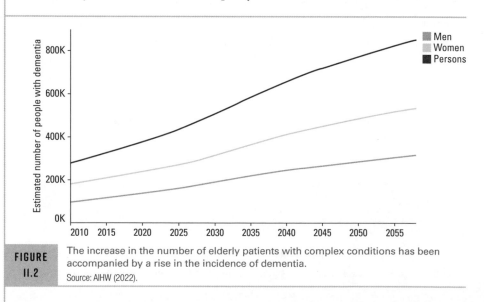

FIGURE 11.2 The increase in the number of elderly patients with complex conditions has been accompanied by a rise in the incidence of dementia.
Source: AIHW (2022).

Nurses and other health-care professionals need to be able to respond to the specific challenges posed by this changing demographic whether in the acute care context of a hospital or community service, or in the context of long-term care in the home or in aged-care facilities.

When dealing with elderly people, nurses are faced with the same legal and ethical issues as when dealing with their usual patients, specifically duty of care, consent, confidentiality, cultural sensitivity and the therapeutic relationship. However, as in the other cases that have been discussed in this book, the precise shape or form of these responsibilities will be coloured by the specific circumstances of this group of people. Because of elderly patients' increasing frailty and reduced physical resources, a greater standard of care in respect of everyday matters will be expected from the nurse. For example, reduced mobility increases risk of thrombosis or bed sores, and where an elderly patient has some symptoms of a reduction in mental capacity, such as mild confusion or disorientation or short-term memory deficits, additional care and attention will need to be given to basic care such as daily hygiene and routine medications.

It is, of course, important when considering the ethical and legal issues facing nurses in an aged-care context to be cognisant of the 'big questions', such as end-of-life decision-making, advance care directives, 'not for resuscitation' orders and the use of treatments that will extend life. The approach of death, and how a person comports themselves in circumstances where questions of life and death are very real (and not simply distant, abstract considerations), are fundamental components of ethics and law. These questions of life and death carry a particular gravitas, and are often the focus of ethical scrutiny and public debate in discussions of ageing. However, as discussed, the focus of this chapter will be on the everyday ethical problems faced by ageing people, and how the nurse can effectively deal with these in a way that promotes the person's capability and supports their autonomy.

Just as the physical and mental conditions that result from ageing affect the content of the nurse's duty of care, the nurse's ethical obligations are given content by these circumstances. In much the same way that the physiological changes in the elderly can focus the nurse's attention on the assistance that may be needed for the aged person to manage everyday activities, it is in everyday interactions that the nurse can recognise and support the significant challenges to autonomy that the elderly can experience. It is in the area of interactions involving activities of daily living that there is the greatest potential for the nurse to have an impact on a person's autonomy – either positively or negatively.

In a pilot study of ethical issues faced by older adult consumers of health care, Katharine V. Smith (2005: 39) notes that:

> the highest ethical concern for older adult consumers [of health care] is how they are attended to and respected, in numerous and multiple interactions on a daily basis.

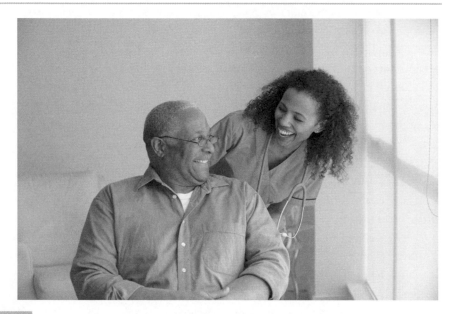

FIGURE 11.3 It is in everyday interactions that the nurse can recognise and support the significant challenges to autonomy that can be experienced by elderly people.

The acknowledgement of this fundamental human need is implicit in the imperative for person-centred care that characterises contemporary nursing practice (ACSQHC 2017). Smith (2005: 39) explains that this approach to care, focusing on attentiveness and respect, has implications for both nursing education and clinical practice, which means nurses' interpersonal skills become critical in responding effectively to the ethical concerns of older patients. This challenge can be difficult because it demands a high level of awareness on the part of the nurse in every interaction, every day, with the aged person. The picture of the nurse that arises here is that of an ethical agent who routinely and habitually employs a form of respectful interaction that promotes dignity and autonomy in elderly people across the spectrum of their abilities.

REFLECTIVE QUESTIONS 11.1

1 What are your views of older persons? How do your views influence how you treat older people?

2 Is health in older age simply a matter of being disease or disability free?

3 List some of the ways that ageing poses a challenge to acting autonomously.

Autonomy building: The nurse as an ethical agent

The experience of losing significant control over one's life as a result of living in an institution (whether short term in a hospital or long term in an aged-care facility) is well known (Williams 1994). Institutional settings such as hospitals and aged-care facilities operate with a huge emphasis on routine and time constraints. For example, in these settings meals are served at set times, medication and wound care are dispensed at specific times of the day, and doctors' rounds, visiting hours, physiotherapy, occupational therapy and cleaning all take place according to a structured timetable. In these kinds of environments, patients' and residents' everyday freedoms are systematically limited. Eating, sleeping, showering and seeing loved ones are all subject to the constraints of the working environment of the institution. Older patients whose autonomy is already challenged by debility or frailty are particularly vulnerable in these settings. While nurses may not always be able to control the broader environment in which they work, they can be conscious of their own interactions with patients and work to minimise the effects of the institution in diminishing the patient's autonomy.

The notion of the nurse as an ethical agent, charged with the significant responsibility of fostering autonomy, stems from the moral obligation to assist patients to acquire the capacities they need for health, and to exercise their rights and freedoms.

So what does it mean to speak of the role of the nurse as capability builder for autonomy – what does this nursing activity look like in practice? Is it simply a matter of encouraging patients to make their own decisions and do things for themselves wherever possible?

LAW AND ETHICS IN PRACTICE

Frank is a 78-year-old man who was admitted to hospital in a frail condition for stabilisation of his heart disease and better control of his diabetes. Frank also has a hearing impairment, requiring that he wear hearing aids. After a fortnight in hospital, Frank's condition improved significantly. With changes to his medication, his blood pressure and blood sugar levels continue to improve and the treating teams are considering discharge. At the final consultation, Frank's endocrine specialist discusses his diabetes management with him, advising Frank of the crucial role of diet and exercise. Frank nods in agreement, saying, 'Yes, Doc, I understand. Thank you, Doc.' Later that day, Brian, who is the nurse on duty, overhears a conversation between Frank and his wife. Frank says that even though the staff had been great, they fussed too much and he was looking forward to getting home to his comfy chair and 'little treats' again, which he said surely couldn't do him too much harm now that they'd got the medication right. Brian shakes his head as he relays the story to the other nurses: 'Can you believe that, after how sick he was and after he's just had that session with the specialist?'

>> **What should Brian do? Has he acted in a way to support Frank to act autonomously? Should he just accept that when acting autonomously some people don't always do what is in their best interests?**

In order to examine how nurses may understand and implement the ideal of capability-building, we will consider the two following options: (1) assessing and enhancing functional ability; and (2) assisted autonomy.

FUNCTIONAL ABILITY

The World Health Organization's report on health and ageing uses the concept of 'functional ability' to describe the goal of healthy ageing (World Health Organization 2015, 2019). A person's functional ability is made up of their:

1 intrinsic mental and physical capacities (physiological, biological)
2 environments (familial, societal, economic, social networks)
3 well-being (happiness, satisfaction, fulfilment).

On this view, the goal of care is to support or improve how the person interacts with their environment and community to foster their well-being as far as possible, given their intrinsic capacities. Effective approaches to health care should aim at developing and maintaining functional ability rather than seeing healthy ageing simply as the absence of disease, and use interventions that help to achieve the goal of a healthy trajectory in old age. Rather than regarding ageing as an inevitable loss of ability, individuals should be appropriately assessed in order to develop a plan of care that matches and improves their functional ability. Care plans should foster a person's interactions in ways that promote not only their well-being but also their autonomy.

The goal of functional ability should also underpin government policies to support a whole-of-community approach to healthy ageing. For example, when an

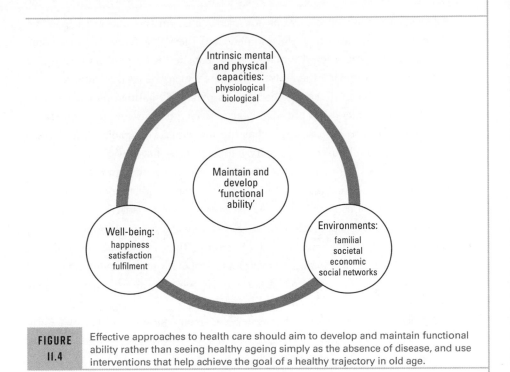

FIGURE II.4 Effective approaches to health care should aim to develop and maintain functional ability rather than seeing healthy ageing simply as the absence of disease, and use interventions that help achieve the goal of a healthy trajectory in old age.

elderly person reaches a point where their ability to live independently becomes exceedingly difficult for them (perhaps they need to consider leaving their home to enter aged-care accommodation), the decision about their future should be shaped by an assessment of their functional ability.

Functional ability is assessed not just by determining the person's mental and physical capacities but by their environmental influences, such as:

→ the effect of government policies, including the level of funding for support services, and the types of services available (for example, are there residential care beds in the local area?)

→ the family and social networks that the person is a part of (for example, can they move in with a family member?)

→ the built environment and its impact on mobility and psychological well-being (for example, does the person live in an apartment building with a lift? Is it easy to get outdoors?)

→ community attitudes to ageing, which can determine whether the elderly are included and how they are valued (for example, what opportunities are there for elderly people to participate in social activities?).

All these factors influence how a person ages by affecting their intrinsic capacities, their interactions with their environment and their experience of satisfaction, happiness and well-being. Ultimately, these constitute the person's health and determine how they view themselves and how they experience their autonomy.

In this approach to ageing, the nurse is part of a multidisciplinary team of health-care providers who promote healthy ageing not just by treating disease or illness, but also by assessing what the individual is capable of, and what government, family and community supports they have available to them. Health-care providers use this information to employ intervention strategies to reduce decline in capacity and optimise personal choice and self-direction (autonomy). Where losses in capacity have occurred in an elderly person, taking a 'functional ability' approach to restoring health will promote not only recovery, but also positive adjustments by the person to their circumstances, bringing psychological and emotional growth. This is particularly important in responding to that feature of ageing noted earlier, namely the person's experience of their own decline and reduced autonomy.

To illustrate this, consider the case of a person who has had a stroke. Early medical intervention minimises the physical impact by reducing the loss of brain tissue, and physical rehabilitation therapies help to reduce the loss of mobility and speech. In a very similar way, mobilisation and strengthening of the person's relationships with their family and their community supports and services can influence the kinds of choices and options available to them, creating new possibilities for their future life.

LAW AND ETHICS IN PRACTICE

Li Chuen has been a keen gardener all her life, but has recently suffered a stroke that greatly weakened the right side of her body. Li Chuen is distressed that she may no longer be able to look after her extensive garden, and has no wish to spend her days indoors watching television.

As part of a rehabilitation program, Li Chuen will join a local community garden project, where she will not only work on improving her physical abilities, but also share her wealth of knowledge with budding gardeners, and participate in a productive social setting. Li Chuen is involved in both a cherished pastime and is also connected to community in the process of physiological, psychological and social rehabilitation.

》》 How can you, as a nurse, assist in changing perceptions of old age from being characterised as an inevitable decline towards death to a more positive ideal that includes a range of options for continuing to live a rich and full life?

Assisted autonomy

In 2020, an extensive literature review, including 46 studies that sought the views of older people, examined older people's perceived autonomy in residential care. The review found that professionals' activities create opportunities for perceived autonomy:

> They said their autonomy was determined by the care atmosphere and whether they had the opportunities to influence decisions, express their will and make their own choices. (Moilanen et al. 2022: 426)

The concept of assisted autonomy means that the nurse interacts with patients in a way that helps to create the conditions for the enhancement and exercise of the patient's autonomy. To do this, the nurse promotes an environment in which the elderly person can access the supports they need to make their own decisions and to act as independently as possible, rather than being merely the passive recipient of care. This may range from something as simple as arranging for a shower chair in the person's home, or connecting the person to support groups in the local community, to ensuring the person's involvement in long-term or complex decision-making about their medical care, such as advanced care planning.

The following four tools can be used by nurses as possible forms of assistance to enhance the exercising of autonomy by the elderly (Whitler 1996):

1   shaping instrumental circumstances
2   using rational persuasion
3   assessing causes of impaired decision-making capacity
4   mentioning opportunities.

SHAPING INSTRUMENTAL CIRCUMSTANCES

The idea of shaping instrumental circumstances means that nurses identify ways to make it easier for the elderly person to express and realise their choices. Nurses might do this by:

→ providing the person with resources (for example, brochures, literacy aids, computer access or a telephone)
→ explaining situations and including giving information about the person's rights
→ creating supportive environments (for example, by putting them in contact with other like-minded people)
→ seeking innovative solutions (for example, through the use of art or music, as in the example at the beginning of this chapter).

If we return to the earlier scenario involving Frank and Brian, it is possible that during his consultation with the endocrinologist, Frank did not hear or properly understand what was being said to him. Was he wearing his hearing aids and were they working properly? Was the specialist communicating in plain English? Had he asked Frank questions that allowed Frank to show his level of comprehension?

It is not uncommon for patients to feel more comfortable speaking to nursing staff about their health and care than they do to doctors. Whether because of the stress they feel and the limited interaction they have with medical staff, in particular with medical specialists, or sometimes because of a lack of familiarity with the technical language that doctors tend to employ, patients can have difficulty retaining or even understanding what is said to them, and may not be prepared to ask questions as a result.

Brian could have ensured that Frank had his hearing aids in and that they were turned on when he was speaking with the doctor. Brian could have taken a proactive role during the conversation to ensure that Frank was aware of issues that might be relevant to his particular circumstances, and be able to voice any questions and clarify anything about which he was unsure.

Rather than judging Frank for not taking responsibility for his diet, Brian could have addressed Frank's concerns regarding the increasing restrictions on his lifestyle. He could make or organise interventions to support Frank to continue to enjoy his life and to avoid seeing taking responsibility for his health as purely involving denying himself enjoyable options. It may be that with the right support regarding diet and nutrition, Frank can continue to have regular food treats and partake in a mobility program that aligns with his interests.

USING RATIONAL PERSUASION

Using rational persuasion involves ensuring that a person is informed by means of providing information, suggestions and reasons that the person can then employ in their own determination of what to do or agree to. The intention of rational persuasion is to provide the person with an appropriate amount of information that will allow them to make an informed decision, rather than to make an effort to persuade the person towards any particular outcome, such as a decision that the nurse prefers. Using reasons to persuade the person to do what the nurse thinks is best would be a form of paternalism, and not supportive of the person's autonomy.

In our scenario, Brian could have provided Frank with information such as the limits of the medication in controlling diabetes and the effects of poorly controlled diabetes on Frank's other conditions. Brian could have taken steps to ensure that family members had information about diet and exercise that could be used to encourage and motivate Frank. Brian could also have discussed what 'treats' Frank enjoyed and then provided him with information about healthy alternatives so that Frank would be able to make a more informed autonomous decision. Of course, it is important to acknowledge that even with all the facts and supports set in place Frank may decide to act in a manner contrary to medical advice. Frank may value his current lifestyle more than the prospect of extending his lifespan. However, in that case Brian would still have assisted Frank in making that decision autonomously by ensuring that he was well informed, knew of and was offered options, and felt that he was supported.

ASSESSING CAUSES OF IMPAIRED DECISION-MAKING CAPACITY

Assessing causes of impaired decision-making capacity involves identifying the causes of the impairment and removing, where possible, the obstacles to the exercise of autonomy and self-determination. Elderly people should not be viewed as being unable to make decisions purely because of their age or illness. Indeed, even people who have dementia may still be well able to make many decisions in a range of settings. For example, a person may have significant memory loss but still be able to make choices about what they want to eat, what clothes they want to wear or how they might like to spend their day. They may even still be able to make some decisions about their health care, such as whether or not to take pain relief for a headache. In this instance, rather than viewing the person as lacking *any* capacity for decision-making, it is essential that the nurse understands any limitations on the person's cognitive capacity, and knows how to put supports in place to assist the person to make decisions. Discussions with close family members about the person's views, likes and dislikes can assist to build a picture of the sorts of decisions that would be consistent with the person's pattern of decision-making.

For example, 92-year-old Mario now lives in an aged-care facility. He has always been a person who enjoys reading and solitude more than the company of others. With the onset of dementia, Mario begins to display aggressive behaviour towards other residents when made to join in activities and so the staff decide to leave Mario to his solitude rather than encourage him to participate. However, following a conversation with a family member, the activities coordinator Anne learns that

Mario loves old films and always made an exception to his tendency to solitude when it came to going to the movies. As a result, Anne implements a weekly movie night to screen old films and the staff are amazed to find that when Mario attends the screenings his behaviour is much more settled. The establishment of an understanding of Mario's preferences and history of behaviour has been aided by Anne's communication with his family. Through this, Anne has not only assisted Mario in influencing what opportunities are available to him, but has also helped him to make decisions about when to participate.

MENTIONING OPPORTUNITIES

The exercise of autonomy is dependent upon there being available opportunities. As discussed earlier, whether they are in a hospital or an aged-care facility, institutional routines often result in seriously reduced opportunities for residents and patients to exercise choice. The opportunity to have input into decisions about daily routines such as when, or even whether, to take a shower or get out of bed, or the opportunity to participate in – and influence – available activities (such as the artists' installation we saw at the beginning of this chapter and as in Mario's case above) can have a significant impact on the person's experience of their autonomy. In order to promote autonomy, it is essential that nurses identify opportunities available (especially in unfamiliar environments such as hospitals) and mention them to their patients.

We can see from the examples above how nurses can equip themselves with tools to assist them in their efforts to promote autonomy in elderly people. However, sometimes there can be disparity between the nurse's belief that they are acting in a way that supports the person's autonomy and the elderly person's experience of those actions (Whitler 1996). This schism can arise when a nurse acts from a position of wanting to protect the person (paternalism), rather than from a genuine disinterested position of supporting the person to exercise *their own* choices. This situation may occur if the nurse becomes too focused on what they think is in the elderly person's best interests. Nurses should always remember to reflect upon and critically assess the effectiveness of the methods they employ to assist in autonomous decision-making, whether it is mentioning options, shaping circumstances or any other communicative tool. This could be as simple as asking the person about their experience of the tool used, where possible. It could also involve having peer discussions and group evaluations as part of the nurse's regular professional development.

REFLECTIVE QUESTIONS 11.2

1 Think of a situation in which you have nursed an elderly person with either physical or cognitive impairment. In what ways did you support them to act autonomously? What might you have done better? Think about which tools you either used or could have used to assist them.

2 Have you ever felt impatient with an elderly patient because of the time constraints of your workplace? How might you approach that situation differently?

3 What is functional ability? Why does it matter?

4 What are four key actions of nurses in providing assisted autonomy?

Responding to abuse of older persons: A rights-based approach to autonomy building

We have discussed so far that the nurse has a moral obligation to build patients' capability to act and decide for themselves. This may involve strategic interventions in an elderly person's life to inform them, to strengthen their connections to community, to support them in autonomous decision-making and, ultimately, to promote healthy ageing. A crucial aspect of putting this obligation into practice is to always act in a way that assists the elderly person to manage the risks that their vulnerabilities may pose. As discussed in Chapter 7, those vulnerabilities can sometimes leave elderly persons open to exploitation by others. As frontline providers of health care, nurses are well positioned to identify the signs of, and respond to, incidents of abuse of older persons.

Some factors that place elderly people at risk of abuse were identified in the *Elder Abuse in New South Wales* report (NSW GPSC 2016):

→ having a disability (particularly cognitive)
→ being socially isolated
→ having a history of previous traumatic events
→ being in contact with a perpetrator who has alcohol or drug dependence.

A further feature that was common to elderly people who had been abused was that these people were dependent upon the perpetrator to meet their daily needs (NSW GPSC 2016: para. 2.10). In other words, elderly people who need high levels of assistance with their basic activities of daily living are particularly vulnerable to abuse.

The combination of abuse, plus the fact that it is occurring within a relationship that is crucial for the vulnerable elderly person, poses a complex ethical challenge for nurses and other health professionals. This is because the elderly person may have strong emotional attachment to the perpetrator. For example, the elderly person may have a long personal history with the perpetrator and feel that they are indebted in some way to that person. As such, a nurse's concerns about possible abuse need to be dealt with carefully so as not to undermine the person's wishes with respect to that relationship, which may involve a family member or friend.

Although the 2007 Amendment to the *Aged Care Act 1997* (Cth) governs mandatory reporting of abuse of older people, this is only with respect to those living in residential aged care or in receipt of services that are funded by the Commonwealth, and it is specific to unlawful sexual contact and unlawful use of force. There is no legislative framework for dealing with elder abuse outside of these contexts – for example, in a public hospital. The law in Australia does not specifically recognise elder abuse. Rather, some of the elements that may constitute elder abuse – such as physical violence constituting assault, theft or unlawful use of a person's property or trespass – can be dealt with under the criminal or civil law. Other aspects of elder abuse, such as manipulation of the elderly person, or restricting access to or isolating the elderly person, are not dealt with in current legislation.[1] In a situation of suspected abuse, nurses must be guided by the following documentation: the Australian Nursing and Midwifery Federation (ANMF) position statement, 'Compulsory Reporting of Abuse in Aged Care Settings for Nurses and Assistants in Nursing' (ANMF 2020), their employer's policy on suspected elder abuse, the Nursing and Midwifery Board of Australia's Code of Conduct for Nurses (NMBA 2018b), and the ICN Code of Ethics for Nurses (ICN 2012, 2021).

In responding to incidents of elder abuse, it can be challenging for nurses to distinguish acting in a paternalistic way from acting in a manner that supports autonomy. However, this distinction is crucial. Witnessing forms of abuse can elicit strong moral outrage and provoke the desire to immediately protect the person suffering the abuse. However, any actions taken with the intention to protect the person (that is, paternalistic actions) must be weighed against the possible impingement on that person's personal autonomy and right to make their own decisions – including bad ones. This challenge is even greater if the elderly person is considered to have diminished capacity in decision-making.[2]

Historically, the law has taken a protective, if not paternalistic, position in relation to vulnerable people, which initially stemmed from the *parens patriae* role of the king: the responsibility to protect those citizens who were incapable of protecting themselves (usually children, the infirm and the seriously mentally ill) (Brereton 2017). Since medieval times people suffering from mental illness and various forms of dementia have been deprived of liberty on the grounds that it is necessary for their own protection. Even today, some legal remedies to exploitation can result in limitations being imposed on the exploited person as much as the perpetrator. For example, where an elderly person has been financially exploited by the person they had appointed as their enduring power of attorney (EPOA) – and who may be their daughter or son – an application can be made to a court or tribunal to take action to protect the person. In this circumstance, a financial management order may be made that would suspend any existing enduring power of attorney. While this outcome should stop the exploitation, it has come at the price of limiting the person's liberty by taking from them the ability to decide who will manage their affairs on their behalf.

In more contemporary debates about personal autonomy, the balance between the responsibility to protect versus the preservation of rights and individual freedoms has shifted to the latter. There is a preference for a rights-based approach that promotes supporting vulnerable people, including the elderly, to make their own decisions where possible, even when the person may be considered to lack capacity in some respects. This has to a large extent been fostered by the United Nations' Convention on the Rights of Persons with Disabilities (UNCRPD), to which Australia is a signatory, and is reflected in the recommendations made by a number of government inquiries that have taken place in respect to elder abuse and the law (United Nations 2006). These include the New South Wales Legislative Council Standing Committee (NSW GPSC 2016), the Australian Law Reform Commission inquiry into elder abuse (ALRC 2016) and the New South Wales Law Reform Commission's review of guardianship legislation (New South Wales Law Reform Commission 2018). Many of the submissions made to all three inquiries emphasised the importance of a rights-based approach that affirms autonomy and self-determination. Professor Wendy Lacey, as Head of the School of Law at the University of South Australia, advised the following in her evidence to the New South Wales Standing Committee:

> It is all too easy to fall into an ageist approach when dealing with older persons and to just see that age alone means that people are automatically vulnerable. In any framework that is adopted for addressing elder abuse it is essential that we put the rights of the older person at the heart of whatever strategy is adopted. That includes respect for dignity, autonomy and the self-determination of the older person and empowering older people to exercise their rights as fully as possible for as long as possible. (Lacey cited in NSW GPSC 2016: para. 3.14)

In response to the ALRC report, the Australian government has developed the National Plan to Respond to the Abuse of Older Australians 2019–2023

(Australian Government, Attorney General's Department 2019). The plan looks at implementing many of the recommendations of the report, including developing a nationally consistent approach that involves promoting autonomy and combating ageism.

The UNCRPD has led the way for the development of a 'new international paradigm', which sees a shift away from substitute decision-making (viewed as paternalistic) towards supported decision-making (Joseph 2015). A substitute decision-making approach, which is the approach employed by current legislation in Australia, involves determining whether a person has legal capacity and, where they are found not to (and there is a need to do so), appointing another person to make decisions on their behalf. The model of supported decision-making, however, necessitates a holistic approach involving the presumption that the person has (decision-making) capacity and early intervention to support the person in exercising that capacity. This approach requires corresponding changes across society consistent with its ideal of supporting people with disabilities to make decisions for themselves rather than having someone appointed to make them for them (Joseph 2015). The New South Wales Law Reform Commission report, *Review of the Guardianship Act 1987* (New South Wales Law Reform Commission 2018) makes recommendations in line with this shift towards supported decision-making, as does the report *Abuse and Neglect of Vulnerable Adults in NSW: The Need for Action – a Special Report to Parliament Under Section 31 of the Ombudsman Act 1974* (NSW Ombudsman 2018: 31).[3]

To illustrate this, we will return to the scenario of the elderly person who was being financially exploited by their EPOA. With the supported decision-making approach, following the cancellation of the EPOA, which stops the abuse, instead of then appointing a new substitute decision-maker or EPOA, measures would be put in place to assist the person to manage their own finances. This international paradigm shift, which is yet to be fully realised in the various legislative regimes in the states and territories, encapsulates the move away from paternalism towards supported autonomy.

Rights-based approaches employ the same concerns regarding paternalism to argue against the introduction of mandatory reporting of elder abuse, explaining that compulsory reporting will not only have negative effects, such as discouraging the elderly to seek help for fear of consequences, but that such an approach is not respectful of elderly people as autonomous adults. Indeed, many submissions to the standing committee characterised mandatory reporting as being inherently paternalistic.

The concerns that stem from a rights-based approach reflect the position on supported or assisted autonomy that has been presented in this chapter. It is important to note that we are not arguing that nurses or other health-care professionals should *not* report elder abuse because it would be a transgression of the elderly person's autonomy. Rather, we are saying that actions taken in response to the abuse should involve placing the elderly person at the centre of decision-making wherever possible by providing the person with information, support and options, and by seeking an understanding of their views and wishes. The nurse's response to abuse should be shaped accordingly, guided by the four principles of bioethics outlined in Chapter 3: non-maleficence, beneficence, respect for autonomy and justice.

Aged care and culturally safe nursing practice

In Chapter 6, we examined the importance of employing culturally safe nursing practices: the need for nurses to be aware of the cultural values that shape their attitudes and the importance of informing themselves of the cultural needs of the patient. Nurses should consider how the elderly person's values and cultural needs might differ from their own. For example, how does the person's culture approach ageing? Remember that while the Western approach to care focuses on the importance of the individual's autonomy in decision-making, other cultures may involve a more collective approach.

ABORIGINAL AND TORRES STRAIT ISLANDER PEOPLE AND AGED CARE

The Aboriginal and Torres Strait Islander population in Australia has a younger age structure, is ageing at a faster rate than the non-Indigenous population and has an incidence of dementia that is three times higher than the non-Indigenous population. Aboriginal and Torres Strait Islander people are also more likely to have chronic conditions. This means that this sector of the population has a greater need for aged care at a younger age (50 years) than other Australians (65 years) (AIHW 2021a, 2021b; Neura 2019).

Nurses need to be aware that an aged care system geared towards the individual patient and their right to privacy is likely to be alienating for Indigenous Australians for whom extended family and community are central (Neura 2019).

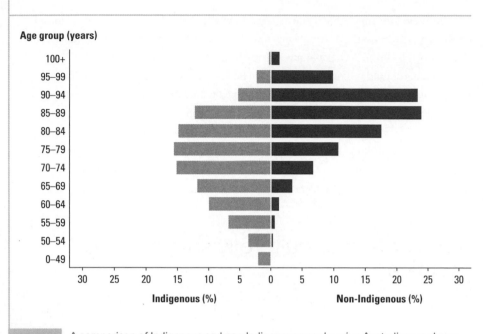

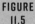

**FIGURE
11.5**

A comparison of Indigenous and non-Indigenous people using Australian aged care services – permanent residential care
Source: AIHW (2021a).

According to the Royal Commission into Aged Care Quality and Safety (2021), 'the aged care system must reflect the fact that for many Aboriginal and Torres Strait Islander people, health is grounded in connection to Country, culture, family and community'.

The National Aboriginal Community Controlled Health Organisation (NACCHO) is the national leadership body for Aboriginal and Torres Strait Islander health in Australia. NACCHO promotes a philosophy of Aboriginal community control and a holistic view of health. NACCHO also emphasises the importance of growing old on country (NACCHO 2022).

While the provision of culture-specific health care is the most appropriate approach for elderly Aboriginal and Torres Strait Islander people, many will still require the services provided by mainstream health care, such as hospitals. In these circumstances, nurses can play an important role in supporting the person to voice their needs and can take steps to ensure they meet those needs in a culturally sensitive way. In order to assist them in providing appropriate care to elderly Aboriginal and Torres Strait Islander patients, nurses should undertake cultural awareness and diversity training, and also familiarise themselves with other resources available, such as contacting their workplace Aboriginal Liaison Officer.

Kali, a community nurse, is attending 87-year-old Omar in his home to assist with wound management. During her visit, she comments on the many family photos that she sees around the house. Omar talks about his sadness at not seeing the rest of his family anymore and, when questioned, explains that it is because there has been a falling out between them and his daughter, Anisa (who is his carer). He is at pains to explain that Anisa is very good to him and only wants what is best, and thinks it is better that other family members don't visit because they will upset things. Omar does not want to go against Anisa's wishes because of all she does for him. Kali also notices that there is no phone in the house and Omar explains that Anisa has a mobile phone and says it is too expensive to pay for two phones.

》》 How should Kali approach this problem? Should she confront Anisa over Omar's isolation? Should she leave the situation alone because Omar has said it is best left alone? What could Kalia do to support Omar to make an autonomous decision? What role might cultural difference play in shaping Kali's approach?

A note on COVID-19

The COVID-19 pandemic posed one of the greatest challenges to the Australian and international health systems in modern times. While the pandemic affected people of all ages, it was the elderly who were most impacted, not only in terms of severity of illness and deaths, but also as a result of the isolation and social distancing policies that were adopted to combat the virus.

Under such circumstances, in which elderly people face serious illness while being isolated from the most important people in their lives, the role of the nurse as a supporter of autonomy becomes pivotal: at the same time that the elderly person's vulnerability intensifies, the resources to overcome that vulnerability are reduced.

Just as the pandemic reinforced the importance of fundamentals in disease management such as hygiene and infection control, it also highlighted the need to return to basic principles when it comes to supporting autonomy. It was the nurse, in their everyday care of elderly patients, who is well positioned to redress the restriction of freedoms and loss of control that that these patients experienced, and in doing so to support both their autonomy and their dignity.

Ethics of aged care overview

Throughout this book we have been working with a concept of autonomy that emphasises its embodied and relational dimensions. That is, autonomy fundamentally involves a relationship between self and others and the physical environment. We have also seen how the law protects and promotes individual freedom by regulating personal behaviour and interpersonal relationships, but that sometimes this falls short of, or even works against, this broader concept of autonomy. It is in this space – between what autonomy requires and what the law permits or protects – that our ethical obligations to promote the autonomy of others exists. In the case of persons who are ageing, the physical and social challenges to their autonomy can increase, and the protection offered by the law can sometimes be either ineffectual or counterproductive (such as when a substitute decision-maker is appointed).

In this chapter, we have examined a number of different ways of thinking about autonomy, as well as practical approaches that highlight the potential of the nurse as a builder of capacity and autonomy. In some ways, the nurse is uniquely placed to assist in redressing the vulnerability faced by the elderly and in making a significant impact on the person's experience of their autonomy. At its core, nursing is a caring profession, with the key value being the care and protection of the vulnerable – that is, the fiduciary relationship. The challenge for nurses in upholding this value is to avoid the paternalism that often results from a desire to protect and to act in a manner that supports the elderly person to exercise their autonomy.

Even though the current legislative frameworks that apply to the elderly have limitations, and are yet to fully implement a rights-based approach, some of their key principles can usefully guide the nurse in interactions with the elderly, such as the presumption of capacity, legal intervention only as a last resort where informal arrangements are not working, freedom of decision-making, freedom of action being limited as little as possible, and the encouragement of self-reliance being employed as far as possible.

LAW AND ETHICS IN PRACTICE

Veronica is an 85-year-old woman who has lived in the same house for more than 40 years. She was recently admitted to hospital after she was found wandering the streets late at night in a confused state. She has also been identified as having complex medical needs. Because of her confused state and agitation, the members of the treatment team are concerned that Veronica is unable to give consent to treatment.

Kay, the Nurse Unit Manager, finds that Veronica is less confused during the day and after speaking with her is able to contact Veronica's long-term partner, Ken. Veronica also tells Kay that she has three adult children, Suzanne, Melanie and Bob, whose father died some years ago. After being contacted by Kay, Ken attends the hospital on a daily basis to help care for Veronica. As Veronica and Ken are obviously very close, the treating team involves Ken in the decision-making process regarding Veronica's medical care. They identify him as her 'person responsible'.[4]

》》 **Consider how this case develops in the box on the next page.**

As discussed earlier, guardianship legislation across the states and territories makes provision for the seeking of substitute consent by health-care professionals. A person responsible or automatic substitute decision-maker is the person from whom health-care professionals can obtain substitute consent for treatment when the patient themself is unable to provide consent. Guardianship legislation sets out a hierarchy of persons responsible who can be considered automatic substitute decision-makers without the need for a formal process to appoint a guardian. This is possible because there is a statutory requirement that legal orders are not to be made unless there is a very real need to do so. It reflects the long-standing fundamental principle that any interference in the liberty of a person must be justified and must be proportionate.

LAW AND ETHICS IN PRACTICE

Kay and the treating team advise Veronica and Ken of her current medical condition and together they decide on a course of treatment. In doing so, they attempt to impinge as little as possible on Veronica's right to make her own decisions. Veronica becomes distressed, however, when the issue of her current accommodation is raised. The team is concerned that she may be at too great a risk if she were to return home unsupported and a meeting is organised to discuss the issues. Prior to the meeting, Kay organises for the social worker to discuss possible options with Veronica and Ken, and Ken encourages Veronica to consider accepting services to support her at home. Veronica is suspicious about having strangers in her home.

In the meantime, Suzanne, Melanie and Bob arrive from interstate and are not happy that Ken is providing substitute consent for Veronica. Suzanne provides the team with a copy of an enduring guardianship appointment identifying her as Veronica's enduring guardian, which includes the authority to make decisions about medical treatment. Suzanne insists on making every decision for Veronica and becomes annoyed with Kay and other staff when they attempt to include Ken in the decision-making at the meeting. Suzanne and her siblings are all very worried about the idea of Veronica going home and Suzanne and Ken argue over what is best for Veronica. Suzanne insists that an aged-care placement should be found.

Veronica, who is already distressed at the prospect of having to leave her home of more than 40 years, is now further upset by the conflict between her partner and her children. She refuses any form of assistance and demands to be discharged home immediately.

》》 What have Kay and the treating team done well in this scenario to support Veronica in decision-making?

》》 What could they have done better?

》》 What might be motivating the actions and behaviours of the family members?

》》 Should anyone lodge an application to the Guardianship Tribunal at this stage?

》》 Given that courts and tribunals across Australia are guided by the principle of taking the least restrictive option (or making orders as a last resort), what steps could be taken to assist with the informal resolution of this situation?

By virtue of the enduring guardianship appointment document, Kay may have made it clear that Suzanne has decision-making authority about health care and accommodation for Veronica. However, medical staff or the social worker can lodge an application with the Guardianship Tribunal because of the level of conflict among the family, and because Veronica is opposed to any of the options offered and continues to insist on going home.

Conclusion

This chapter has provided an understanding of the challenges that ageing poses to autonomy, in particular at the level of everyday interaction. It has reiterated the idea that, in protecting equality, the law includes an inbuilt bias towards promoting the capacity of people and subsequently has developed an understanding of the role of the nurse as a builder of capacity for autonomy. The chapter has demonstrated some ideas and techniques that can be employed by nurses in the provision of support for, and the promotion of autonomy in, aged persons. Finally, we have seen that the idea of capacity-building for autonomy reflects both national and international shifts in thinking around ethics and the law regarding people with decision-making disabilities (including the elderly).

REFLECTIVE QUESTIONS 11.3

1 List some of the particular ways in which elderly people are vulnerable to abuse. What can a nurse do to reduce those vulnerabilities?

2 Does the law in Australia specifically recognise elder abuse? How is elder abuse dealt with under current Australian law?

3 In responding to incidents of elder abuse, how can the nurse distinguish between acting in a paternalistic manner and acting in a manner that supports the autonomy of the person?

4 What is the role of a 'person responsible' or 'automatic substitute decision-maker'? Is a guardianship order necessary to appoint a 'person responsible' or 'automatic substitute decision-maker'?

Further reading

Australian Law Reform Commission (2016). *Protecting the rights of older Australians from abuse.* ALRC. www.alrc.gov.au/inquiries/elder-abuse

——(2017, 14 June). *Elder abuse – a national legal response.* ALRC. www.alrc.gov.au/publication/elder-abuse-a-national-legal-response-alrc-report-131/

Joosten, M. (2016). *A long time coming: Essays on old age.* Scribe.

NSW Ombudsman (2018, 2 November). *Abuse and neglect of vulnerable adults in NSW – the need for action: a special report to Parliament under section 31 of the Ombudsman Act 1974.* www.ombo.nsw.gov.au/__data/assets/pdf_file/0005/138155/Abuse-and-neglect-of-vulnerable-adults-in-NSW-November-2018.pdf

Smith, K.V. (2005). Ethical issues related to health care: The older adult's perspective. *Journal of Gerontological Nursing, 31*(2), 32–9.

World Health Organization (2022). *Ageing and health.* WHO. www.who.int/news-room/fact-sheets/detail/ageing-and-health

Notes

1 It should be noted here that this gap in the law in relation to elder abuse is to some extent being addressed by: (1) the Australian Government's *National Plan to Respond to the Abuse of Older Australians 2019–2023*, www.ag.gov.au/rights-and-protections/publications/national-plan-respond-abuse-older-australians-elder-abuse-2019-2023; (2) the Australian Government's decision, following the Royal Commission into Aged Care Quality and Safety, to replace the *Aged Care Act 1997* with a new Act, planned to come into effect 1 July 2023; (3) the establishment in South Australia of an Adult Safeguarding Unit, subsequent to the *Office of the Ageing (Adult Safeguarding) Amendment Act 2018*; and (4) the establishment in New South Wales of an Ageing and Disability Commissioner from 1 July 2019, to investigate and respond to allegations of abuse of older people and people with disability in home and community settings.

2 The NSW government's interagency policy, *Preventing and Responding to Abuse of Older People (Elder Abuse)* (Family and Community Services, NSW Government 2018: 17) sets out a five-step good practice approach to identifying and responding to suspected elder abuse. The following is an extract from that policy:

Identify abuse: Consider whether a risk assessment is appropriate. Where you suspect, have witnessed or have had abuse disclosed, gather information. Always take an account directly from the victim rather than the 'carer' or family member.

Assess immediate safety: Evaluate the urgency of safety concerns. Contact emergency services where appropriate. Protect evidence. Report via internal channels.

Provide support: Listen, acknowledge and validate. Offer information to support fully informed decision-making. Refer to other services as appropriate.

Inform manager and document: Report suspected, witnessed or disclosed abuse in accordance with agency procedures. Document the abuse and response according to your agency's policies and procedures. Document where the older person has made an informed decision not to accept intervention.

Respond and refer: Discuss the available options with the older person (not an intermediary). If the person does not have decision-making capacity, discuss the available options with the older person and their lawful substitute decision-maker. Offer information in an easily understood way. Seek consent from the older person or their substitute decision-maker for referral, then make the referrals. Where the older person makes an informed decision to not accept assistance, assess whether their safety is at risk or there is criminal activity. Be aware of the need for additional resources such as language or culture-specific supports. Understand when it is important to act without the consent of the older person. Understand when to refer to the NSW Police – staff should refer to internal policies clarifying situations when police must be called for reports of violence, abuse and neglect. Coordinate and monitor as appropriate.

3   The guardianship legislation of all states and territories sets out a hierarchy of 'persons responsible' or 'automatic substitute decision-makers' with respect to medical and dental treatment. This hierarchy is to be consulted by health-care professionals when determining from whom they should seek substitute consent when a patient is incapable of providing consent to treatment. In New South Wales, the hierarchy, as outlined in section 33A(4) of the NSW *Guardianship Act 1987*, is as follows (in descending order):

   (a)   the person's guardian, if any, but only if the order [e.g. guardianship order made by a court or tribunal] or instrument appointing the guardian [e.g. Enduring Guardianship Appointment] provides for the guardian to exercise the function of giving consent to the carrying out of medical or dental treatment on the person,

   (b)   the spouse of the person, if any, if:

   (i)   the relationship between the person and the spouse is close and continuing, and

   (ii)   the spouse is not a person under guardianship,

   (c)   a person who has the care of the person, [unpaid carer who supports and assists the person regularly]

   (b)   a close friend or relative of the person.

The term 'person responsible' is often interchanged with 'next of kin'; however, there is a significant difference. A 'person responsible' may be, but is not necessarily, a family member. Closeness and continuity of contact is key rather than a sole focus on familial relations. Nurses should consult the legislation of their respective state or territory to familiarise themselves with the hierarchy. They should also consult the legislation with respect to what treatments a 'person responsible' may or may not consent to.

   Even where a 'person responsible' or an 'enduring guardian/enduring power of attorney' is readily identifiable, conflict among family members and close friends over decision-making can pose a significant challenge to health-care workers. In cases where conflict cannot be informally resolved and is having negative impacts on the person and their care, health-care professionals can contact the Guardianship Tribunal or Board of their respective state or territory for guidance in determining whether there is a need to lodge an application with them (see *Guardianship Act 1987* (NSW), s 33A).

4   While changes in legislation have been recommended by various reports – in order for Australia to comply with its obligations as a signatory to the UNCRPD – and those recommendations have been accepted by the Australian Government (as with the ALRC Report), it may take some time for those legislative changes to be implemented. However, the commitment to shifting to a supported decision-making model is reflected in current practices/policy employed by key government and non-government agencies in Australia: see NDIS (2019, 2022).

APPENDIX

TABLES OF LEGISLATION

Chapter 2

LAWS PERTAINING TO THE INTERPRETATION OF LEGISLATION

Cth	*Acts Interpretation Act 1901*
	Judiciary Act 1903
ACT	*Legislation Act 2001*
NSW	*Interpretation Act 1987*
NT	*Interpretation Act 1978*
Qld	*Acts Interpretation Act 1954*
SA	*Acts Interpretation Act 1915*
Tas	*Acts Interpretation Act 1931*
Vic	*Interpretation of Legislation Act 1984*
WA	*Interpretation Act 1984*

CORONERS ACTS

ACT	*Coroners Act 1997*
NSW	*Coroners Act 2009*
NT	*Coroners Act 1993*
Qld	*Coroners Act 2003*
SA	*Coroners Act 2003*
Tas	*Coroners Act 1995*
Vic	*Coroners Act 2008*
WA	*Coroners Act 1996*

Chapter 4

LAWS PERTAINING TO CONSENT

ACT	*Medical Treatment (Health Directions) Act 2006*
NSW	*Children and Young Persons (Care and Protection) Act 1998, No. 157*
	Guardianship Act 1987
	Guardianship Regulation 2016
NT	*Advance Personal Planning Act 2013*
	Guardianship of Adults Act 2016

Qld	*Voluntary Assisted Dying Act 2021*
	Guardianship and Administration Act 2000 Powers of Attorney Act 1988
SA	*Consent to Medical and Dental Procedures Act 1985*
	Consent to Medical Treatment and Palliative Care Act 1995
	Guardianship and Administration Act 1993 Natural Death Act 1983
Tas	*Criminal Code Act 1924* (section 124 relates to consent to sexual interaction)
	Guardianship and Administration Act 1995
	End-of-Life Choices (Voluntary Assisted Dying) Act 2021 will come into effect in October 2022
Vic	*Guardianship and Administration Act 2019*
	Medical Treatment Planning and Decisions Act 2016
WA	*Acts Amendment (Consent to Medical Treatment) Act 2008*
	Guardianship and Administration Act 1990

LAWS PERTAINING TO BLOOD TRANSFUSIONS FOR CHILDREN

ACT	*Transplantation and Anatomy Act 1978*
NSW	*Children and Young Persons (Care and Protection) Act 1998, No. 157*
	Human Tissue Act 1983
NT	*Emergency Medical Operations Act 1973*
Qld	*Transplantation and Anatomy Act 1979*
SA	*Consent to Medical Treatment and Palliative Care Act 1995*
	Transplantation and Anatomy Act 1983
Tas	*Human Tissue Act 1985*
Vic	*Coroners and Human Tissue Acts (Amendment) 2006*
	Medical Treatment Planning and Decisions Act 2016
WA	*Human Tissue and Transplant Act 1982*

LAWS PERTAINING TO DETENTION OF CHILDREN

ACT	*Children and Young Persons Act 2008*
NSW	*Children and Young Persons (Care and Protection) Act 1998, No. 157*
NT	*Care and Protection of Children Act 2007*
Qld	*Child Protection Act 1999*
SA	*Children and Young People (Safety) Act 2017*
Tas	*Children, Young Persons and Their Families Act 1997*
Vic	*Children, Youth and Families Act 2005*
WA	*Children and Community Services Act 2004*

MENTAL HEALTH LEGISLATION

ACT	*Mental Health Act 2015*
NSW	*Mental Health Act 2007*, No. 8
NT	*Guardianship of Adults Act 2016*
	Mental Health and Related Services Act 1998
	Cross-border Justice Act 2009
Qld	*Mental Health Act 2016*
SA	*Mental Health Act 2009*
Tas	*Mental Health Act 2013*
Vic	*Mental Health Act 2014*
WA	*Mental Health Act 2014*

LEGISLATION PERTAINING TO ADVANCE CARE DIRECTIVES

Cth	*Euthanasia Laws Act 1997*
ACT	*Medical Treatment (Health Directions) Act 2006*
NT	*Advanced Personal Planning Act 2013*
Qld	*Powers of Attorney Act 1998*
	Voluntary Assisted Dying Act 2021
SA	*Consent to Medical Treatment and Palliative Care Act 1995*
	Advance Care Directives Act 2013
Tas	Advanced care planning is possible under common law. The *Guardianship and Administration Amendment (Advance Care Directives) Act 2021* was still to come into effect at the time of writing.
Vic	*Medical Treatment Planning and Decisions Act 2016*
WA	*Guardianship and Administration Act 1990*
	Advanced care planning is possible under common law.

Chapter 5

POISONS LEGISLATION

Cth	*Drugs of Dependence Act 1989*
	Narcotic Drugs Amendment Act 2016
	National Health Act 1953 (amended 2015 and 2016)
	Therapeutic Goods Act 1989
ACT	*Medicines, Poisons and Therapeutic Goods Act 2008*
NSW	*Poisons and Therapeutic Goods Act 1966*
	Poisons and Therapeutic Goods Regulations 2008
NT	*Medicines, Poisons and Therapeutic Goods Act 2012*

Qld	Health Act 1937
SA	Health (Drugs and Poisons) Regulation 1996 (amended 2011)
	Controlled Substances Act 1984
	Controlled Substances (Poisons) Regulations 2011
	Controlled Substances (Controlled Drugs, Precursors and Plants) Regulations 2014
Tas	Poisons Act 1971
	Poisons Regulations 2008 (amended 2010)
	Therapeutic Goods Act 2001
Vic	Drugs, Poisons and Controlled Substances Act 1981
	Drugs, Poisons and Controlled Substances Regulations 2017
WA	Medicines and Poisons Act 2014

LEGISLATION PERTAINING TO NEGLIGENCE

ACT	Civil Law (Wrongs) Act 2002 (amended 2006)
NSW	Civil Liability Act 2002
NT	Personal Injuries (Liabilities Damages) Act 2003
Qld	Civil Liability Act 2003
SA	Civil Liability Act 1936
Tas	Civil Liability Act 2002
Vic	Wrongs Act 1958
WA	Civil Liability Act 2002

Chapter 6

Cth	Marriage Amendment (Definition and Religious Freedoms) Act 2017, No. 129

HUMAN RIGHTS AND ANTI-DISCRIMINATION LEGISLATION

Cth	Age Discrimination Act 2004
	Australian Human Rights Commission Act 1986
	Disability Discrimination Act 1992
	Disability Discrimination and Other Human Rights Legislation Amendment Act 2009
	Racial Discrimination Act 1975
	Sex Discrimination Act 1984
	Sex Discrimination Amendment (Sexual Orientation, Gender Identity and Intersex Status) Act 2013
ACT	Discrimination Act 1991
	Human Rights Act 2004
	Human Rights Commission Act 2005
NSW	Anti-Discrimination Act 1977, No. 48
NT	Anti-Discrimination Act 1992

»

》

Qld	*Anti-Discrimination Act 1991*
SA	*Equal Opportunity Act 1984*
	Racial Vilification Act 1996
Tas	*Anti-Discrimination Act 1998*
	Equal Opportunity Act 2010
Vic	*Charter of Human Rights and Responsibilities 2006*
	Equal Opportunity Act 2010
	Racial and Religious Tolerance Act 2001
WA	*Equal Opportunity Act 1984*

Chapter 7

PRIVACY LEGISLATION

Cth		*Freedom of Information Act 1982*
		Privacy Act 1988
		Public Interest Disclosure Act 2013
		Surveillance Devices Act 2004
ACT	Administered by the Commonwealth government Privacy Commissioner, who acts on behalf of the ACT government	*Australian Capital Territory Government Service (Consequential Provisions) Act 1994*
		Privacy Amendment (Enhancing Privacy Protection) Act 2012
		Right to Information Act 2009
		Health Records (Privacy and Access) Act 1997
		Human Rights Act 2004
		Freedom of Information Act 1989
		Territory Records Act 2002 (public records)
		Spent Convictions Act 2000
		Listening Devices Act 1992
		Crimes (Forensic Procedures) Act 2000
NSW	Administered by the office of the New South Wales Privacy Commissioner. On 1 July 2010, the *Government Information (Public Access) Act 2009* replaced sections of the *Freedom of Information Act 1989* (NSW) and section 12 of the *Local Government Act 1993* (NSW).	*Criminal Records Act 1991* (spent convictions)
		Crimes (Forensic Procedures) Amendment Act 2009
		Government Information (Public Access) (Consequential Amendments and Repeal) Act 2009
		Health Records and Information Privacy Act 2002
		Privacy and Personal Information Protection Act 1998
		State Records Act 1998
		Surveillance Devices Act 2007
		Telecommunications (Interception and Access) (New South Wales) Act 1987
		Workplace Surveillance Act 2005
NT	Administered by the Information Commissioner for the Northern Territory	*Criminal Records (Spent Convictions) Act 1992*
		Northern Territory Information Act 2002
		Surveillance Devices Act 2007
		Telecommunications (Interception) Northern Territory Act 2001

Qld	Administered by the Queensland government. The *Right to Information Act 2009* and the *Information Privacy Act 2009* replaced Freedom of Information (FOI) laws to provide safeguards for the way the public sector handles an individual's personal information.	*Criminal Law (Rehabilitation of Offenders) Act 1986* (spent convictions) *Information Privacy Act 2009* *Invasion of Privacy Act 1971* (listening devices, invasion of privacy of the home) *Police Powers and Responsibilities Act 2000* (Chapter 4 deals with covert evidence-gathering powers.) *Private Employment Agents (Code of Conduct) Regulation 2015* (Provisions 14 and 15 deal with job-seekers' information and the need to ensure it is not disclosed or improperly used.) *Public Records Act 2002* *Right to Information Act 2009* *Whistleblowers Protection Act 1994*
SA	Administered by the South Australian government, which follows the Commonwealth Information Privacy Principles and has a privacy committee	*Freedom of Information Act 1991* *Listening and Surveillance Devices Act 2016* *State Records Act 1997* *Telecommunications (Interception) Act 2012*
Tas	Administered by the Tasmanian Department of Justice	*Annulled Convictions Act 2003* (spent convictions) *Archives Act 1983* *Listening Devices Act 1991* *Freedom of Information Act 1991* *Personal Information Protection Act 2004* *Police Powers (Surveillance Devices) Act 2006* *Right to Information Act 2009* *Telecommunications (Interception) Tasmania Amendment Act 2010*
Vic	Administered by the Victorian Equal Opportunity and Human Rights Commission	*Charter of Human Rights and Responsibilities Act 2006* *Freedom of Information Act 1982* *Health Records Act 2001* *Information Privacy Act 2000* *Public Records Act 1973* *Privacy and Data Protection Act 2014* *Surveillance Devices Act 1999* *Telecommunications (Interception) (State Provisions) (Amendment) Act 2002*
WA	Western Australia is in the process of establishing an Information and Privacy Commissioner (encompassing the current Information Commissioner).	*Freedom of Information Act 1992* *Health Services (Conciliation and Review) Act 1995* *State Records Act 2000* *Spent Convictions Act 1988* *Surveillance Devices Act 1998* *Telecommunications (Interception) Western Australia Amendment Act 2011*

MANDATORY REPORTING REQUIREMENTS

	WHO IS MANDATED TO REPORT?	WHAT IS TO BE REPORTED?	ABUSE AND NEGLECT TYPES THAT MUST BE REPORTED	LEGAL PROVISIONS
ACT	A person who is: a doctor; a dentist; a nurse; an enrolled nurse; a midwife; a psychologist; a teacher at a school; a person authorised to inspect education programs, materials or other records used for home education of a child or young person under the *Education Act 2004*; a police officer; a person employed to counsel children or young people at a school; a person caring for a child at a child care centre; a person coordinating or monitoring home-based care for a family day care scheme proprietor; a public servant who, in the course of employment as a public servant, works with, or provides services personally to children and young people or families; the public advocate; an official visitor; minister of religion, religious leader or member of the clergy of a church or religious denomination; a person who, in the course of the person's employment, has contact with or provides services to children, young people and their families and is prescribed by regulation.	A belief, on reasonable grounds, that a child or young person has experienced or is experiencing sexual abuse or non-accidental physical injury; and the reasons for the belief arise from information obtained by the person during the course of, or because of, the person's work (whether paid or unpaid)	Physical abuse Sexual abuse	Section 356 of the *Children and Young People Act 2008* (ACT)
NSW	A person who, in the course of his or her professional work, or other paid employment, delivers health care, welfare, education, children's services, residential services or law enforcement, wholly or partly, to children. A person who holds a management position in an organisation, the duties of which include direct responsibility for, or direct supervision of, the provision of health care, welfare, education, children's services, residential services or law enforcement, wholly or partly, to children. A person in religious ministry, or a person providing religion-based activities to children. A registered psychologist providing a professional service as a psychologist. *Note*: Children's services means either or both of the following (subject to the regulations): (a) an education and care service within the meaning of the Children (Education and Care Services) National Law (NSW); (b) a State regulated education and care service within the meaning of the *Children (Education and Care Services) Supplementary Provisions Act 2011*.	Suspicion on reasonable grounds, obtained during the course of or from the person's work, that a child is at risk of significant harm because of the presence to a significant extent of circumstances of: neglect, physical abuse, sexual abuse, psychological abuse, risk of harm through exposure to domestic violence, and failure to engage with services after a pre-natal report.	Physical abuse Sexual abuse Emotional or psychological abuse Neglect Exposure to domestic violence	Sections 23 and 27 of the *Children and Young Persons (Care and Protection) Act 1998* (NSW)

	Person	Threshold	Type of abuse	Legislation
NT	Any person	A belief on reasonable grounds that a child has suffered or is likely to suffer harm or exploitation.	Physical abuse Sexual abuse or other exploitation of the child Emotional/ psychological abuse Neglect Exposure to physical violence (e.g. a child witnessing violence between parents at home)	Sections 15, 16 and 26 of the *Care and Protection of Children Act 2007* (NT)
	A health practitioner or someone who performs work of a kind that is prescribed by regulation	Reasonable grounds to believe a child aged 14 or 15 years has been or is likely to be a victim of a sexual offence and the age difference between the child and offender is greater than two years.	Sexual abuse	Section 26(2) of the *Care and Protection of Children Act 2007* (NT)
Qld	An authorised officer, a public service employee employed by the department, a person employed in a departmental care service or licensed care service	A reasonable suspicion that a child in care (a child placed in the care of an entity conducting a departmental care service or a licensee) has suffered, is suffering, or is at unacceptable risk of suffering, significant harm caused by physical or sexual abuse.	Physical abuse Sexual abuse	Part 1AA, section 13 F of the *Child Protection Act 1999* (Qld)
	Doctors; registered nurses; teachers; a police officer who, under a direction given by the commissioner of the police service under the Police Service Administration Act 1990, is responsible for reporting under this section; a person engaged to perform a child advocate function under the *Public Guardian Act 2014*, early childhood education and care professionals.	A reasonable suspicion that a child has suffered, is suffering or is at an unacceptable risk of suffering, significant harm caused by physical or sexual abuse; and may not have a parent able and willing to protect the child from the harm.	Physical abuse Sexual abuse	Part 1AA, section 13E of the *Child Protection Act 1999* (Qld)

»

	WHO IS MANDATED TO REPORT?	WHAT IS TO BE REPORTED?	ABUSE AND NEGLECT TYPES THAT MUST BE REPORTED	LEGAL PROVISIONS
	School staff	Awareness or reasonable suspicion that a child has been or is likely to be sexually abused; and the suspicion is formed in the course of the person's employment.	Sexual abuse	Sections 364, 365, 365A, 366, 366A of the *Education (General Provisions) Act 2006* (Qld)
SA	Medical practitioners; pharmacists; registered or enrolled nurses; dentists; psychologists; police officers; community corrections officers under the *Correctional Services Act 1982*; social workers; ministers of religion; employees of, or volunteers in, an organisation formed for religious or spiritual purposes; teachers employed as such in a school (within the meaning of the *Education and Early Childhood Services (Registration and Standards) Act 2011)* or a preschool or kindergarten; employees of, or volunteers in, an organisation that provides health, welfare, education, sporting or recreational, child care or residential services wholly or partly for children and young people, being a person who – (i) provides such services directly to children and young people; or (ii) holds a management position in the organisation, the duties of which include direct responsibility for, or direct supervision of, the provision of those services to children and young people	Reasonable grounds to suspect a child or young person is, or may be, at risk; and the suspicion was formed in the course of the person's employment.	Physical abuse Sexual abuse Mental and emotional abuse Neglect	Sections 17, 18, 30 and 31 of the *Children and Young People (Safety) Act 2017* (SA) Section 11 of the *Children's Protection Act 1993* (SA)
Tas	Medical practitioners; registered or enrolled nurses; persons registered under the Health Practitioner Regulation National Law (Tasmania) in the midwifery, dental (dentists, dental therapist, dental hygienist or oral health therapist) or psychology professions; police officers; probation officers; principals and teachers in any educational institution including kindergartens; persons who provide child care or a child care service for fee or reward; persons concerned in the management of an approved education and care service, within the meaning of the Education and Care Services National Law (Tasmania) or a child care service licensed under the *Child Care Act 2001*; a member of the clergy of any church or religious denomination; a member of the Parliament of this State; any	Knowledge, or a belief or suspicion on reasonable grounds that: a child has been or is being 'abused' or 'neglected' or is an affected child within the meaning of the *Family Violence Act 2004* (a child whose safety, psychological wellbeing or interests are affected or likely to be affected by family violence) or there is a reasonable likelihood of a child being killed or abused or neglected by a person with whom the child resides; or while a woman is pregnant, that there is reasonable likelihood that after the birth of the child: the child will suffer abuse	Sexual abuse (any) Physical abuse Emotional/ psychological abuse Neglect Exposure to family violence	Sections 3, 4 and 14 of the *Children, Young Persons and Their Families Act 1997* (Tas)

	other person who is employed or engaged as an employee for, of, or in, or who is a volunteer in, a government agency that provides health, welfare, education, child care or residential services wholly or partly for children, and an organisation that receives any funding from the Crown for the provision of such services; and any other person of a class determined by the Minister by notice in the Gazette to be prescribed persons.	or neglect, or may be killed by a person with whom the child is likely to reside; or that the child will require medical treatment or other intervention as a result of the behaviour of the woman or another person with whom the woman resides or is likely to reside, before the birth of the child. Note on extent of harm required to activate the duty (section 3(1) definition of 'abuse and neglect': for all forms except sexual abuse, reports must be made where: (i) the injured, abused or neglected person has suffered, or is likely to suffer, physical or psychological harm detrimental to the person's wellbeing; or (ii) the injured, abused or neglected person's physical or psychological development is in jeopardy. All instances of suspected sexual abuse must be reported.	
Vic	Registered medical practitioners, nurses, midwives, a person registered as a teacher or an early childhood teacher under the *Education and Training Reform Act 2006* or teachers granted permission to teach under that Act; principals of government or non-government schools within the meaning of the *Education and Training Reform Act 2006*; police officers, a person in religious ministry, out-of-home care workers (excluding voluntary foster and kinship carers), early childhood workers, youth justice workers and registered psychologists.	Belief on reasonable grounds that a child is in need of protection on a ground referred to in section 162(1)(c) or 162(1)(d), formed in the course of practising his or her profession or carrying out the duties of his or her office, position or employment as soon as practicable after forming the belief and after each occasion on which he or she becomes aware of any further reasonable grounds for the belief	Physical abuse Sexual abuse Note that technically, under section 162, the duty is limited to instances of physical injury and sexual abuse where 'the child's parents have not protected, or are unlikely to protect, the child from harm of that type'.	Sections 182(1), 184 and 162(1)(c)–(d) of the *Children, Youth and Families Act 2005* (Vic)

>>

	WHO IS MANDATED TO REPORT?	WHAT IS TO BE REPORTED?	ABUSE AND NEGLECT TYPES THAT MUST BE REPORTED	LEGAL PROVISIONS
WA	Doctors; nurses and midwives; teachers and boarding supervisors; and police officers	Belief on reasonable grounds that child sexual abuse has occurred or is occurring, where this belief is formed in the course of the person's work, whether paid or unpaid	Sexual abuse	Sections 124A and 124B of the *Children and Community Services Act 2004* (WA)
	The Principal Registrar, a registrar or a deputy registrar; family counsellors; family consultants; family dispute resolution practitioners, arbitrators or legal practitioners independently representing the child's interests	Reasonable grounds for suspecting that a child has been: abused, or is at risk of being abused; ill-treated, or is at risk of being ill-treated; or exposed or subjected to behaviour that psychologically harms the child	Physical abuse Sexual abuse Neglect Psychological harm including (but not limited to) harm caused by being subjected or exposed to family violence	Sections 5 and 160 of the *Family Court Act 1997* (WA)

Source: Higgins et al. (2010), updated Australian Institute of Family Studies (AIFS) (2020).

LEGISLATION PERTAINING TO COMMUNICABLE DISEASES

Cth	*Biosecurity (Consequential Amendments and Transitional Provisions) Act 2015*
ACT	*Public Health Act 1997*
NSW	*Public Health Act 2010*
NT	*Notifiable Diseases Act 1999*
Qld	*Public Health Act 2005*
SA	*Public Health Act 2011*
Tas	*Public Health Act 1997*
Vic	*Public Health and Well-being Act 2008*
WA	*Public Health Act 2016* *Public Health (Consequential Provisions) Act 2016*

CORONERS ACTS

See table for Chapter 2.

Chapter 8

LEGISLATION REGULATING NURSING PRACTICE

ACT	*Health Practitioner Regulation National Law (ACT) Act 2010*
NSW	*Health Practitioner Regulation National Law and Other Legislation Amendment Act 2017*
NT	*Health Practitioner Regulation National Law (NT) Act 2010*
Qld	*Health Practitioner Regulation National Law and Other Legislation Amendment Act 2019*
SA	*Health Practitioner Regulation National Law (South Australia) (Amendment of Law) Regulations 2017)*
Tas	*Health Practitioner Regulation National Law (Tasmania) Act 2010*
Vic	*Health Practitioner Regulation National Law (Victoria) Act 2009*
WA	*Health Practitioner Regulation National Law (WA) Amendment Act 2018*

Chapter 9

WHISTLEBLOWER PROTECTION LEGISLATION

Cth	*Public Interest Disclosure Act 2013*
	The *Corporations Act 2001* and the *Taxation Administration Act 1953* contain some protections for whistleblowers.
ACT	*Public Interest Disclosure Act 2013 (Cth)*

»

NSW	*Protected Disclosure Act 1994*
NT	*Public Interest Disclosure Act 2008*
Qld	*Public Interest Disclosure Act 2010* (previously the *Whistleblowers Protection Act 1994*)
SA	*Whistleblowers Protection Act 1993* *Public Interest Disclosure Act 2018*
Tas	*Public Interest Disclosure Act 2002*
Vic	*Protected Disclosure Act 2012*
WA	*Public Interest Disclosure Act 2003*

Chapter 10

ABORTION LEGISLATION

ACT	*Medical Practitioners (Maternal Health) Amendment Act 2002* Abortion is defined under section 80 of the *Health Act 1993*
NSW	*Abortion Law Reform Act 2019*
NT	*The Termination of Pregnancy Law Reform Act 2017*
Qld	*Termination of Pregnancy Act 2018*
SA	*Termination of Pregnancy Act 2021*
Tas	*Reproductive Health (Access to Terminations) Act 2013*
Vic	*Abortion Law Reform Act 2008*
WA	*Acts Amendment (Abortion) Act 1998*, s 119 *Health Act 1911*, ss 334 and 335 *Criminal Code*, s 290

EUTHANASIA LEGISLATION

Cth	*Criminal Code Amendment (Suicide Related Material Offences) Act 2005* *Euthanasia Laws Act 1997*
NSW	*Voluntary Assisted Dying Act 2022* This Act is expected to come into effect in November 2023.
Qld	*Voluntary Assisted Dying Act 2021*
SA	*Voluntary Assisted Dying Act 2021* There is a task force working to establish processes for implementation of the Act.
Tas	*End-of-Life Choices (Voluntary Assisted Dying) Act 2021* This Act is expected to come into effect in October 2022.
Vic	*Voluntary Assisted Dying Act 2017*
WA	*Voluntary Assisted Dying Act 2019*

Chapter 11

AGED CARE

See also legislation relating to torts, the criminal code, mandatory reporting, anti-discrimination, guardianship and domestic violence.

Cth	*Aged Care Act 1997* (and subsequent amendments) concerns the provision of aged care and its funding from the Commonwealth government.

REFERENCES

ABC News (2016, 22 November). Maligned EPAS patient record software system suffers two more outages in Adelaide. www.abc.net.au/news/2016-11-22/maligned-epas-software-system-suffers-two-more-outages/8044698

ACQSC *see* Aged Care Safety and Quality Commission

ACSQHC *see* Australian Commission on Safety and Quality in Health Care

Aged Care Safety and Quality Commission (ACQSC) (2022). *Quality Standards.* www.agedcarequality.gov.au/providers/standards

AHPRA *see* Australian Health Practitioner Regulatory Agency

AIFS *see* Australian Institute of Family Studies

AIHW *see* Australian Institute of Health and Welfare

Alcorn, G. (1997, 7 January). Confusion over law as second person takes life. *Sydney Morning Herald.*

ALRC *see* Australian Law Reform Commission

Anda, R.F., Felitti, V.J., Bremner, M.D. et al (2006). The enduring effects of abuse and related adverse experiences in childhood: A convergence of evidence from neurobiology and epidemiology. *European Archives of Psychiatry and Clinical Neuroscience, 256*(3), 174–86.

Anesi, G. (2012). The 'decrepit concept' of confidentiality, 30 years later. *American Medical Association Journal of Ethics, 14*(9), 708–11.

ANMAC *see* Australian Nursing and Midwifery Accreditation Council

ANMF *see* Australian Nursing and Midwifery Federation

APNA *see* Australian Primary Health Nurses Association

Ashby, M. (1997). The fallacies of death causation in palliative care. *Medical Journal of Australia, 166*(4), 176–7.

Atkins, K. (ed.) (2004). *Self and subjectivity: A reader with commentary.* Blackwell.

——(2005). *Re Alex* – narrative identity and the case of gender dysphoria. *Griffith Law Review, 14*(1), 1–16.

——(2008) *Narrative identity and moral identity: A practical perspective.* Routledge.

Australian Bureau of Statistics (2016). *Personal Safety Survey.* www.abs.gov.au/statistics/people/crime-and-justice/personal-safety-australia/latest-release

——(2018a). Estimates of Aboriginal and Torres Strait Islander Australians. www.abs.gov.au/ausstats/abs@.nsf/mf/3238.0.55.001

——(2018b). Population aged over 85 to double in the next 25 years. www.abs.gov.au/articles/population-aged-over-85-double-next-25-years

Australian Commission on Safety and Quality in Health Care (ACSQHC) (2010). *Consensus statement: Essential elements for recognising and responding to clinical deterioration – consultation report.* ACSQHC.

——(2013). Australian open disclosure framework. www.safetyandquality.gov.au/our-work/open-disclosure/the-open-disclosure-framework

——(2017). Patient and consumer-centred care. www.safetyandquality.gov.au/our-work/patient-and-consumer-centred-care

——(2018). Partnering with consumers standard. www.safetyandquality.gov.au/standards/nsqhs-standards/partnering-consumers-standard

——(2021a). *Incident management guide.* www.safetyandquality.gov.au/publications-and-resources/resource-library/incident-management-guide

——(2021b). Informed consent. www.safetyandquality.gov.au/our-work/partnering-consumers/informed-consent

——(2022a). Action 6.07. Clinical handover. www.safetyandquality.gov.au/standards/nsqhs-standards/communicating-safety-standard/communication-clinical-handover/action-607

——(2022b). Person-centred care. www.safetyandquality.gov.au/our-work/partnering-consumers/person-centred-care

Australian Council of Professions (2003). What is a profession? www.professions.org.au/what-is-a-professional

Australian Digital Health Agency (2019a). Benefits of My Health Record for healthcare professionals. www.myhealthrecord.gov.au/for-healthcare-professionals/what-is-my-health-record/benefits-my-health-record-for-healthcare

——(2019b). Learn about My Health Record system security. www.myhealthrecord.gov.au/for-you-your-family/learn-about-my-health-record-system-security

Australian Government (2008). Apology to Australia's Indigenous people. www.australia.gov.au/about-australia/our-country/our-people/apology-to-australias-indigenous-peoples

——(2022a). Gender and sexual diversity. *Style Manual.* www.stylemanual.gov.au/accessible-and-inclusive-content/inclusive-language/gender-and-sexual-diversity

——(2022b). Immunisation coverage rates for all children. www.health.gov.au/health-topics/immunisation/childhood-immunisation-coverage/immunisation-coverage-rates-for-all-children

Australian Government, Attorney General's Department (2019). *National Plan to Respond to the Abuse of Older Australians (Elder Abuse) 2019–2023.* www.ag.gov.au/rights-and-protections/publications/national-plan-respond-abuse-older-australians-elder-abuse-2019-2023

Australian Health Practitioner Regulatory Agency (AHPRA) (2018). Legislation. www.ahpra.gov.au/about-ahpra/what-we-do/Legislation.aspx

——(2020a). *Guidelines for mandatory notifications.* www.nursingmidwiferyboard.gov.au/Codes-Guidelines-Statements/Codes-Guidelines/Guidelines-for-mandatory-notifications.aspx

——(2020b). *Regulatory guide.* www.ahpra.gov.au/Publications/Corporate-publications.aspx

——(2021a) English language skills. www.nursingmidwiferyboard.gov.au/Registration-Standards/English-language-skills.aspx

——(2021b). Cancelled, disqualified and/or prohibited health practitioners. www.ahpra.gov.au/Registration/Registers-of-Practitioners/Cancelled-Health-Practitioners/PHY0001321474.aspx

——(2021c). The National Registration and Accreditation Scheme. www.ahpra.gov.au/About-AHPRA/What-We-Do/AHPRA-in-numbers.aspx

——(2021d). How we manage concerns. www.ahpra.gov.au/Notifications/How-we-manage-concerns.aspx

——(2021e). Tribunal suspends nurse after misogynistic social media posts. www.nursingmidwiferyboard.gov.au/News/2021-09-22-Tribunal-suspends-nurse-after-misogynistic-social-media-posts.aspx

——(2021f). Professional indemnity insurance arrangements. www.ahpra.gov.au/Registration/Registration-Standards/PII.aspx

——(2021g). Mandatory notifications. www.ahpra.gov.au/Notifications/Make-a-complaint/Mandatory-notifications.aspx

Australian Human Rights Commission (2022a) What responsibilities do I have when exercising my human rights during COVID-19? https://humanrights.gov.au/about/covid19-and-human-rights/what-responsibilities-do-i-have-when-exercising-my-human-rights-during

——(2022b). What are human rights? www.humanrights.gov.au/our-work/stories-discrimination

Australian Institute of Family Studies (AIFS) (2020). *Mandatory reporting of child abuse and neglect.* CFCA resource sheet. https://aifs.gov.au/sites/default/files/publication-documents/2006_mandatory_reporting_of_child_abuse_and_neglect_0.pdf

Australian Institute of Health and Welfare (AIHW) (2019). *Admitted patient care 2017–18: Australian hospital statistics.* AIHW

——(2020a). Suicide and intentional self-harm. www.aihw.gov.au/reports/australias-health/suicide-and-intentional-self-harm

——(2020b). *Indigenous health and wellbeing.* AIHW. www.aihw.gov.au/reports/australias-health/indigenous-health-and-wellbeing

———(2021a). Older Aboriginal and Torres Strait Islander people. www.aihw.gov.au/reports/older-people/older-australians/contents/population-groups-of-interest/older-aboriginal-and-torres-strait-islander-people

———(2021b). Aged care for Indigenous Australians. www.aihw.gov.au/reports/australias-welfare/aged-care-for-indigenous-australians

———(2022). *Dementia in Australia: Prevalence of dementia*. www.aihw.gov.au/reports/dementia/dementia-in-aus/contents/population-health-impacts-of-dementia/prevalence-of-dementia

Australian Law Reform Commission (ALRC) (2016). *Protecting the rights of older Australians from abuse*. www.alrc.gov.au/inquiries/elder-abuse

Australian Nursing and Midwifery Accreditation Council (ANMAC) (2021). Accreditation Policy and Procedure. www.anmac.org.au/document/accreditation-policy-and-procedure

Australian Nursing and Midwifery Federation (ANMF) (2020). Compulsory reporting of abuse in aged care settings for nurses and assistants in nursing. www.anmf.org.au/media/ocwbnrvf/ps_compulsory_reporting_of_abuse_in_aged_care_settings.pdf

Australian Primary Health Nurses Association (APNA) (2019). *Nurses' scope of practice*. www.apna.asn.au

Austroads (2022). *Assessing fitness to drive*. https://austroads.com.au/drivers-and-vehicles/assessing-fitness-to-drive

Baier, A. (1986). Trust and anti-trust. *Ethics*, *96*, 231–60.

———(1994). *Moral prejudices*. Harvard University Press.

Banks, S. & Gallagher, A. (2009). *Ethics in professional life: virtues for health and social care*. London: Palgrave Macmillan.

Barnable, A., Cunning, G. & Parcon, M. (2018). Nursing students' perceptions of confidentiality, accountability, and E-professionalism in relation to Facebook. *Nurse Educator*, *43*(1), 28–31.

Bayles, M. (1989). *Professional ethics*. Wadsworth Cengage.

———(2009, 16 March). Professional–client relationship. *Professional Ethics*. http://pl311.blogspot.com/2009/03/professional-client-relationship.html

Bearskin, L. (2011). A critical lens on culture in nursing practice. *Nursing Ethics*, *18*(4), 548–59.

Beauchamp, T.L. & Childress, J.F. (2019). *Principles of biomedical ethics*, 8th ed. Oxford University Press.

Beltran-Aroca, C.M., Girela-Lopez, E., Collazo-Chao, E., Montero-Pérez-Barquero, M. & Muñoz-Villanueva, M.C. (2016). Confidentiality breaches in clinical practice: What happens in hospitals? *BMC Medical Ethics*, *17*(1), 52.

Bennett, B. & Freckleton, I. (eds) (2021). *Pandemics, public health emergencies and government powers: Perspectives on Australian law*. Federation Press.

Benson, P. (2000). Feeling crazy. In N. Stoljar & C. Mackenzie (eds), *Relational autonomy: Feminist perspectives on autonomy, agency and the social self*. Oxford University Press.

Berghout, M., van Exel, J., Leensvaart, L. & Cramm, J.M. (2015). Healthcare professionals' views on patient-centered care in hospitals. *BMC Health Services Research*. www.ncbi.nlm.nih.gov/pmc/articles/PMC4572638/0

Berglund, C. (2012). *Ethics for health care*, 4th ed. Oxford University Press.

Berkich, D. (2007). A fallacy in potentiality. *Dialogue: Canadian Philosophical Review*, *46*(1), 137–50.

Bird, S. (2018). Children and consent for medical treatment. *News GP*. www1.racgp.org.au/newsgp/professional/what-is-too-young-children-and-consent-for-medical

Blue Knot Foundation (2021). Understanding trauma and abuse. https://blueknot.org.au/resources/understanding-trauma-and-abuse

Blumenthal, D. & Tavenner, M. (2010). The 'meaningful use' regulation for electronic health records. *New England Journal of Medicine*, *363*(6), 501–4.

Bogle, A. & Willis, O. (2018, 21 August). Lax security culture in hospitals could affect My Health Record privacy, insiders fear. *ABC News*. www.abc.net.au/news/health/2018-08-21/lax-hospital-security-culture-could-undermine-my-health-record/10128274

Brereton, P.L.G. (2017, 5 May). The Origins and evolution of the *parens patriae* jurisdiction. AM RFD Lecture on Legal History Sydney Law School. www.supremecourt.justice.nsw.gov.au/Documents/Publications/Speeches/2017%20Speeches/Brereton_050517.pdf

Burnard, P. & Chapman, C. (2004). *Professional and ethical issues in nursing.* Ballière Tindall.

Burns, K. & Belton, S. (2012). 'Click first, care second' photography. *Medical Journal of Australia, 197,* 265–6.

Burton, N. (2015, 22 May). Empathy vs sympathy. *Psychology Today.* www.psychologytoday.com/au/blog/hide-and-seek/201505/empathy-vs-sympathy

Calhoun, C. (2008). Losing oneself. In K. Atkins & C. Mackenzie (eds), *Practical identity and narrative agency.* Routledge.

Campbell, P. (2021). Recent WA trends in medical negligence and professional regulation. *Health Blog.* www.pmlawyers.com.au/blog/2021/05/health-blog/recent-wa-trends-in-medical-negligence-and-professional-regulation

Cancer Council of Victoria (2022). Treatment types. https://www.cancervic.org.au/cancer-information/treatments/treatments-types

Carnes, B.A, Staats, D.O. & Sonntag, W.E. (2008). Does senescence give rise to disease? *Mechanisms of Ageing and Development, 129*(12), 693–9.

Cass, A., Lowell, A., Christie, M., Snelling, P., Flack, M., Marrnganyin, B. & Brown, I. (2002). Sharing the true stories: Improving communication between Aboriginal patients and healthcare workers. *Medical Journal of Australia, 176,* 466–70.

CATSINaM (2021). *Close the Gap Campaign Report.* https://apo.org.au/node/311463

CEC *see* Clinical Excellence Commission

Centre for Remote Health (2017). *CARPA standard treatment manual,* 7th ed. www.crh.org.au/the-manuals/carpa-standard-treatment-manual-7th-edition

Chiarella, M. & Staunton, P. (2020). *Law for nurses and midwives,* 9th ed. Elsevier.

Chiarella, M. & White, J. (2013). 'Which tail wags which dog? Exploring the interface between professional regulation and professional education'. *Nurse Education Today, 33,* 1274–8.

Chochinov, H.M. (2007) Dignity and the essence of medicine: The A, B, C, and D of dignity conserving care. *BMJ, 335*(7612), 184–7.

——(2013). The secret is out: Patients are people with feelings that matter. *Palliative Support and Care, 11*(4), 287–8.

Chochinov, H.M., Schoppee, T., Scarton, L., et al. (2022). Dignity therapy intervention fidelity: A cross-sectional descriptive study with older adult outpatients with cancer. *BMC Palliative Care, 21*(8). https://bmcpalliatcare.biomedcentral.com/articles/10.1186/s12904-021-00888-y

Clinical Excellence Commission (CEC) (2018). *Between the flags.* www.cec.health.nsw.gov.au/keep-patients-safe/between-the-flags/overview

——(2020a). Brief bites. www.cec.health.nsw.gov.au/keep-patients-safe/human-factors/brief-bites

——(2020b). Clinical incident data. www.cec.health.nsw.gov.au/Review-incidents/Biannual-Incident-Report/Clinical-incident-data

——(2020c). System factors – clinical management. www.cec.health.nsw.gov.au/Review-incidents/Biannual-Incident-Report/saer-data/system-factors-clinical-management

Coady, M. & Bloch, S. (eds). (1996). *Codes of ethics and the professions.* Melbourne University Press.

Cohen, R. (1978). *Tarasoff v Regents of the University of California:* The duty to warn – common law and statutory problems for California psychotherapists. *California Western Law Review, 14,* 153–82.

Coombes, J., Cullen, P., Bennett-Brook, K., Longbottom, M., Mackean, T., Field, B. & Parry, V. (2022). Culturally safe and integrated primary health care: A case study of Yerin Eleanor Duncan Aboriginal Health Services' holistic model. *Journal of the Australian Indigenous HealthInfoNet, 3*(1). https://ro.ecu.edu.au/aihjournal/vol3/iss1/5

Coon, D. & Mitterer, J.O. (2010). *Introduction to psychology: Gateways to mind and behaviour.* Wadsworth Cengage.

Coroner's Court of New South Wales (2017). *Inquest into the death of Ahlia Raftery.* https://coroners.nsw.gov .au/coroners-court/download.html/documents/findings/2017/RAFTERY%20Ahlia%20-%20Findings%20 -%20redacted.pdf

——(2020a). Inquests and inquiries. www.coroners.justice.nsw.gov.au/Pages/coroner_role/coroner_role.aspx

——(2020b). Role of the Coroner. www.coroners.nsw.gov.au/coroners-court/how-the-coroners-court-work/ role-of-the-coroner.html

Cox, A., Perry, B. & Frederico, M. (2020). Resourcing the system and enhancing relationships: Pathways to positive outcomes for children impacted by abuse and neglect. *Child Welfare, 98*(6), 177–202.

Crameri, P. et al. (2015). It is more than sex and clothes: Culturally safe services for older lesbian, gay, bisexual, transgender and intersex people. *Australasian Journal on Ageing, 34*(Supp. 2), 21–5.

Creature Tales Tasmania (2012). *Animated anthologies.* http://creaturetales.com.au/project/animated- anthologies

Croke, E.M. (2003). Nurses, negligence and malpractice: An analysis based on more than 250 cases against nurses. *American Journal of Nursing, 103*(9), 54–63.

Crouch, B. & Wills, D. (2016, 25 February). SA Health staff sacked, disciplined as 21 caught spying on patient records. *The Advertiser.* www.adelaidenow.com.au/news/south-australia/sa-health-staff-sacked- disciplined-as-21-caught-spying-on-patient-records/news-story/790103a3482c0259c926023692752ccc

Dale, S. (2021). Personhood, critical interests, and the moral imperative of advance directives in Alzheimer's cases. *Voices in Bioethics, 7.* https://doi.org/10.7916/vib.v7i.7818

Department of Health and Human Services, Victoria (2016). *Medical Treatment Planning and Decisions Act 2016.* www.health.vic.gov.au/patient-care/medical-treatment-planning-and-decisions-act-2016?msclkid= ab2760e0a97211ecb681ad41e8d9b16c

——(2018). Advance care planning forms. www2.health.vic.gov.au/hospitals-and-health-services/patient- care/end-of-life-care/advance-care-planning/acp-forms

DeSousa, R. (2008). Wellness for all: the possibilities of cultural safety and cultural competence in New Zealand. *Journal of Research in Nursing, 13*(2), 125–35.

Dillon, R. (1992). How to lose your self-respect. *American Philosophical Quarterly, 29*(2), 125–39.

——(2001). Self-forgiveness and self-respect. *Ethics, 112*(1), 53–83.

——(2013). Self-respect and self-esteem. In H. LaFollette (ed.), *International encyclopedia of ethics.* Wiley Blackwell.

Dunn, M.C., Clare, I.C.H. & Holland, A.J. (2008). To empower or to protect? Constructing the 'vulnerable adult' in English law and public policy. *Legal Studies, 28*(2), 234–53.

Dworkin, G. (1993). *Life's dominion: An argument about abortion, euthanasia, and individual freedom.* Knopf.

EMAP Publishing Limited (2010, 30 November). Confidentiality breach as nurse tells teen's family of secret abortion. *Nursing Times.* www.nursingtimes.net/whats-new-in-nursing/news-topics/ethics-and-law-in- nursing/confidentiality-breach-as-nurse-tells-teens-family-of-secret-abortion/5010932.article

Evans, N. (2012, 5 December). Security scare: Kate Middleton nurse reveals medical details to DJ impersonating the Queen in radio prank call. *Mirror News.* www.mirror.co.uk/news/uk-news/kate- middleton-nurse-reveals-medical-1473720

Fallon, A., Kennelly, S. & O'Neill, D. (2016). Frailty in emergency departments. *The Lancet, 387*(10029), 1720.

Family and Community Services, NSW Government (2018). *Preventing and responding to abuse of older people (Elder Abuse): NSW Interagency Policy June 2018.* www.elderabusehelpline.com.au/uploads/pdf/NSW_ Interagency_Policy_Abuse_of_Older_People.pdf

Forrester, K. & Griffiths, D. (2014). *Essentials of law for health professionals,* 4th ed. Mosby Elsevier.

Foucault, M. (1997). Subjectivity and truth. In P. Rabinow (ed.), *The Essential Works of Michel Foucault 1954– 1984. Ethics, Subjectivity, and Truth. Vol. 1.* The New Press.

Frankel, T. (2011). *Fiduciary law*. Oxford University Press.

Freud, S. (1991). *On Metapsychology*. Penguin.

Gallagher, S. (2005). *How the body shapes the mind*. Clarendon Press.

———(2017). *Enactivist interventions: Rethinking the mind*. Oxford University Press.

Gallagher, S. & Hutto, D.D. (2007). Primary interaction and narrative practice. In J. Zlatev, T. Racine, C. Sinha & E. Itkonen (eds), *The shared mind: Perspectives on intersubjectivity*. John Benjamins.

Gallagher, S. & Meltzoff, A. (1996). The earliest sense of self and others: Merleau-Ponty and recent developmental studies. *Philosophical Psychology*, *9*, 213–36.

Gentile, M. (2010). *Giving voice to values: How to speak your mind when you know what's right*. Yale University Press.

Gillett, G. (1995). Ethical aspects of the Northern Territory euthanasia legislation. *Journal of Law and Medicine*, *3*, 145–51.

Glick, S.M. (1997). Unlimited human autonomy – a cultural bias? *New England Journal of Medicine*, *336*(13), 954–6.

Gligorov, N. (2017). Don't worry, this will only hurt a bit: The role of expectation and attention in pain intensity. *Monist: An International Quarterly Journal of General Philosophical Inquiry*, *100*(4), 501–13.

Glover, J. (1977). *Causing death and saving lives*. Penguin.

The Guardian Australia (2018, 30 October). German nurse admits to killing 100 patients as trial opens. www.theguardian.com/world/2018/oct/30/german-nurse-serial-killer-niels-hoegel-on-trial-100-patients-deaths

Gunn, M.A. & McDonald, F.J. (2021). COVID-19, rationing and the right to health: Can patients bring legal actions if they are denied access to care? *Medical Journal of Australia*, *214*(5), 207–8.

Habermas, J. (1996). *Between Facts and Norms*. MIT Press.

Hambrick, E., Seedat, S. & Perry, B. (2021, 6 September). Editorial: How the timing, nature, and duration of relationally positive experiences influence outcomes in children with adverse childhood experiences. *Frontiers in Behavioral Neuroscience*. https://doi.org/10.3389/fnbeh.2021.755959

Hamlyn, C. (2018, 6 May). The final move. *ABC News*. www.abc.net.au/news/2018-05-05/david-goodall-trip-to-switzerland-for-voluntary-euthanasia/9716354

Hammer, J., Springer, J., Beck, N., Menditto, A. & Coleman, J. (2011). The relationship between seclusion and restraint use and childhood abuse among psychiatric inpatients. *Journal of Interpersonal Violence*, *26*(3), 567–79.

Hancock, B.H. (2018). Michel Foucault and the problematics of power: Theorizing DTCA and medicalized subjectivity. *Journal of Medicine and Philosophy*, *43*, 439–68.

Hershenov, D. & Hershenov R. (2015). Morally relevant potential. *Journal of Medical Ethics*, *3*, 268–71.

Higgins, D., Bromfield, L., Richardson, N., Holzer, P. & Berlyn, C. (comp.) (2010), updated by Commerford, J. (2017). *Mandatory reporting of child abuse*. Australian Institute of Family Studies and National Child Protection Clearinghouse.

Holst-Wolf, J., Yeh, I.L. & Konczak, J. (2016). Development of proprioceptive acuity in typically developing children: Normative data on forearm position sense. *Frontiers of Human Neuroscience 10*, 436. https://doi.org/10.3389/fnhum.2016.00436

Howatson-Jones, L. (2016). *Reflective practice in nursing*, 3rd ed. Sage.

International Confederation of Midwives (ICM) (2014). *The International Code of Ethics for Midwives*. www.internationalmidwives.org/our-work/policy-and-practice/international-code-of-ethics-for-midwives.html

International Council of Nurses (ICN) (2012). *The ICN Code of Ethics for Nurses*.

———(2021). *The ICN Code of Ethics for Nurses: Revised 2021*. www.icn.ch/system/files/2021-10/ICN_Code-of-Ethics_EN_Web_0.pdf

Isaacs, D. (2003). Moral status of the fetus: Fetal rights or maternal autonomy? *Journal of Paediatric Child Health Care, 39*(1), 58–9.

Jethwa, S., Bryant, P., Singh, S., Jones, M., Berlin, A. & Rosenthal, J. (2009). Your life in their pocket: Students' behaviours regarding confidential patient information. *Family Medicine, 41*, 327–31.

Johnson, M. (2013, 17 April). Hospital staff disciplined over eel case. *New Zealand Herald*. www.nzherald .co.nz/lifestyle/news/article.cfm?c_id=6&objectid=10878003

Jones, C. & Hayter, M. (2013). Editorial: Social media use by nurses and midwives: A recipe for disaster or a 'force for good'? *Journal of Clinical Nursing, 22*, 1495–6.

Jones, K. (2017, 30 October). The benefits of Magnet status for nurses, patients and organisations. *Nursing Times*. www.nursingtimes.net/roles/nurse-managers/the-benefits-of-magnet-status-for-nurses-patients-and-organisations/7021852.article

Jones, K., Arneil, M., Coventry, L., et al. (2019). Benchmarking nurse outcomes in Australian Magnet® hospitals: Cross-sectional survey. *BMC Nursing, 18*, 62. https://doi.org/10.1186/s12912-019-0383-6

Joseph, L. (2015). Guardianship and litigation: Legal capacity and litigation guardians in NSW. *Law Society of NSW Journal, 13*. https://lsj.com.au/articles/legal-capacity-and-litigation-guardians-in-nsw

Joyce, A. (2010). Transference. *The Corsini Encyclopedia of Psychology*. John Wiley & Sons.

Jung, C.G. (1946). The psychology of the transference. In *Collected Works*. Princeton University Press.

Kahneman, D. (2011). *Thinking fast and slow*. Allen Lane.

Kaspiew, R., Carson, R. & Rhoades, H. (2016). Elder abuse in Australia. *Family Matters, 98*, 64–73.

Keast, K. (2017, 21 June). Push for cultural safety into legislation. *HealthTimes*. https://healthtimes.com.au/hub/aboriginal-health/32/news/kk1/push-for-cultural-safety-into-legislation/2662

Keenan, T., Evans, S. & Crowly, K. (2016). *An introduction to child development*, 3rd ed. Sage.

Kelly, M. (2003). Trust me, I'm a doctor: The role and function of trust in clinical practice. PhD thesis, Macquarie University.

Kemp, K., Arnold, B. & Vaile, D. (2018, 2 August). My Health Record still isn't safe enough to proceed. It needs more than a band-aid fix. *ABC News*. www.abc.net.au/news/2018-08-02/my-health-record-still-not-safe/10063026

Kennett, J. & Cocking, D. (1998). Friendship and the self. *Ethics, 108*, 502–27.

Kim, J. (2018, 20 July). Cyberattack on Singapore health database steals details of 1.5 million including PM. *Reuters News Agency*. www.reuters.com/article/us-singapore-cyberattack/cyberattack-on-singapore-health-database-steals-details-of-1-5-million-including-pm-idUSKBN1KA14J

Korsgaard, C. (1996). *Creating the kingdom of ends*. Cambridge University Press.

Kucukkelepce, G., Kucukkelepce, D. & Aslan, S. (2021). Investigation of the relationship between nursing students' privacy consciousness and attitudes towards patient privacy. *International Journal of Caring Sciences, 14*(3), 1713–23.

Kuczewski, M. & McCruden, P. (2001). Informed consent: Does it take a village? The problem of culture and truth telling. *Cambridge Quarterly of Healthcare Ethics, 10*, 34–46.

Laceulle, H. (2018). Narrative identity and moral agency. In *Aging and self-realization: Cultural narratives about later life*. Transcript Verlag.

Lagerwey, M.D. (2010). Ethical vulnerabilities in nursing history: Conflicting loyalties and the patient as 'other'. *Nursing Ethics, 15*(5), 590–602.

Li, E. et al. (2021). Electronic health records, interoperability and patient safety in health systems of high-income countries: A systematic review protocol. *BMJ Open, 11*(7). https://pubmed.ncbi.nlm.nih.gov/34261679

Lilienfeld, S., Lynn, S.J., Ruscio, J. & Beyerstein, B. (2010). *50 great myths of popular psychology: Shattering widespread misconceptions about human behavior*. Wiley-Blackwell.

Lizza, J. (2007). Potentiality and human embryos. *Bioethics, 27*(1), 379–85.

Luper, S. (2009). Death. In E.W. Zalta (ed.), *Stanford encyclopedia of philosophy*, Summer ed. Stanford University Press. http://plato.stanford.edu/archives/sum2009/entries/death

MacIntyre, A. (1985). *After virtue: A study in moral theory*. Duckworth.

Mackenzie, C. (1992). Abortion and embodiment. *Australasian Journal of Philosophy*, *70*(2), 136–55.

———(2020). Vulnerability, insecurity and the pathologies of trust and distrust. *International Journal of Philosophical Studies*, *28*(5), 624–43.

Marsh, P. & Kelly, L. (2018). Dignity of risk in the community: A review of and reflections on the literature. *Health, Risk and Society*, *20*(5–6), 297–311.

McIlwraith, J. & Madden, B. (2014). *Health care and the law*, 6th ed. Law Book Co.

McKinstry, B., Watson, P., Pinnock, H., Heaney, D. & Sheikh, A. (2009). Confidentiality and the telephone in family practice: A qualitative study of the views of patients, clinicians and administrative staff. *Family Practice Advance Access*, *26*(5), 344–50.

Merleau-Ponty, M. (1961). *Phenomenology of perception* (C. Smith, trans.). Macmillan.

Mestre, J.M. & Barchard, K.A. (2017, 12 April). Four signs you have high emotional intelligence. *The Conversation*. https://theconversation.com/four-signs-you-have-high-emotional-intelligence-71165

Meyers, D. (1989). *Self, society and personal choice*. Westview Press.

———(2004). *Being yourself: Essays on identity, action, and social life*. Rowman & Littlefield.

Michel, J.-P., Lynn, B., Beattie, L., Martin, F. & Walston, J. (eds) (2018). *Oxford textbook of geriatric medicine*, 3rd ed. Oxford University Press.

Mill, J.S. (1975). On liberty. In *Three essays*. Oxford University Press.

Miller, A. (1974). *The crucible: A play in four acts*. Penguin.

Moilanen, T., Kangasniemi, M., Papinaho, O., Mynttinen, M., Siipi, H., Suominen, S. & Suhonen, R. (2022). Older people's perceived autonomy in residential care: An integrative review. *Nursing Ethics*, *28*(3), 414–34.

Nagel, T. (1979). *Mortal questions*. Cambridge University Press.

Naren, T., Burzacott, J., West, C. & Widdicombe, D. (2021). Role of Aboriginal health practitioners in administering and increasing COVID-19 vaccination rates in a Victorian Aboriginal Community Controlled Health Organisation. *Rural Remote Health*, *21*(4), 163–6.

National Aboriginal Community Controlled Health Organisation (NACCHO) (2022). Website. www.naccho.org.au

National Aboriginal and Torres Strait Islander Health Worker Association (NATSIHWA) (2016). *Cultural Safety Framework*. www.natsihwa.org.au/sites/default/files/natsihwa-cultural_safety-framework_summary.pdf

———(2022). *Support for decision making: Consultation summary report*. www.ndis.gov.au/community/we-listened/support-decision-making-consultation-summary-report

National Disability Insurance Scheme (NDIS) (2019). *People with disability and supported decision-making: A guide for NDIS providers in NSW*. https://www.nds.org.au/images/resources/People_with_Disability_and_SDM-guide_for_NDIS_Providers_in_NSW.pdf

National Health and Medical Research Council (NHMRC) (2018). *National Statement on Ethical Conduct in Human Research 2007 (Updated 2018)*. www.nhmrc.gov.au/about-us/publications/national-statement-ethical-conduct-human-research-2007-updated-2018

NATSIHWA *see* National Aboriginal and Torres Strait Islander Health Worker Association

Negayama, K., Dellafield-Butt, J., Mimose, K. et al. (2015, 27 February). Embodied intersubjective engagement in mother–infant tactile communication: A cross-cultural study of Japanese and Scottish mother–infant behaviors during infant pick-up. *Frontiers of Psychology*. https://doi.org/10.3389/fpsyg.2015.00066

Neura (2019). Aboriginal ageing health information. www.neura.edu.au/health/aboriginal-ageing/?gclid=CjwKCAjwt7SWBhAnEiwAx8ZLahFIvCz23SRmLB3PEVu56YlqP_cE2wBYfb2oT629PT-GCXAXu4b2cRoCj70QAvD_BwE

New South Wales Communities & Justice (2020). Supported decision making. https://www.justice.nsw.gov
.au/diversityservices/Pages/divserv/ds_capacity_tool/ds_capa_decision.aspx

New South Wales Government (2020). *Capacity toolkit.* www.justice.nsw.gov.au/diversityservices/Pages/
divserv/ds_capacity_tool/ds_capacity_tool.aspx

New South Wales Health (2021). Record $30.2 billion for health care in NSW. www.health.nsw.gov.au/news/
Pages/20210622_04.aspx

New South Wales Law Reform Commission (2002). *Issues Paper 24 (2004) – minors' consent to medical
treatment.* www.lawlink.nsw.gov.au/__4a2565b5001b20d1.nsf/0/a0f52f107a4423c7ca256e970028817c?
OpenDocument

—— (2018). *Review of the Guardianship Act 1987.* www.lawreform.justice.nsw.gov.au/Pages/lrc/lrc_current_
projects/Guardianship/Report-145.aspx

New South Wales Legislative Council General Purpose Standing Committee (NSW GPSC) (2016). *Elder
abuse in NSW.* www.parliament.nsw.gov.au/committees/DBAssets/InquiryReport/ReportAcrobat/6063/
Report%2044%20-%20Elder%20abuse%20in%20New%20South%20Wales.pdf

NHMRC *see* National Health and Medical Research Council

NMBA *see* Nursing and Midwifery Board of Australia

NSW GPSC *see* New South Wales Legislative Council General Purpose Standing Committee

NSW Ombudsman (2018, 2 November). *Abuse and neglect of vulnerable adults in NSW: The need for
action – a special report to parliament under section 31 of the Ombudsman Act 1974.* www.ombo.nsw
.gov.au/__data/assets/pdf_file/0003/62139/Abuse-and-neglect-of-vulnerable-adults-in-NSW-
November-2018.pdf

Nursing and Midwifery Board of Australia (NMBA) (2016). *Registered Nurse Standards of Practice.* www.cdu
.edu.au/sites/default/files/health/docs/nmba_registered_nurse_standards_for_practice.pdf

——(2017). Newsletters. www.nursingmidwiferyboard.gov.au/News/Newsletters.aspx

——(2018a). *Code of Conduct for Midwives.* www.nursingmidwiferyboard.gov.au/Codes-Guidelines-
Statements/Professional-standards.aspx

——(2018b) *Code of Conduct for Nurses.* www.nursingmidwiferyboard.gov.au/Codes-Guidelines-
Statements/Professional-standards.aspx

——(2018c, 28 March). Cultural safety: Nurses and midwives leading the way for safer healthcare. Joint
Statement. www.nursingmidwiferyboard.gov.au/News/2018-03-23-joint-statement.aspx

——(2020). Newsletters. www.nursingmidwiferyboard.gov.au/News/Newsletters.aspx

——(2021a). *Registration Standards.* https://www.nursingmidwiferyboard.gov.au/Registration-Standards
.aspx

——(2021b). *Functions of the board.* www.nursingmidwiferyboard.gov.au/About.aspx#functions

Office of the Australian Information Commissioner (2022a). *Privacy Act.* www.oaic.gov.au/privacy-law/
privacy-act/

——(2022b). Communication with patients. www.oaic.gov.au/privacy/privacy-for-health-service-providers/
communications-with-patients

O'Neill, M. (2006, 20 February). Allegations of abuse at aged care facility. [Radio broadcast transcript].
Lateline. ABC TV. www.abc.net.au/lateline/content/2006/s1574385.htm

O'Neill, N. & Peisah, C. (2011). *Capacity and the law.* Sydney University Press.

Oral, R., Ramirez, M., Coohey, C., Nakada, S., Walz, A., Kuntz, A., Benoit, J. & Peek-Asa, C. (2016). Adverse
childhood experiences and trauma informed care: The future of health care. *Pediatric Research, 79*(1–2),
227–33.

Pain, C., Green, M., Duff, C., Hyland, D., Pantle, A., Fitzpatrick, K. & Hughes, C. (2017). Between the flags:
Implementing a safety-net system at scale to recognise and manage deteriorating patients in the New
South Wales Public Health System'. *International Journal for Quality in Health Care, 29*(1), 130–6.

Palliative Care Australia (2022). Facts about morphine and other opioid medicines in palliative care. https://palliativecare.org.au/resource/resources-facts-about-morphine-and-other-opioid-medicines-in-palliative-care

Pang, C.L. McKay, D., Chang, S., Chen, Q., Zhang, X. & Cui, L. (2020). Privacy concerns of the Australian My Health Record: Implications for other large-scale opt-out personal health records. *Information Processing & Management*, *57*(6). www.sciencedirect.com/science/article/pii/S0306457320308591

Papps, E. & Ramsden, I. (1996). Cultural safety in nursing: The New Zealand experience. *International Journal for Quality in Health Care*, *8*(5), 491–7.

Parliament of Victoria, Legal and Social Issues Committee (2016). Submissions. *Inquiry into End of Life Choices*. www.parliament.vic.gov.au/lsic/article/2759

Perera, G., Holbrook, A., Thabane, L., Foster, G. & Willison, D. (2011). Views on health information sharing and privacy from primary care practices using electronic medical records. *International Journal of Medical Informatics*, *80*, 94–101.

Perry, B. (2013). The death of empathy? In D. Narvaez, J. Panksepp, N. Schore & T. Gleason (eds), *Evolution, early experience and human development: From research to practice and policy*. Oxford University Press.

Peter, E. & Morgan, K. (2001). Explorations of a trust approach for nursing ethics. *Nursing Inquiry*, *8*, 3–10.

Petersen, K. (2011). Abortion laws and medical developments: A medico-legal anomaly in Queensland. *Journal of Law and Medicine*, *18*(3), 594–600.

Petherbridge, D. (2021). Recognition, vulnerability and trust. *International Journal of Philosophical Studies*, *29*(1), 1–23.

Porteous, J., Stewart-Wynne, E.G., Connolly, M. & Crommelin, P.F. (2009). iSoBAR – a concept and handover checklist: The National Clinical Handover Initiative. *Medical Journal of Australia*, *190*(11), 152.

Presz, P., Preisz, A., Daley, S. & Farzad, J. (2022). 'Dalarinji': A flexible clinic, belonging to and for the Aboriginal people, in an Australian emergency department. *Emergency Medicine Australasia*, *34*(1), 4651.

Queensland Health (2016). Inala Indigenous Health Service. https://www.health.qld.gov.au/iihs

Quill, T. & Greenlaw, J. (2008). Physician-assisted death. In M. Crowley (ed.), *From birth to death and bench to clinic: Hasting Centre bioethics briefing book for journalists, policymakers, and the campaigns*. The Hastings Centre.

Rachels, J. (1994). Active and passive euthanasia. In T.L. Beauchamp & J.F. Childress (eds), *Principles of biomedical ethics*, 4th ed. Oxford University Press.

Ravens, T. (2007, 14 November). Aboriginal elder died 'alone, thirsty'. *Sydney Morning Herald*. http://news.smh.com.au/national/aboriginal-elder-died-alone-thirsty-20071114-1a5l.html

Ricoeur, P. (1992). *Oneself as another* (K. Blamey, trans.). University of Chicago Press.

Robinson, G. (2010, 23 December). Power balance wristbands a sham: ACCC. *Sydney Morning Herald*. www.smh.com.au/small-business/power-balance-wristbands-a-sham-accc-20101222-1960g.html

Royal Commission into Aged Care Quality and Safety (2020). *Aged care and COVID-19: A special report*. https://agedcare.royalcommission.gov.au/sites/default/files/2020-12/aged-care-and-covid-19-a-special-report.pdf

——(2021). *Final report*. https://agedcare.royalcommission.gov.au/publications/final-report

Royal Commission into Violence, Abuse and Exploitation of People with Disability (2022). *Fifth progress report*. https://disability.royalcommission.gov.au/publications/fifth-progress-report

Rutherford, M. (2014). The value of trust to nursing. *Nursing Economics*, *32*(6), 283–8. www.proquest.com/openview/20691fadd117514d5e5ccce6523c862c/1?pq-origsite=gscholar&cbl=30765

SA Health (2012). Firearms notifications – mandatory reporting by health professionals. www.sahealth.sa.gov.au/wps/wcm/connect/public+content/sa+health+internet/clinical+resources/health+notifications/firearm+notifications

Sacks, O. (1985). *The man who mistook his wife for a hat*. Picador.

Sanson, M. & Anthony, A. (2018). *Connecting with law*, 4th ed. Oxford University Press.

Santana, M., Manalili, K., Jolley, R., Zelinsky, S., Quan, H. & Lu. M. (2017). How to practice person-centred care: A conceptual framework. *Health Expectations*, *21*(2). https://doi.org/10.1111/hex.12640

Sebag-Montefiore, P. (2019). Touch. *Granta*, *146*. https://granta.com/touch

Seedhouse, D. (2009). *Ethics: The heart of health care*. Wiley-Blackwell.

Siegler, M. (1994). Biomedical ethics. In T.L. Beauchamp & J.F. Childress (eds), *Principles of biomedical ethics*, 4th ed. Oxford University Press.

Singer, P. (1993). *Practical ethics*, 2nd ed. Cambridge University Press.

——(1995). Abortion. In T. Honderich (ed.), *The Oxford companion to philosophy*. Oxford University Press.

——(2005). Decisions about death. *Free Inquiry*. www.secularhumanism.org/index.php?section=library&page=singer_25_5

Singer, P. & Dawson, K. (1988). IVF technology and the argument from potential. *Philosophy and Public Affairs*, *17*(2), 87–104.

Skene, L. (1997). When can doctors treat patients who cannot or will not consent? *Monash University Law Review*, *23*(1), 77–91.

Smith, E., Jones, T., Ward, R. et al. (2014). *From blues to rainbows: The mental health and well-being of gender diverse and transgender young people in Australia*. Australian Research Centre in Sex, Health and Society (ARCSHS), La Trobe University. https://apo.org.au/sites/default/files/resource-files/2014-09/apo-nid41426.pdf

Smith, K.V. (2005). Ethical issues related to health care: The older adult's perspective. *Journal of Gerontological Nursing*, *31*(2), 32–9.

Spooner, R. (2012, 21 November). Mercy killer didn't want political debate. *WA Today*. www.watoday.com.au/wa-news/mercy-killer-didnt-want-political-debate-20121120-29o21.html

Statista (2022). Number of monthly active Facebook users worldwide as of 4th quarter 2018 (in millions). www.statista.com/statistics/264810/number-of-monthly-active-facebook-users-worldwide

Staunton, P. & Chiarella, M. (2013). *Law for nurses and midwives*, 7th ed. Churchill Livingston/Elsevier.

Stein-Parbury, J. (2009). *Patient and person: Interpersonal skills in nursing*. Elsevier.

Studdert, D.M. & Richardson, M.W. (2010). Legal aspects of open disclosure: A review of Australian law. *Medical Journal of Australia*, *193*, 273–6.

Tasmanian Government (2021). *Health – 'delivering better health, mental health and preventative health services in hospital, in the community and in the home'.* www.premier.tas.gov.au/budget_2021/health

Tatz, C. (2003). *With intent to destroy: Reflecting on genocide*. Verso.

Taylor, K. & Guerin, P. (2019). *Health care and Indigenous Australians: Cultural safety in practice*, 3rd ed. Bloomsbury.

Thomson, J.A.K. (1966). *The Ethics of Aristotle. The Nichomachean Ethics translated*. Penguin.

Tooley, M. (1972). Abortion and infanticide. *Philosophy and Public Affairs*, *2*, 37–65.

Twomey, A. (2020). Multi-level government and COVID-19: Australia as a case study. Melbourne Forum on Constitution Building. https://law.unimelb.edu.au/__data/assets/pdf_file/0003/3473832/MF20-Web3-Aust-ATwomey-FINAL.pdf

United Nations (1948). *Universal Declaration of Human Rights.* www.un.org/sites/un2.un.org/files/2021/03/udhr.pdf

——(1991). *Principles for people with mental illness and the improvement of health care.* www.mhrt.nsw.gov.au/files/mhrt/pdf/UN_Principles.pdf

——(2006). *United Nations Convention on the Rights of Persons with Disabilities.* www.un.org/disabilities/convention/conventionfull.shtml

Ussher, J.M., Hawkey, A., Perz, J., Liamputtong, P., Marjadi, B., Schmied, V., Dune, T., Sekar, J.A., Ryan, S., Charter, R., Thepsourinthone, J., Noack-Lundberg, K. & Brook, E. (2020). *Crossing the line: Lived experience of sexual violence among trans women of colour from culturally and linguistically diverse (CALD) backgrounds in Australia*.ANROWS. www.anrows.org.au/publication/crossing-the-line-lived-experience-of-sexual-violence-among-trans-women-of-colour-from-culturally-and-linguistically-diverse-cald-backgrounds-in-australia

Verbunt, E., Luke, L., et al. (2021). Cultural determinants of health for Aboriginal and Torres Strait Islander people – a narrative overview of reviews. *International Journal for Equity in Health, 20*(1), 1–9.

Victoria Health (2018). *Voluntary assisted dying*. www.health.vic.gov.au/patient-care/voluntary-assisted-dying

Victoria State Government (2018a). *Patient-centred care explained*. Better Health Channel. www.betterhealth.vic.gov.au/health/servicesandsupport/patient-centred-care-explained.

——(2018b). *Voluntary assisted dying*. Better Health Channel. www.betterhealth.vic.gov.au/health/ServicesAndSupport/voluntary-assisted-dying

Vincini, S., Jhang, Y., Buder, E. & Gallagher, S. (2017). Neonatal imitation: Theory, experimental design, and significance for the field of social cognition. *Frontiers of Psychology*. https://doi.org/10.3389/fpsyg.2017.01323

WA Health (2019). Table 1: WA health system Severity Assessment Codes (SAC) – Summary. In *Clinical incident management guideline*, Government of Western Australia. ww2.health.wa.gov.au/~/media/Files/Corporate/general-documents/patient-safety/PDF/WA-Health-Severity-Assessment-Codes.pdf

Wakerman, J., Humphreys, J., Russell, D. et al. (2019). Remote health workforce turnover and retention: What are the policy and practice priorities? *Human Resources for Health, 19*(99).

Waller, K. (1994). *Coronial law and practice in NSW*, 3rd ed. Butterworths.

Warren, M.A. (1989). The moral significance of birth. *Hypatia: A Journal of Feminist Philosophy, 4*(3), 46–65.

Whitler, J.M. (1996). Ethics of assisted autonomy in the nursing home: Types of assisting among long-term care nurses. *Nursing Ethics, 3*, 224–35.

WHO *see* World Health Organization

Williams, B. (1981). *Moral luck*. Cambridge University Press.

Williams, L. (2018). Medical assistance in dying: A disruption of therapeutic relationships. *Medical Journal of Australia, 209*(7), 286–7.

Williams, S.M. (1994). *Environment and mental health*. John Wiley & Sons.

Willmot, L., Christensen, S., Butler, D. & Dixon, B. (2013). *Contract law*, 4th ed. Oxford University Press.

World Health Organization (WHO) (2015). *World report on ageing and health*. www.who.int/ageing/events/world-report-2015-launch/en

——(2019). *Decade of Healthy Ageing 2020–2030, Update 1*. www.who.int/docs/default-source/documents/decade-of-health-ageing/decade-healthy-ageing-update-march-2019.pdf?sfvrsn=5a6d0e5c_2

——(2021). Abuse of older people. www.who.int/news-room/fact-sheets/detail/abuse-of-older-people

——(2022). Ageing and health. www.who.int/news-room/fact-sheets/detail/ageing-and-health

Legal cases cited

Albrighton v Royal Prince Alfred Hospital [1980] 2 NSWLR 542

Bawa-Garba v General Medical Council [2018] EWCA Civ 1879

Bolam v Friern Hospital Management Committee [1957] 1 WLR 582

Boxell & Ors v Peninsula Health [2019] VSC 830

Breen v Williams [1996] HCA 57; (1996) 186 CLR

Brightwater Care Group (Inc) v Rossiter [2009] WASC 229 CIV 2406/09

Ces v Superclinics Australia Pty Ltd [1995] 38 NSWLR 47

Dept Health and Community Services v JWB and SMB (*Marion*'s case) [1992] HCA 15; (1992) 175 CLR 218

Donoghue v Stevenson (1932) SC (HL) 31

Gillick v West Norfolk AHA (1986) 1 AC 150

Harriton v Stephens (2006) 226 CLR 52

Health Care Complaints Commission v Do [2014] NSWCA 307

Health Care Complaints Commission v Litchfield [1997] NSWCA 264

Health Care Complaints Commission v Ndiweni, Professional Standards Committee Inquiry, 23368/22, 29 March 2022

Health Care Complaints Commission v Shrimpton [2019] NSWCATOD 25

Hollis v Vabu Pty Ltd (2001) 207 CLR 21

Hunter and New England Area Health Service v A [2009] 74 NSWLR 88

Inquest into the death of Ahlia Raftery, State Coroner's Court (NSW), 9 June 2017

K v Minister for Youth and Community Services [1982] NSWLR 311

Lipohar v The Queen [1999] HCA 65; (1999) 200 CLR 485

Mabo v Queensland (No 2) (1992) 175 CLR 1

Malette v Shulman (1990) 2 Med LR 162

Naidoo v Brisbane Waters Administration Pty Ltd [2017] NSWDC 372

Nepean Blue Mountains Local Health District v Starkey [2016] NSCA 114

New South Wales v Lepore (2003) 212 CLR 511

Prince Alfred College Incorporated v ADC (2016) 258 CLR 134

R v Bayliss and Cullen (1986) 9 Qld Lawyer Reps 8

R v Davidson [1969] VR 667

R v Leach and Brennan [2010] QDC (Cairns), unreported 14 October Everson DCJ

R v Wald [1971] 3 NSWDCR 25

Re Alex [2004] FamCA 297

Re Isabel Amaro; Findings of the Conduct and Competence Committee, Nursing and Midwifery Council (UK), 4 August 2016

Rogers v Whitaker [1992] HCA 58; (1992) 175 CLR 479

Sidaway v Governors of Bethlem Royal Hospital [1985] AC 871

State of Queensland v Masson (2020) 94 ALJR 785

Tarasoff v Regents of the University of California 551 P 2d 334 (1974)

Wallace v Kam (2013) 250 CLR 375

Wang v Central Sydney Area Health Services & 2 Ors [2000] NSWSC 515

Watson v Marshall [1971] HCA 33; (1971) 24 CLR 621

X v The Sydney Children's Hospitals Network [2013] NSWCA 320

INDEX